Advanced Practitioner Respiratory Care Review

WRITTEN REGISTRY
AND CLINICAL SIMULATION EXAM

Advanced Practitioner Respiratory Care Review

WRITTEN REGISTRY AND CLINICAL SIMULATION EXAM

Gary Persing, BS, RRT

Director of Clinical Education
Respiratory Therapy Program
Tulsa Junior College
Tulsa, Oklahoma

W.B. SAUNDERS COMPANY
A Division of Harcourt Brace & Company
Philadelphia   London   Toronto   Montreal   Sydney   Tokyo

W.B. Saunders Company
A Division of Harcourt Brace & Company

The Curtis Center
Independence Square West
Philadelphia, Pennsylvania 19106

Library of Congress Cataloging-in-Publication Data

Persing, Gary.
 Advanced practitioner respiratory care review: written registry and clinical simulation exam / Gary Persing.
  p. cm.
 ISBN 0-7216-4963-7
 1. Respiratory therapy—Examinations, questions, etc. I. Title.
 [DNLM: 1. Respiratory Therapy—examination questions.
 2. Respiratory Tract Diseases—examination questions. WF 18 P466a 1994]
 RC735.I5P449 1994
 616.2′0076—dc20
 DNLM/DLC   93-20774

Advanced Practitioner Respiratory Care Review:
Written Registry and Clinical Simulation Exam   ISBN 0-7216-4963-7

Printed in the United States of America.

Last digit is the print number: 9   8   7   6   5

This book is dedicated to the most important people in my life:
My wife, Debbie, for her love, patience and support;
my daughter, Lindsey, the apple of my eye;
my Mom and Dad, for their loving kindness;
and to my Lord and Savior Jesus Christ
for His guidance and forgiveness.

PREFACE

One of the most satisfying accomplishments that may be achieved by respiratory care practitioners is the successful completion of the Advanced Practitioner Written Registry/ Clinical Simulation Examination offered by the National Board for Respiratory Care (NBRC). Being awarded the credential of Registered Respiratory Therapist (RRT) is indeed a great accomplishment. Becoming a registered respiratory therapist requires passing the Entry Level Certification Examination (CRTT), as well as a 100-question multiple-choice written test and a clinical simulation examination composed of 10 problems.

The purpose of this text is to prepare the individual to successfully complete both the Written Registry Examination and the Clinical Simulation Examination. The NBRC provides a test matrix that indicates the areas that will be tested on these examinations. I have used this matrix as a guideline to provide the material in this text in order to better prepare you for the examination. Because the NBRC examinations may exclude more current types of therapy or equipment, the clinical practices reflected in this book are not necessarily the most current in your region.

As I have done with my *Entry Level Respiratory Care Review* textbook, I divided this book into a Study Guide section and a Workbook section. The Study Guide section consists of 16 chapters, each preceded by pretest questions. These questions should be answered prior to studying the chapter to best determine your knowledge in this area and then the chapter should be studied carefully.

Once you have completed a Study Guide chapter, begin working the corresponding Workbook chapter. Answer all the questions you can without referring to the Study Guide. When you come to questions you cannot answer, turn back to the corresponding Roman numeral heading in the Study Guide chapter to find the information to that question. Do not get discouraged if you find yourself frequently turning back and forth between the Study Guide and the Workbook. By going back and reviewing the material in the Study Guide and then writing it down in the Workbook, you will increase your retention of this material. That is my main objective for including Workbook chapters — to increase your retention by reading the material and also writing it down.

Once you have completed all 16 Study Guide chapters and their corresponding Workbook chapters, a 100-question Posttest, provided at the end of the book, should be taken. Take this test as though it were the real thing. Find a quiet place. The time limit is 2 hours, the same as for the NBRC examination. After taking the test, you may grade it using the answer sheet found on the page immediately following the last page of the examination. The correct answers are provided, as is the Study Guide section where the information regarding the answer can be found. After grading the test, determine your strongest and weakest areas. Review chapters in which you missed the most questions.

Following the Workbook section, you will find three clinical simulations similar to those offered on the NBRC Clinical Simulation Examination. A score sheet is provided so that you may determine your score on each simulation.

Proper preparation is a must in passing the NBRC Advanced Practitioner Examinations. The NBRC provides excellent material to help study for the credentialing examinations. I highly recommend their self-assessment examinations and practice clinical simulations. I am sure you will find them very helpful. Certainly, over the course of your education in the field of respiratory care you have accumulated many excellent textbooks that will be invaluable in your examination preparation. What I have attempted to do with this text is to summarize, in a comprehensive and understandable way, the most important material necessary for you to understand in order to pass the NBRC Registry Examinations. It is my sincere hope that you will find this textbook beneficial in your preparation for the NBRC Registry examinations and that you will soon be awarded the credential of Registered Respiratory Therapist.

GARY PERSING, BS, RRT

ACKNOWLEDGMENTS

A very special thanks to Lisa Biello, Vice-President and Editor-in-Chief, Health Related Professions, at the W.B. Saunders Company, who has been so helpful to me along the way in preparing this text.

I also want to thank all of my students who have made teaching a wonderful and rewarding experience for me.

GARY PERSING, BS, RRT

CONTENTS

CHAPTER 15

Respiratory Home Care . . . .

CHAPTER 16

Pulmonary Function Testing . . . .

SECTION II   **WORKBOOK**

CHAPTER 17

Oxygen and Medical Gas Therapy . . . .

CHAPTER 18

Humidity and Aerosol Therapy . . . .

CHAPTER 19

Cardiopulmonary Patient Assessment . . . . .

CHAPTER 20

Management of the Airway . . . .

CHAPTER 21

Special Respiratory Care Procedures . . . . . .

Study Guide

CHAPTER 1

Oxygen and Medical Gas Therapy

PRETEST QUESTIONS*

1. How long will an E cylinder run before it becomes empty if it contains 1900 pounds per square inch gauge (psig) of oxygen with a 4 L/min nasal cannula connected to the outlet of the regulator?

A. 47 minutes
B. 1.7 hours
C. 2.2 hours
D. 3.6 hours
E. 4.2 hours

$$\frac{1900 \times .28}{4} = \frac{}{60}$$

2. After fitting a patient with a partial rebreathing mask set for a liter flow of 8 L/min, you notice the reservoir bag collapses before the patient is finished inspiring. Which of the following should the respiratory therapist do to help correct this situation?

A. Change to a 6 L/min nasal cannula
B. Decrease the flow
C. Change to a nonrebreathing mask
D. Increase the flow
E. Make no change, since this is a normal occurrence

3. A patient with carbon monoxide poisoning can be treated best with which of the following therapies?

A. Nasal cannula at 6 L/min
B. Simple oxygen mask
C. Continuous positive airway pressure (CPAP)
D. Nonrebreathing mask
E. Hyperbaric oxygen

4. The following blood gas measurements have been obtained from a patient breathing 60% oxygen through an aerosol mask:

pH   7.47 ↑
$PaCO_2$ 31 torr ↓
PaO_2 58 torr

What should the respiratory therapist recommend at this time?

A. Start patient on CPAP.
B. Increase to 70% aerosol mask.
C. Intubate patient and start mechanical ventilation.
D. Start patient on nonrebreathing mask.
E. Start incentive spirometry every 2 hours.

5. What is the patient's total arterial oxygen content given the following data?

pH	7.41
$PaCO_2$	37 torr
HCO_3	26 mEq/L
PaO_2	88 torr
SaO_2	95%
Hemoglobin (Hb)	14 vol%

$(14 \times 1.34).95 \times 37 (.003)$

A. 12 vol%
B. 14 vol%
C. 16 vol%
D. 18 vol%
E. 20 vol%

6. A patient breathing 30% oxygen through a Venturi mask with an oxygen flow of 5 L/min is receiving a total flow of which of the following?

A. 36 L/min
B. 45 L/min
C. 54 L/min
D. 60 L/min
E. 64 L/min

$\frac{100}{21} \frac{9}{30} \frac{9}{70}$

---

*See answers at the end of the chapter

3

CHAPTER 1

Oxygen and Medical Gas Therapy

I. STORAGE AND CONTROL OF MEDICAL GASES

A. Storage of medical gases and cylinder characteristics
1. Cylinders are constructed of **chrome molybdenum steel.**
2. Gas cylinders are stored at high pressures, with a **full oxygen cylinder containing 2200 psig pressure.**
3. Cylinders are constructed in various sizes with the most common size for oxygen storage being the "H" cylinder and the "E" cylinder.
   a. The **H cylinder holds 244 cubic feet (6900 liters) of oxygen.**
   b. The **E cylinder, used for transport, holds 22 cubic feet (622 liters) of oxygen.**

NOTE: There are 28.3 liters in 1 cubic foot.

4. Cylinder valves allow attachment of regulators in order to remove the gas from the cylinder at various flowrates
5. The valves are constructed in such a way as to allow connection of only one type of gas regulator—that is, an oxygen regulator will not attach to a helium cylinder. This is prevented by the use of cylinder/regulator safety systems.
   a. **Large cylinders use the American Standard Safety System (ASSS).** Each type of gas cylinder outlet has a specific number of threads per inch and a different thread size and may require a turn to the right or to the left for attachment of the regulator.
   b. **Small cylinders use the Pin Index Safety System (PISS).** Each cylinder valve has two holes drilled into specific positions that will line up only with corresponding pins on the appropriate regulator. There are six different hole placement positions. **Oxygen cylinders have hole placements in the 2 and 5 positions.**
6. Safety relief devices on cylinder valves allow for the escape of excess gas if the pressure in the cylinder should increase. There are two types of safety relief devices:
   a. Frangible disk—breaks at 3000 psig
   b. Fusible plug—melts at 170°F
7. The Compressed Gas Association (CGA) developed a color-coded system for cylinders to distinguish the various gases.

Gas	Color of Cylinder
Oxygen	Green
	White (internationally)
Helium	Brown
Carbon dioxide	Gray
Nitrous oxide	Light blue
Cyclopropane	Orange
Ethylene	Red
Air	Yellow
Carbon dioxide/oxygen	Gray and green
Helium/oxygen	Brown and green

8. Cylinder markings

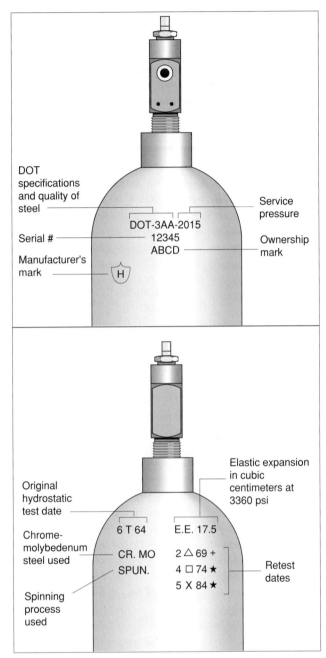

From Persing G. *Entry Level Respiratory Care Review*. Philadelphia: WB Saunders; 1992.

9. Cylinder testing
   a. Cylinders are visually tested by dropping a lightbulb inside to look for corrosion.
   b. Cylinders are **hydrostatically tested every 5 or 10 years, depending on the cylinder marking. **A star next to the latest test date denotes a 10-year period before the next test must be done.**
   c. Hydrostatic testing determines:
      (1) Wall stress
      (2) Cylinder expansion
      (3) Leaks
10. Liquid gas systems
    a. One cubic foot of liquid oxygen expands

860 times as it changes to a gas. Liquid oxygen is much more economical.
   b. The liquid oxygen is stored in insulated containers at a pressure not to exceed 250 psig and a temperature less than −**297°F** (−183°C) (boiling point of oxygen).
   c. Liquid oxygen is most commonly produced by the process of **fractional distillation.
B. Control of medical gases
   1. Regulators are devices attached to the cylinder valve to:
      a. Regulate flow
      b. Reduce cylinder pressure to working pressure (50 psig)
   2. The reducing valve may be:
      a. Single-stage—reduces the cylinder pressure directly to 50 psig; has one safety relief device
      b. Double-stage—reduces the cylinder pressure to approximately 150 psig, then to 50 psig; has two safety relief devices
      c. Triple-stage—reduces the cylinder pressure to approximately 300 psig, then to 150 psig and 50 psig; has three safety relief devices
   3. Regulators may be preset or adjustable.
   4. Operation of a **preset regulator:**

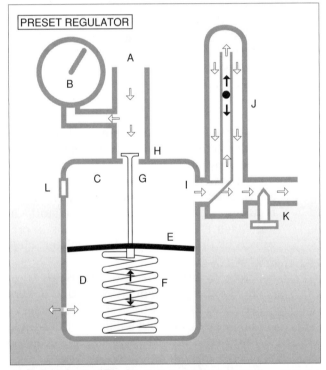

From Persing G. *Entry Level Respiratory Care Review*. Philadelphia: WB Saunders; 1992.

   a. High cylinder pressure enters the inlet (A) of the reducing valve past an inlet valve (H) into the pressure chamber (C). The valve stem (G) is also shown.
   b. Gas pushes down on the diaphragm (E). As

the gas pressure overcomes the pressure on the spring (F) attached to the diaphragm it moves downward, pulling with it the valve that closes off gas flow into the pressure chamber. The spring is located in the ambient chamber (D).

c. As gas exits the pressure chamber through the outlet (I), pressure again drops in the chamber, and the spring, diaphragm, and valve move upward to allow gas to enter the chamber again.

d. In essence, the spring and diaphragm are continually moving up and down as gas leaves the chamber and goes through the flowmeter and needle valve (K).

e. Excessive pressure in the pressure chamber is vented through a pressure relief valve (L).

f. The spring tension on this regulator is **preset** at **50 psig.**

5. **Adjustable regulator**

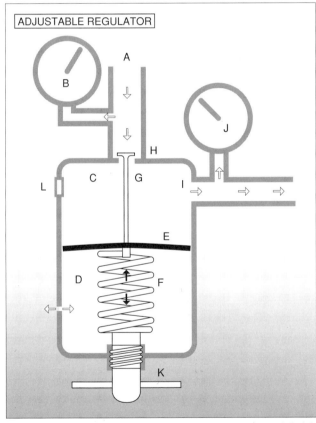

ADJUSTABLE REGULATOR

From Persing G. *Entry Level Respiratory Care Review.* Philadelphia: WB Saunders; 1992.

a. Works the same as the preset regulator except the spring tension is adjustable by the user

b. This is an example of a Bourdon gauge regulator.

6. Technical problems associated with reducing valves and regulators:

a. Dust or debris from the cylinder valve entering the regulator may rupture the diaphragm. **Always "crack" the cylinder prior to attaching a regulator.**

b. Constant pressure "trapped" in the pressure chamber after the cylinder is turned off may rupture the diaphragm. Always vent out pressure in the regulator by opening the needle valve after the cylinder is turned off.

c. A hole in the diaphragm will result in a continuous leak into the ambient chamber and through the vent hole, causing failure of the regulator.

d. A weak spring could result in the diaphragm vibrating, causing inadequate flow because of premature closing of the inlet valve.

e. When attaching a regulator to a small cylinder, make sure the plastic washer is in place or gas will be heard leaking around the cylinder valve outlet and regulator inlet.

7. **Calculating how long cylinder contents will last:**

minutes remaining in cylinder =
$$\frac{\text{cylinder pressure} \times \text{cylinder factor}}{\text{flowrate}}$$

Cylinder factors:
H cylinder = 3.14 L/psig
E cylinder = 0.28 L/psig

EXAMPLE: Calculate how long a full H cylinder will last running at 8 L/min.

$$\frac{2200 \text{ psig} \times 3.14 \text{ L/psig}}{8 \text{ L/min}} = \frac{6908}{8} =$$

$$\frac{863.5 \text{ minutes}}{60} = \textbf{14.39 hours}$$

EXAMPLE: An E cylinder of oxygen contains 1800 psig. If the respiratory care practitioner runs the cylinder at 4 L/min through a nasal cannula, how long will the contents last until the cylinder reaches 200 psig?

$$\frac{(1800 \text{ psig} - 200 \text{ psig}) \times 0.28 \text{ L/psig}}{4 \text{ L/min}} =$$

$$\frac{448}{4} = \textbf{112 minutes}$$

$$\frac{\textbf{112 minutes}}{\textbf{60}} = \textbf{1.9 hours}$$

8. **Flowmeters**
   a. **Uncompensated flowmeter**

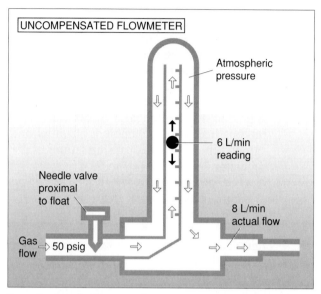

From Persing G. *Entry Level Respiratory Care Review*. Philadelphia: WB Saunders; 1992.

   (1) Needle valve is located proximal to (before) the float; therefore, atmospheric pressure is in the tube. Any back pressure in the tube affects the rise of the float.
   (2) When a restriction such as a humidifier or nebulizer is attached to the outlet, the reading on the flowmeter is not accurate. The flowmeter reading is lower than the flow the patient actually receives.
   (3) Should not be used clinically
   b. **Compensated flowmeter**

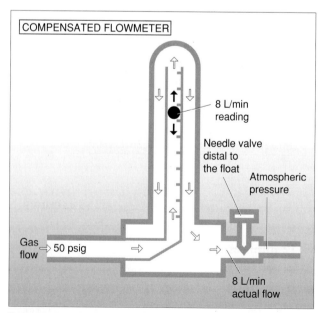

From Persing G. *Entry Level Respiratory Care Review*. Philadelphia: WB Saunders; 1992.

   (1) The needle valve is located distal to (after) the float; therefore, 50 psig is in the tube, and only back pressure exceeding that will affect the rise of the float.
   (2) The flowmeter reads accurately with an attachment such as a humidifier or nebulizer on the outlet.
   (3) There are three ways to determine if a flowmeter compensates for pressure:
       (a) Labeled as such on the flowmeter
       (b) Needle valve is located after the float
       (c) Float jumps when the flowmeter is plugged into wall outlet while turned off.
   (4) Flowmeter outlets use the **Diameter Index Safety System (DISS),** as does all gas-administering equipment that operates at **less than 200 psig,** to avoid attachment to the wrong gas source.
 (5) If the flowmeter is turned completely off, but gas is still bubbling through the humidifier or gas is still heard coming from the flowmeter, this indicates a **faulty valve seat, and the flowmeter should be replaced.
   c. **Bourdon gauge**

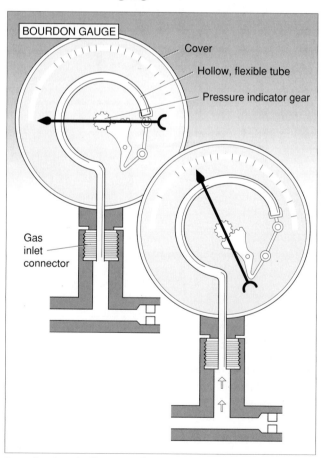

From Persing G. *Entry Level Respiratory Care Review*. Philadelphia: WB Saunders; 1992.

(1) The Bourdon gauge is actually a pressure gauge that has been calibrated in liters per minute. **It does not compensate for back pressure.**

(2) When a humidifier or nebulizer is attached to its outlet, back pressure is generated into the gauge (which measures pressure) and **readings are higher than the flow the patient is actually receiving.**

(3) The gauge's working mechanism operates by gas entering the hollow, flexible, question mark–shaped tube. The tube tends to straighten as pressure is applied to it. A gear mechanism is attached to the tube, and as the tube straightens it rotates a needle indicator denoting the pressure (flow).

(4) The advantage of the Bourdon gauge is that it is not position-dependent as are Thorpe tube flowmeters.

9. Air compressors

  a. Used to provide medical air through either portable compressors or large medical air piping systems

  b. Three types of air compressors generally used

    (1) Piston type

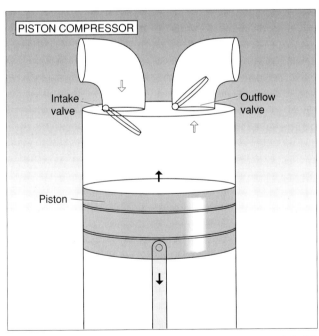

From Persing G. *Entry Level Respiratory Care Review*. Philadelphia: WB Saunders; 1992.

(a) As piston drops, gas is drawn in through a one-way intake valve. On the upstroke, the intake valve closes and gas exits through an outflow one-way valve.

(b) Seen most commonly on large medical air piping systems

(c) Air is drawn into the compressor and travels to a reservoir tank. From this tank the air passes through a drier to remove the moisture and on to a pressure-reducing valve that reduces the pressure to 50 psig to power the compressed air wall outlet.

    (2) Diaphragm type

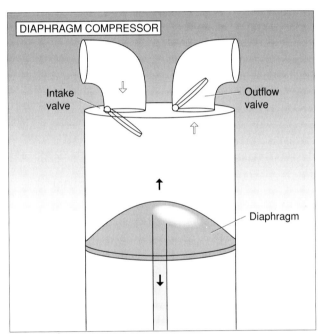

From Persing G. *Entry Level Respiratory Care Review*. Philadelphia: WB Saunders; 1992.

(a) A diaphragm is used instead of a piston.

(b) On the downstroke, the flexible diaphragm bends downward drawing air in through a one-way intake valve. Air is forced out the one-way outflow on the upstroke.

(c) Used commonly on oxygen concentrators

(3) Rotary type

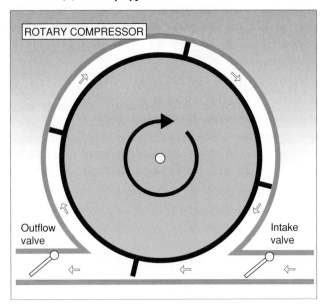

From Persing G. *Entry Level Respiratory Care Review*. Philadelphia: WB Saunders; 1992.

    (a) The rotor acts like a fan pushing air from one area to another. As the rotor turns counterclockwise, gas is drawn into one side and forced out the other.
    (b) Used in the MA-1 ventilator

II. OXYGEN THERAPY

A. **Indications for oxygen therapy**
  1. Treat hypoxemia
  2. Decrease the work of breathing
  3. Reduce myocardial work
B. **Signs and symptoms of hypoxemia**
  1. Tachycardia
  2. Dyspnea
  3. Cyanosis
  4. Impairment of special senses
  5. Headache
  6. Mental disturbance
  7. Slight hyperventilation
C. **Complications of oxygen therapy**
  1. Respiratory depression—most affected is the chronic obstructive pulmonary disease (COPD) patient breathing on "hypoxic drive" mechanism. **Maintain PaO_2 between 50 and 60 torr**.
  2. Atelectasis—high oxygen concentrations in the lung wash out nitrogen in the lung and reduce the production of surfactant, leading to atelectasis. Maintain FIO_2 at less than 0.5 to 0.6.
  3. Oxygen toxicity—high oxygen concentrations result in toxicity to lung tissue because of increased oxygen free radicals. This leads to adult

respiratory distress syndrome (ARDS). Maintain FIO_2 at less than 0.5 to 0.6.
  4. Retrolental fibroplasia (neonatal retinopathy) is caused by **high PaO_2 levels** in infants, resulting in blindness. It is more common in premature infants. **Maintain PaO_2 at less than 100 torr.** Normal PaO_2 value in infants is 50 to 70 torr.
  5. Reduced mucociliary activity—maintain FIO_2 at less than 0.5 to 0.6
D. Normal PaO_2 values by age

Age	*Normal PaO_2*
<60 years	80 torr
70 years	70 torr
80 years	60 torr
90 years	50 torr

E. **Four types of hypoxia**
  1. **Hypoxemic hypoxia**
    a. Caused by lack of oxygen in the blood owing to:
      (1) Inadequate oxygen in the inspired air—giving oxygen is beneficial
      (2) Alveolar hypoventilation—oxygen alone may not be beneficial
      (3) Atelectasis—oxygen alone not beneficial
      (4) Pulmonary edema—high-percentage oxygen may be beneficial
      (5) Ventilation/perfusion mismatch—oxygen may be beneficial
      (6) Anatomic right-to-left shunt—oxygen not beneficial
    b. If a normal PaO_2 cannot be maintained with a 60% oxygen mask, a large shunt is probable and should not be treated with higher oxygen concentrations. **CPAP should be administered (if the $PaCO_2$ is normal). If the $PaCO_2$ is elevated along with hypoxemia, mechanical ventilation should be initiated.**
  2. **Anemic hypoxia**
    a. The capacity of blood to carry oxygen is decreased owing to:
      (1) Decreased hemoglobin level
        (a) Normal level is 12 to 16 g/100 ml blood
NOTE: g/100 ml of blood may also be expressed as g/dl, or vol %.
        **(b) The patient's PaO_2 may be normal, but with a diminished capacity of the blood to carry oxygen, the tissues may be deprived of it. The hemoglobin value must be deter-

mined in order to assess the patient's oxygenation status.

    (c) The hemoglobin content may be increased by giving the patient red blood cells.

  (2) Carbon monoxide poisoning

    (a) Carbon monoxide combines with hemoglobin 200 to 250 times faster than oxygen does; therefore, it occupies the iron sites on hemoglobin before oxygen can. This causes tissue hypoxia.

    (b) Since hemoglobin will release the carbon monoxide more readily when high PaO_2 values are present, the patient should immediately be started on a nonrebreathing mask that delivers close to 100% oxygen.

    (c) Elevating the PaO_2 even higher to further increase the dissociation of hemoglobin from carbon monoxide may be achieved with **hyperbaric oxygen therapy** (discussed later in this chapter).

    (d) Patients who have been involved in fires or who have breathed car fumes must be treated immediately for carbon monoxide poisoning.

  **(e) PaO_2 and oxygen saturation (SaO_2) readings (discussed later in this chapter) may be within normal range, but the patient may be severely hypoxic.

  ** (f) The level of carbon monoxide bound to hemoglobin (carboxyhemoglobin) may be determined by the use of a co-oximeter (discussed later in this chapter).

  **(g) The patient will usually present with normal PaO_2 and low or normal $PaCO_2$ values. The pH is usually low because of lactic acidosis (metabolic acidosis).

  (3) Excessive blood loss—treated by giving blood

  (4) Methemoglobinemia—results most commonly from nitrite poisoning, treated by administering ascorbic acid or methylene blue, which removes the chemical (nitrite) from the system

  (5) Iron deficiency—treated by increasing iron intake and giving blood

b. Oxygen is carried in the blood in two ways:

  (1) Bound to hemoglobin (1.34* $\times$ Hb$\times$ SaO_2)

  (2) Dissolved in plasma (0.003† $\times PaO_2$)

NOTE: The sum of these two values equals the total oxygen content in ml/dl of blood or ml/100 ml of blood

EXAMPLE: Given the following information calculate the patient's total arterial oxygen content.

Arterial Blood Gas (ABG) Results
pH   7.42
PCO_2 41 torr
PO_2 90 torr
SaO_2 98%
Hb   15 ml/dl

Oxygen bound to hemoglobin =
$$1.34 \times 15 \times 0.98 = 19.7 \text{ ml/dl}$$

Oxygen dissolved in plasma =
$$0.003 \times 90 = 0.27 \text{ ml/dl}$$

Total arterial oxygen content =
$$19.7 \text{ ml} + 0.27 \text{ ml} = \textbf{19.97 ml/dl}$$

May also be expressed as **19.97 vol %.

  3. **Stagnant (circulatory) hypoxia**

    a. The oxygen content and carrying capacity are normal, but capillary perfusion is diminished owing to:

     (1) Decreased heart rate

     (2) Decreased cardiac output

     (3) Shock

     (4) Emboli

    b. May be seen as a localized problem as peripheral cyanosis due to exposure to cold weather

  4. **Histotoxic hypoxia**

    a. The oxidative enzyme mechanism of the cell is impaired owing to:

     (1) Cyanide poisoning

     (2) Alcohol poisoning

    b. Rarely accompanied by hypoxemia; increased venous PO_2 levels present

F. **Oxygen Delivery Devices**

  1. **Low-flow oxygen systems** are oxygen delivery devices that do not meet the patient's in-

---

*1.34 ml of oxygen is capable of combining with 1 g of hemoglobin

†0.003 ml of oxygen dissolves in the plasma for 1 torr of oxygen tension (Pa_{O_2})

spiratory flow demands; therefore, room air is entrained by the patient to make up the difference. The normal inspiratory flowrate is 25 to 30 L/min. The following devices are connected to **humidifiers.** (In some areas humidifiers are not used if less than 5 L/min is delivered.)

a. **Nasal catheter**

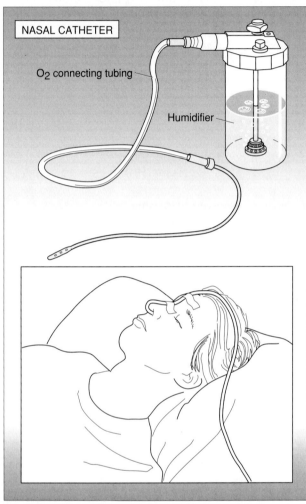

From Persing G. *Entry Level Respiratory Care Review.* Philadelphia: WB Saunders; 1992.

(1) Delivers oxygen percentages of 24% to 44% at flowrates of 1 to 6 L/min (about 4% increase for every liter)

(2) The catheter should be lubricated with water-soluble gel and inserted nasally to just above the uvula. The catheter may be measured from the patient's nose to ear to place it at that position.

(3) If catheter is inserted too far, swallowing of air and gastric distention may result.

(4) Change catheter to alternate nostril every 8 hours.

b. **Transtracheal oxygen catheter**

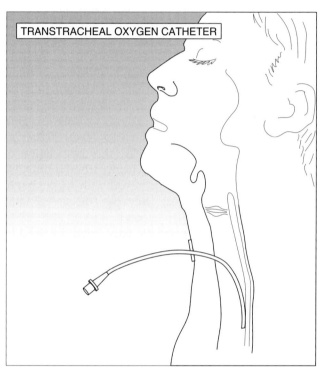

From Persing G. *Entry Level Respiratory Care Review.* Philadelphia: WB Saunders; 1992.

(1) A catheter inserted directly into the trachea to deliver low flowrates (1 to 3 L/min) of continuous oxygen

(2) Conserves oxygen for home patients by bypassing anatomic deadspace, which results in reduced work of breathing

(3) Possible complications include accidental removal of the catheter and irritation or infection at the insertion site and in trachea.

c. **Nasal cannula**

d. **Simple oxygen mask**

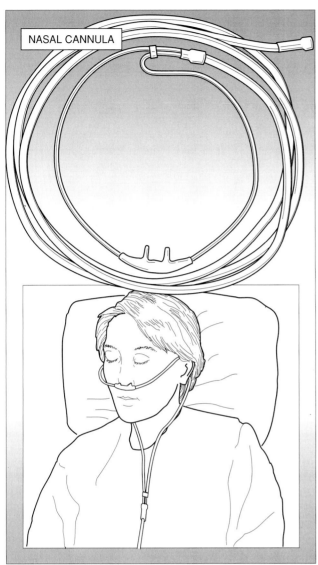

From Persing G. *Entry Level Respiratory Care Review*. Philadelphia: WB Saunders; 1992.

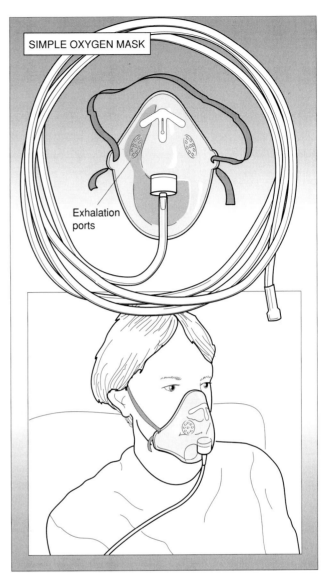

From Persing G. *Entry Level Respiratory Care Review*. Philadelphia: WB Saunders; 1992.

(1) Delivers oxygen percentages of 24% to 44% at flowrates of 1 to 6 L/min (about 4% increase per liter)

(2) Much better tolerated by the patient than a nasal catheter

(1) Delivers oxygen percentages of 35% to 55% at flowrates of 6 to 10 L/min

(2) Minimum flowrate of 6 L/min is needed to prevent buildup of exhaled carbon dioxide in the mask.

e. **Partial rebreathing mask**

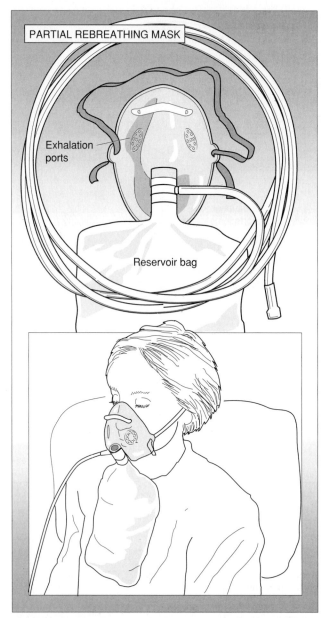

From Persing G. *Entry Level Respiratory Care Review.* Philadelphia: WB Saunders; 1992.

(1) Delivers oxygen percentages of 35% to 60% at flowrates of 8 to 15 L/min
(2) Flowrate must be sufficient to keep the reservoir bag at least one-third to one-half full at all times.
(3) Need to ensure that the patient is not positioned so that the reservoir bag gets kinked off; lower percentage of oxygen would result

f. **Nonrebreathing mask**

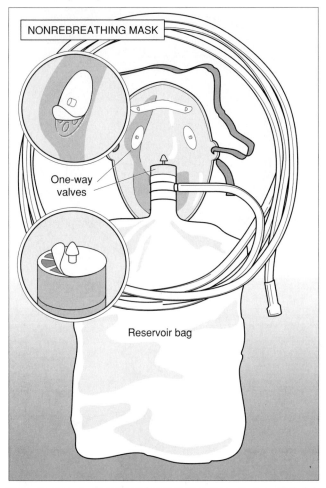

From Persing G. *Entry Level Respiratory Care Review.* Philadelphia: WB Saunders; 1992.

(1) Delivers oxygen percentages of 75% to 100% at flowrates of 8 to 15 L/min
(2) Flowrate must be sufficient to keep the reservoir bag at least one-third to one-half full at all times.
(3) The nonrebreathing mask is equipped with a one-way flutter valve between the mask and the reservoir bag that will not allow exhaled gases into the reservoir bag.
(4) One-way flutter valves are located on side ports of the mask to prevent room air entrainment. If one valve is used, FIO_2 decreases and the mask is considered to be of the low-flow type, but if both valves are used, FIO_2 increases, no air entrainment can occur, and the mask is considered a high-flow device.
(5) Must ensure that the reservoir bag does not kink off, especially if both exhalation ports have one-way flutter valves, as no room air would be available to the

patient (for this reason one flutter valve is often left off)

**g. Low-flow oxygen devices are adequate for use only if the following criteria are met:
    (1) **Tidal volume of 300 to 700 ml**
    (2) **Respiratory rate of less than 25 breaths/min**
    (3) **Regular and consistent ventilatory pattern**

Any patient requiring supplemental oxygen who does not meet these criteria should be placed on a high-flow oxygen delivery device (see further on).

**The percentage of oxygen delivered by a low-flow device is variable, depending on the patient's tidal volume, respiratory rate, inspiratory time, and ventilatory pattern.

2. **High-flow devices** provide all of the total inspiratory flow required by the patient. They provide relatively accurate and consistent oxygen percentages. With the exception of the Venturi mask, these devices are attached to **nebulizers.**

   a. **Venturi mask (air entrainment mask) — 24% to 50% oxygen delivery**

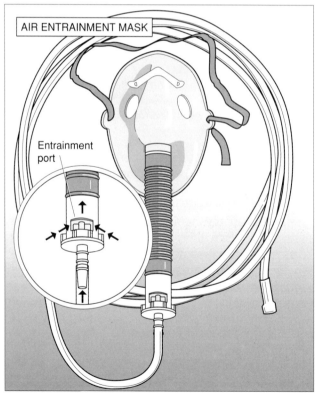

From Persing G. *Entry Level Respiratory Care Review.* Philadelphia: WB Saunders; 1992.

   (1) Increasing the flowrate on the device will not alter the FIO_2. The jet size and entrainment port alter the FIO_2:

Larger entrainment port→more air entrained→lower FIO_2
Smaller entrainment port→less air entrained→higher FIO_2
Larger jet size→less air entrained→higher FIO_2
Smaller jet size→more air entrained→lower FIO_2

NOTE: It is important to prevent the entrainment port from becoming occluded (e.g., by patient's hand, bedsheet), as this will decrease the amount of air entrainment and thus increase the delivered oxygen percentage.

   (2) Air:oxygen entrainment ratios

Air:Oxygen Ratio	Oxygen Percentage
25:1	24%
10:1	28%
8:1	30%
5:1	35%
3:1	40%
1.7:1	50%
1:1	60%

These ratios may be calculated by the following formula:

$$\frac{100 - x}{x - 20*} = \frac{\text{parts air entrained}}{1 \text{ part oxygen}}$$

EXAMPLE: Calculate the air:oxygen ratio for 40%

$$\frac{100 - 40}{40 - 20} = \frac{60}{20} = \frac{3}{1} \text{ or } \textbf{3:1 ratio}$$

This means that for *every liter of oxygen* (source gas) delivered from the flowmeter, *3 liters of air* are entrained into the device.

   (3) **Calculating total flow**
If a Venturi mask is set on 40% with a flowrate of 12 L/min, the total flow delivered would be:

12 L/min of oxygen
36 L/min of air (12 × 3)
48 L/min total flow

FASTER METHOD: Add the ratio parts together and multiply by the flow.

---

*Use 21 on percentages of less than 40%

40% (3:1 air:oxygen ratio)
3 + 1 = 4   **4 × 12 = 48 L/min**

EXAMPLE: A Venturi mask is set on 24% with a flow of 4 L/min. Calculate the total flow.

$$\frac{100 - 24}{24 - 21} = \frac{76}{3} = \frac{25}{1} = \textbf{25:1} \text{ air:oxygen ratio}$$

4 L/min oxygen   sum of ratio parts × flow
100 L/min of air   *or*
104 L/min total flow

$$(25 + 1) =$$
$$26 \times 4 = 104 \text{ L/min}$$

EXAMPLE: The physician has ordered a 40% aerosol mask to be placed on a patient who has a total inspiratory flow of 44 L/min. What is the minimum flow we must set the flowmeter on to meet this patient's inspiratory flow demands?

Since the air:oxygen ratio for 40% is 3:1, add the ratio parts together.

$$3 + 1 = 4$$

We now must set the flowmeter on the lowest liter flow that when multiplied by 4 delivers a total flow of at least 44 L/min. In other words, 4 × ? = 44

The flowmeter must be set at a minimum of 11 L/min.

b. **Aerosol mask**

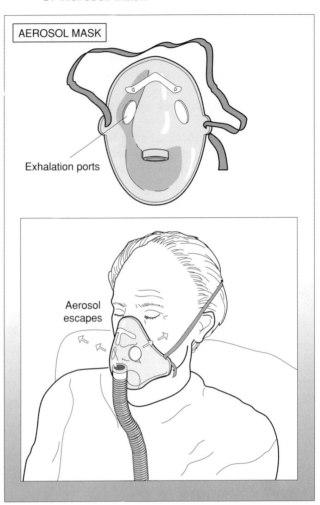

From Persing G. *Entry Level Respiratory Care Review*. Philadelphia: WB Saunders; 1992.

(1) Delivers oxygen percentages of 21% to 60% (depending on nebulizer setting) at flowrates of 8 to 15 L/min (on flowmeter)
(2) If the nebulizer is set on 100%, more than likely the device would not meet the patient's inspiratory flow demands. Room air would be entrained, decreasing FIO_2.
**(3) Mist should be visible flowing from the exhalation ports at all times to ensure adequate flowrates.

c. **Face tent**

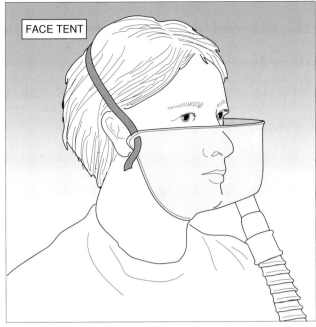

FACE TENT

From Persing G. *Entry Level Respiratory Care Review*. Philadelphia: WB Saunders; 1992.

(1) Delivers oxygen percentages of 21% to 40% (depending on nebulizer setting) at flowrates of 8 to 15 L/min
(2) Used primarily on patients with facial trauma or burns or those who cannot tolerate a mask

d. **T-tube flow-by or Briggs' adaptor**

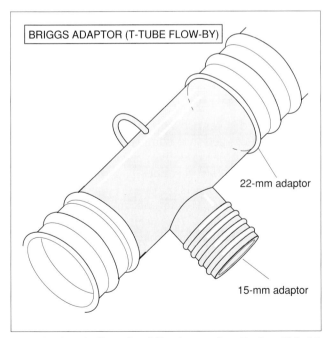

BRIGGS ADAPTOR (T-TUBE FLOW-BY)

22-mm adaptor

15-mm adaptor

From Persing G. *Entry Level Respiratory Care Review*. Philadelphia: WB Saunders; 1992.

(1) Delivers oxygen percentages of 21% to 100% (depending on nebulizer setting) at flowrates of 8 to 15 L/min
(2) Used on the intubated or tracheostomy patient
(3) A piece of 50-cc reservoir tubing should be attached to the opposite end of the T-tube. This prevents air entrainment during inspiration, and if the reservoir falls off, FIO_2 may **decrease.**
**(4) Adequate flowrates ensured by visualizing mist flowing out of the 50-cc reservoir at all times.

e. **Tracheostomy mask (collar)**

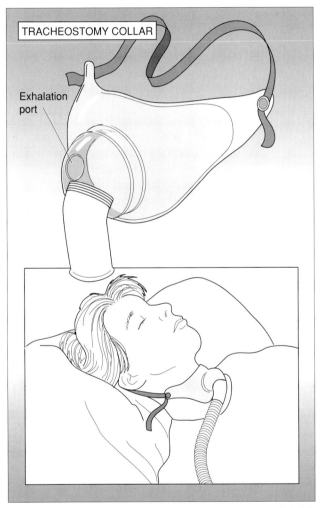

TRACHEOSTOMY COLLAR

Exhalation port

From Persing G. *Entry Level Respiratory Care Review*. Philadelphia: WB Saunders; 1992.

(1) Delivers oxygen percentages of 35% to 60% (depending on nebulizer setting) at flowrates of 10 to 15 L/min
**(2) Adequate flowrates are ensured by visualizing mist flowing out of the exhalation port at all times.
(3) Mask should fit directly over the tracheostomy tube.

f. **Oxygen tent**

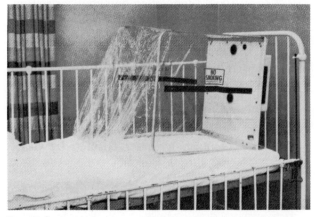

From Safar P, ed. *Respiratory Therapy.* Philadelphia: FA Davis; 1965

(1) Delivers oxygen percentages of 21% to 50% at flowrates of 15 L/min or higher
(2) Used primarily on children with croup or pneumonia.
(3) Not an ideal oxygen delivery device because of high source of leaks and reduced oxygen percentage when the tent is opened for patient care
(4) A fire hazard exists if electrical devices or friction toys that may spark are left in the tent.

G. **Important points concerning high-flow devices**

1. High-flow devices set on 60% or higher may deliver a total flow of less than 25 to 30 L/min; thereby not meeting the patient's inspiratory flow demands. It essentially acts as a low-flow device, with the patient breathing in room air to make up the difference. This means the oxygen setting on the device is no longer accurate, and the patient is receiving less oxygen.
2. To ensure adequate flowrates on a device set on 60% or higher, use two flowmeters connected in-line together.
3. In order to ensure adequate flow, set the flowmeter to a rate that will deliver a total flow of **at least 40 L/min.**
**4. A restriction, such as kinked aerosol tubing or water in the tubing, causes back pressure into the nebulizer, decreasing the amount of air entrainment and therefore increasing the oxygen percentage.
5. Increasing the flowrate on a high-flow device will not increase the FIO_2 delivered. It will only increase the total flow.

H. **Calculating FIO_2**

$$FIO_2 = \frac{\text{oxygen flow} + (\text{air flow} \times 0.2)}{\text{total flow}}$$

EXAMPLE: A nebulizer set on the 40% dilution mode and connected to an oxygen flowmeter running at 10 L/min has an air bleed-in of 6 L/min downstream. Calculate the FIO_2.

Oxygen flow = 10 L/min
    Air flow = 30 L/min (entrained through nebulizer)
    Air flow = <u>6 L/min</u> (bleed-in)
  Total flow = 46 L/min

$$FIO_2 = \frac{10 + (36 \times 0.2)}{46} = \frac{10 + 7.2}{46} = \frac{17.2}{46} = \mathbf{0.37}$$

I. **Oxygen blenders**

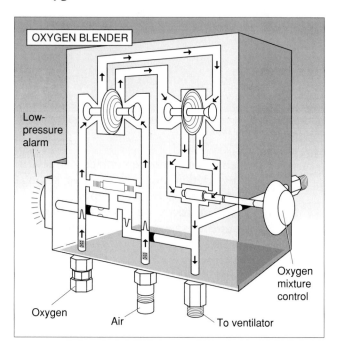

1. These devices use 50 psig gas sources to mix or blend oxygen and compressed air proportionately in order to deliver oxygen percentages of 21% to 100% at flowrates of 2 to 100 L/min.
2. A blender consists of pressure-regulating valves that regulate oxygen and air inlet pressure, a mixture control (precision metering device), and an audible alarm system that sounds when a drop in inlet pressure occurs.
3. Blenders provide a stable FIO_2 as long as the outlet flow exceeds the patient's inspiratory flow demands.

III. MIXED GAS THERAPY

A. **Helium/oxygen therapy**
   1. Helium is the second lightest gas and, therefore, when combined with oxygen will decrease the total density of the gas. This allows the gas to pass through obstructions more easily.
   2. Helium/oxygen mixtures (Heliox) are stored in brown and green cylinders.
   3. Helium does not support life; therefore, it must be mixed with oxygen. Two common mixtures are:
      a. 80% helium/20% oxygen
      b. 70% helium/30% oxygen
   4. Running these gas mixtures through an oxygen flowmeter will give inaccurate readings, since the gas is lighter than pure oxygen. A correction factor may be used to make the reading accurate.
      a. 80:20 mixture of helium/oxygen— **multiply the flowmeter reading by 1.8** to determine the correct flow; divide the flowrate by 1.8 if you want to deliver a specific flow

EXAMPLE: An 80:20 mixture of helium/oxygen is running through an oxygen flowmeter at 10 L/min. What is the actual flowrate?

$$10 \times 1.8 = \textbf{18 L/min}$$

EXAMPLE: You want to deliver 12 L/min of an 80:20 mixture of helium/oxygen to the patient. What must you set the oxygen flowmeter on to deliver this flow?

$$\frac{12}{1.8} = \textbf{6.6 L/min}$$

      b. 70:30 mixture of helium/oxygen— **multiply the flowmeter reading by 1.6;** divide by 1.6 to obtain a specific flow (see preceding problem and substitute 1.6)
   5. Helium/oxygen mixtures must be delivered in a tightly closed system such as a nonrebreathing mask, endotracheal tube, or tracheostomy tube to prevent this lighter gas from leaking out.
   6. The only side effect of helium/oxygen therapy is distortion of the voice.
   7. Extreme caution must be used when mixing Heliox from a helium cylinder and an oxygen cylinder. Inaccurate flow readings may result in the patient receiving less than 21% oxygen. A premixed helium/oxygen cylinder is recommended.
   8. Helium/oxygen mixtures are safe and may be of benefit in the treatment of:
      a. Obstruction from secretions
      b. Asthma (during episode of bronchospasm)

B. **Carbon dioxide/oxygen therapy**

NOTE: In the past, the field of respiratory care has used carbon dioxide/oxygen gas mixtures for a variety of reasons. Although at present it is used only sparingly, the concepts behind its use are important for the practitioner to understand.
   1. **Physiologic actions of carbon dioxide**
      a. Respiratory stimulant in concentrations of up to 10%, resulting in increased respiratory rate and tidal volume
      b. Respiratory depressant in concentrations greater than 10%, resulting in decreased respiratory rate and tidal volume
      c. Increased blood pressure, resulting from systemic vasoconstriction
      d. Increased heart rate
      e. Increased cerebral blood flow, resulting from cerebral vasodilation
      f. Vasodilation of capillary beds
      g. Central nervous system (CNS) depressant in low concentrations (5% to 10%), resulting in mental depression or unconsciousness
      h. CNS stimulant in high concentrations (>30%, resulting in seizures)
**NOTE: The carbon dioxide/oxygen mixture most commonly used consists of 95% oxygen and 5% carbon dioxide. This is commonly referred to as a "95/5 treatment."
   2. **Indications for carbon dioxide therapy**
      a. To improve cerebral blood flow
         (1) Stroke patients
         (2) Fainting spells
      b. To stimulate deep breathing
         (1) Prevent or treat atelectasis
         (2) Since there is more frequently an increase in respiratory rate than in tidal volume, this is not effective. Tidal volume may increase, but not as significantly as rate.
      c. To treat hiccoughs
         (1) May interfere with the spasms of the phrenic nerve, thereby stopping the hiccoughs
      d. To stop seizure activity
         (1) Low concentrations (5%) cause CNS depression
      e. To treat carbon monoxide poisoning
         (1) Low concentrations (3% to 7%) enhance the release of carbon monoxide from hemoglobin.
   3. **Side effects of carbon dioxide therapy**
      a. Dyspnea
      b. Dizziness

   c. Muscle tremors

   d. Nasal irritation

   e. Paresthesia

   f. Headache

   g. Nausea (carbon dioxide toxicity)

   h. Vomiting (carbon dioxide toxicity)

   i. Disorientation (carbon dioxide toxicity)

   j. Severe elevation in blood pressure (carbon dioxide toxicity)

4. **Important points concerning carbon dioxide**

   a. No more than 5% carbon dioxide should be used.

   b. The treatment should not exceed 10 minutes.

   c. The treatment should be given with a nonrebreathing mask that is held over the face and is not strapped on so that it can be easily removed if needed.

   d. The treatment is contraindicated in patients who have compromised central respiratory centers, such as those with severe COPD.

   e. Carbon dioxide/oxygen therapy is not the treatment of choice to stimulate deep breathing. Other methods are much more effective, as well as much safer.

IV. HYPERBARIC OXYGEN THERAPY

A. Hyperbaric chambers

  1. Fixed multiplace chamber

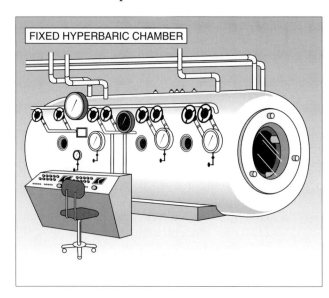

FIXED HYPERBARIC CHAMBER

  2. Portable monoplace chamber

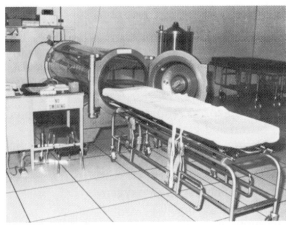

From Davis JC, Hunt TK. *Hyperbaric Oxygen Therapy.* Bethesda MD: Undersea Medical Society; 1977.

B. Hyperbaric oxygen therapy is the delivery of oxygen at a pressure greater than atmospheric pressure and is accomplished by placing the patient in a hyperbaric chamber.

C. The multiplace chamber is a walk-in unit that will accommodate several people.

D. The monoplace unit will accommodate only one person at a time.

E. The chambers are usually pressurized to 3 atmospheres (atm), or three times atmospheric pressure, as the patient breathes 100% oxygen.

F. This increased pressure likewise increases the amount of oxygen in the blood and tissues. While breathing room air at 1 atm, the PaO_2 is about 100 torr with about 0.3 vol% oxygen dissolved in the plasma; while breathing 100% oxygen at 3 atm, the PaO_2 is about 1800 torr with 6.2 vol% of oxygen dissolved in the plasma.

G. **Physiologic effects of hyperbaric oxygen**

  1. Elevated PaO_2 levels

  2. Vasoconstriction

  3. New capillary bed formation

  4. Metabolic alteration of aerobic and anaerobic organisms

  5. Reduction of nitrogen bubbles in the blood

H. **Indications for hyperbaric oxygen therapy**

  1. Carbon monoxide poisoning

  2. Cyanide poisoning

  3. Decompression sickness (''bends'')

  4. Gas gangrene

  5. Gas embolism

I. Hyperbaric oxygen treatments, or ''dives'' as they are often called, usually require 90 minutes at 2 to 3 atm, two to four times a day.

V. OXYGEN ANALYZERS

A. **Physical analyzers (paramagnetic)**
   1. Uses the Pauling principle
   2. Measures partial pressure of oxygen more closely
   3. Reading is affected by higher altitude.
   4. The Beckman D-2 is an example of a physical analyzer.
B. **Electrical analyzer**
   1. Uses the "wheatstone bridge" and the principle of thermal conduction
   2. Measures oxygen percentage more closely
   3. Has a slow response time
   4. Mira is an example of an electrical analyzer.
C. **Electrochemical Analyzers**
   1. Galvanic cell type
      a. Electrolyte gel is used to chemically reduce oxygen to electron flow.
      b. Uses a Clark electrode and measures partial pressure.
      c. Reading is affected by water, positive pressure, high altitude, a torn membrane, or lack of electrolyte gel.
      d. The Teledyne and Hudson are examples of galvanic cell electrochemical analyzers.
   2. **Polarographic type**
      a. A battery polarizes the electrodes to allow oxygen reduction to occur, giving off electron flow.
      b. Uses the Clark electrode and more accurately measures partial pressures.
      c. Reading is affected by water, positive pressure, high altitude, a torn membrane, or lack of electrolyte gel.
      d. Electrodes last longer on the galvanic cell, but the polarographic analyzer has a quicker response time.
      e. IL and Ohio are examples of the polarographic electrochemical analyzer.

VI. OXYGEN SATURATION MONITORING (PULSE OXIMETRY)

A. Use of the pulse oximeter
   1. Pulse oximeters are devices that measure oxygen saturation (SaO_2) by the principle of **spectrophotometry.**
   2. Light from the probe is directed through a capillary bed to be absorbed in different amounts, depending on the amount of oxygen bound to hemoglobin. The result is displayed on the monitor as a percentage of saturation.
   3. The probe is noninvasive and may be attached to the finger, toe, or ear in adults and the ankle or foot of infants.
   4. Pulse oximeters seem to be quite accurate, although some studies show they may be less accurate when used for "spot checks" rather than continuous monitoring.
B. **Causes of inaccurate readings**
   1. Low blood perfusion
   2. Carbon monoxide poisoning
   3. Severe anemia
   4. Hypotension
   5. Hypothermia
   6. Cardiac arrest

VII. CO-OXIMETRY

A. This procedure requires arterial blood to be obtained, and the oximeter is able to measure the amount of hemoglobin, oxyhemoglobin, and carboxyhemoglobin.
B. This procedure uses the principle of spectrophotometry.
**C. The level of carbon monoxide bound to hemoglobin (carboxyhemoglobin) may be measured by this method.
   1. Carboxyhemoglobin is usually expressed as a percentage of total hemoglobin.
   2. Carboxyhemoglobin in concentrations as high as 10% may be seen in heavy smokers, but higher levels are measured in victims who have inhaled large amounts of car fumes or smoke.
   3. Patients with carboxyhemoglobin levels of less than 20% are usually asymptomatic.
   4. Carboxyhemoglobin levels of greater than 20% will result in nausea and vomiting, with fatal levels being 60% to 80%.

REFERENCES

1. Eubanks D, Bone R. *Comprehensive Respiratory Care.* 2nd ed. St. Louis: CV Mosby; 1990.
2. Malley W. *Clinical Blood Gases: Application and Noninvasive Alternatives.* Philadelphia: WB Saunders; 1990.
3. McPherson SP. *Respiratory Therapy Equipment.* 4th ed. St. Louis: Mosby; 1990.
4. Scanlan C, Spearman C, Sheldon R. *Egan's Fundamentals of Respiratory Care.* 5th ed. St. Louis: CV Mosby; 1990.

PRETEST ANSWERS

1. C

2. D

3. E

4. A

5. D

6. B

Humidity and Aerosol Therapy

PRETEST QUESTIONS*

1. Secretions will tend to become thicker if the inspired air has which of the following characteristics?

A. A relative humidity of 100% at body temperature
B. 32 mg of water per liter of gas
C. A water vapor pressure of 47 torr
D. 48 mg of water per liter of gas
E. A body humidity of 100%

2. A patient receiving 38 mg of water per liter of gas from a nebulizer has a humidity deficit of which of the following?

A. 6 mg/L
B. 9 mg/L
C. 12 mg/L
D. 18 mg/L
E. 20 mg/L

3. After connecting a nasal cannula to the humidifier outlet you kink the tubing and hear a whistling noise coming from the humidifier. Which of the following has most likely caused this occurrence?

A. The humidifier jar is cracked.
B. The capillary tube in the humidifier is disconnected.
C. The humidifier has no leaks.
D. The top of the humidifier is not screwed on tightly.
E. The flow is too low.

4. You notice that the patient's secretions have become thicker and more difficult to suction since replacing the ventilator humidifier with a heat moisture exchanger. The respiratory therapist should recommend which of the following?

A. Increase inspiratory flowrate.
B. Increase the temperature of the heat moisture exchanger.
C. Replace with a new heat moisture exchanger.
D. Rinse the heat moisture exchanger with sterile water and reconnect to the circuit.
E. Replace the heat moisture exchanger with a conventional heated humidifier.

5. Which of the following are indications for aerosol therapy?

I. To induce cough for sputum collection
II. To improve the mobilization of secretions
III. To treat postextubation inflammation of the upper airway

A. I only
B. II only
C. I and III only
D. II and III only
E. I, II, and III

6. You notice very little mist is being produced by a nebulizer attached to an aerosol mask. Which of the following could be responsible for this?

I. The liter flow is too high.
II. The nebulizer jet is clogged with soap residue.
III. The filter on the capillary tube is obstructed.

A. I only
B. II only
C. I and III only
D. II and III only
E. I, II, and III

---

*See answers at the end of the chapter.

CHAPTER **2**

Humidity and Aerosol Therapy

I. HUMIDITY THERAPY

A. **Humidity**—water in a gaseous state or vapor; also called "molecular water" or "invisible moisture"
B. **Clinical uses of humidity**
  1. To humidify dry therapeutic gases
  2. To provide 100% body humidity of the inspired gas for patients with endotracheal tubes or tracheostomy tubes
NOTE: The objective of humidity therapy is to make up for water loss that occurs when dry gas is delivered or when the upper airway is bypassed. Adding "liquid" water or mist to the airway to thin secretions is accomplished by **aerosol therapy** (discussed later in this chapter).
C. **Normal airway humidification**
  1. Nose—it warms, humidifies, and filters inspired air.
  2. Pharynx, trachea, and bronchial tree—also warms, humidifies, and filters inspired air.
  3. By the time inspired air reaches the oropharynx, it has been warmed to approximately 34°C and is 80% to 90% saturated.
  4. By the time the inspired air reaches the carina, it has been warmed to body temperature (37°C) and is 100% saturated.
5. When the inspired air is fully saturated (100%), it holds **44 mg of water per liter of gas and exerts a **water vapor pressure of 47 torr**.
D. **Absolute and relative humidity**
  1. **Absolute humidity**—the amount of water in a given volume of gas; expressed in milligrams per liter (mg/L)
  2. **Relative humidity**—a ratio of the amount of water in a given volume of gas to the amount it is capable of holding at that temperature; **expressed as a percentage; it is measured with the use of a hygrometer.**
  3. **Relative humidity =**
$$\frac{\textbf{absolute humidity}}{\textbf{capacity}} \times \textbf{100}$$

EXAMPLE: The amount of moisture in a given volume of gas at 31°C contains 24 mg of water per liter of gas. Calculate the relative humidity. (At 31°C, the air can hold 32.01 mg of water per liter of gas.)

$$\text{Relative humidity} = \frac{24 \text{ mg/L}}{32.01 \text{ mg/L}} =$$
$$0.75 \times 100 = \textbf{75\%}$$

EXAMPLE: A gas at 22°C has a relative humidity of 54%. Calculate the absolute humidity. (At 22°C the air can hold 19.42 mg of water per liter of gas.)

Absolute humidity = relative humidity ×
capacity = 0.54 × 19.42 mg/L = **10.5 mg/L**
E. **Body humidity**
  1. The relative humidity at body temperature expressed as a percentage
  2. Body humidity $= \dfrac{\text{absolute humidity}}{44 \text{ mg/L}} \times 100$
    (capacity at body temperature)

EXAMPLE: If the patient's inspired gas contains 21 mg of water per liter of gas, what is the body humidity?

$$\text{Body humidity} = \frac{21 \text{ mg/L}}{44 \text{ mg/L}} = 0.48 \times 100 = \textbf{48\%}$$

  3. A 48% body humidity indicates that the inspired air is holding only 48% of the water it takes to fully saturate the gas in the airway at body temperature. The body's humidification system will make up the other 52% by the time the air reaches the carina.
F. **Humidity deficit**
  1. Inspired air that is not fully saturated at body temperature creates a humidity deficit. This deficit is made up by the body's own humidification system.
  2. Humidity deficit may be expressed in milligrams per liter or as a percentage.

3. **Humidity deficit =**

$$\textbf{44 mg/L} - \textbf{absolute humidity}$$

or

when expressed as a percentage:

$$\frac{\textbf{Humidity deficit (mg/L)}}{\textbf{44 mg/L}} \times \textbf{100}$$

EXAMPLE: A patient on T-tube flow-by is inspiring air from an Ohio nebulizer that contains 18 mg of water per liter of air. What is this patient's humidity deficit?

44 mg/L
−18 mg/L and as a percentage:
26 mg/L

$$\frac{26 \text{ mg/L}}{44 \text{ mg/L}} = 0.48 \times 100 = \textbf{59\%}$$

4. This is why it is important to deliver humidified gas at body temperature to patients with artificial airways that bypass the patient's upper airway.

**5. If adequate humidity is not provided, the patient's airway can dry out, leading to thickening of secretions that result in increased airway resistance.

6. Gas being delivered to a patient with an endotracheal tube or tracheostomy tube that contains **less than 44 mg of water per liter of gas or a water vapor pressure of less than 47 torr will tend to dry secretions out, making them thicker and more difficult to mobilize.

G. **Efficiency of humidifiers**—dependent upon three important factors:
   1. The time of contact between the gas and water (longer contact time → increased humidity)
   2. The surface area involved in gas/water contact (greater surface area involved → increased humidity)
   3. The temperature of the gas and water (increased temperature of gas or water → increased humidity)

H. **Types of humidifiers**

1. **Pass-over humidifier** (nonheated humidifier)

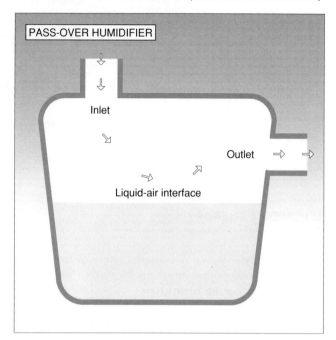

a. Gas simply passes over the surface of the water picking up moisture and delivering it to the patient.
b. Produces a low-humidity output because of the limited time of gas/water contact and surface area involved
c. Provides a body humidity of approximately 25%

2. **Bubble humidifier** (nonheated humidifier)

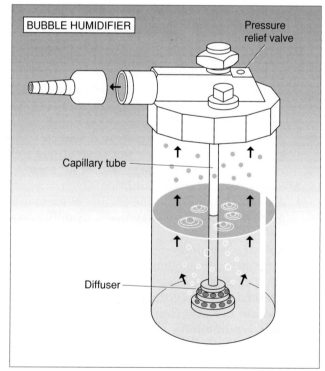

From Persing G. *Entry Level Respiratory Care Review*. Philadelphia: WB Saunders; 1992.

a. The most common type of humidifier used on oxygen delivery devices

b. Gas flows out of the flowmeter through a tube under the surface of the water and exits through a diffuser at the lower end of the tube.

c. **Provides a body humidity of 35% to 40%**

3. **Jet humidifier** (nonheated humidifier)

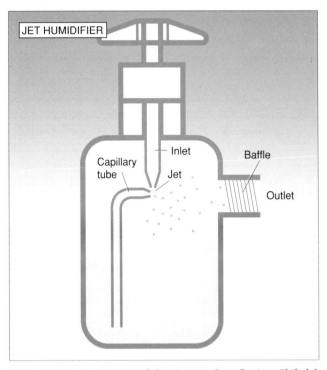

From Persing G. *Entry Level Respiratory Care Review*. Philadelphia: WB Saunders; 1992.

a. An aerosol is actually produced as water is drawn up the capillary tube into the flow of gas. The aerosol is baffled, leaving only molecular moisture to be delivered to the patient.

b. An underwater jet is another type of jet humidifier. Gas from the flowmeter travels through a capillary tube under the surface of the water and through a restriction (jet) that draws water into the tube. Gas bubbles containing aerosol float to the surface of the water, delivering higher humidity to the patient.

c. These humidifiers have a greater potential for water output than the bubble or pass-over humidifiers.

4. **Wick humidifier** (heated humidifier)

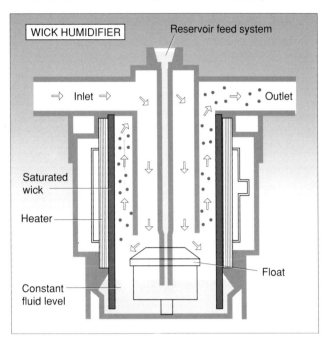

From Persing G. *Entry Level Respiratory Care Review*. Philadelphia: WB Saunders; 1992.

a. Gas from the flowmeter or ventilator enters the humidifier and is exposed to the wick (made of cloth, sponge, or paper), which is partially submerged under the surface of the water.

b. As gas passes the wick, it absorbs water and is delivered to the patient.

c. Because the water bath or the gas is heated, a body humidity approaching 100% is delivered to the patient. It is ideal to use on patients with artificial airways and those on mechanical ventilators.

5. **Cascade humidifier** (heated humidifier)

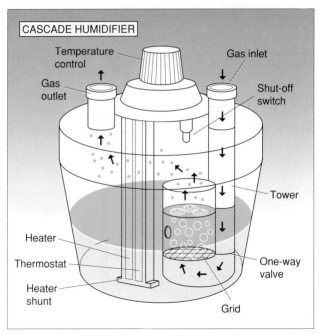

From Persing G. *Entry Level Respiratory Care Review*. Philadelphia: WB Saunders; 1992.

    a. Gas travels down the tower and hits the bottom of the jar, which displaces the water upward over a grid, forming a liquid film. The gas travels back up through the grid (from underneath) picking up moisture and delivering it to the patient.

    b. Since it is heated, it is capable of delivering the gas at **100% body humidity**.

  **c. If the Cascade is allowed to run dry, the thermostat will automatically turn the heater off, preventing the reservoir from being damaged or allowing hot, dry gas to be delivered to the patient.

I. Important points concerning humidifiers

  1. Most nonheated humidifiers have a pressure pop-off valve set at 2 pounds per square inch (psi). After the device is set up, the tubing of the oxygen delivery device (cannula, mask, and so on) should be kinked to obstruct flow. If the pop-off valve makes a sound, there are no leaks. If no sound is heard, all connections should be tightened, as should the humidifier top.

  2. Water in all humidifiers should be maintained at the levels marked on the humidifier jar to ensure maximum humidity output.

  3. Condensation will occur in the tubing of heated humidifiers. This water should be discarded in a trash container or basin and **never** back into the humidifier.

  4. Inspired gas temperatures should be monitored continuously with an in-line thermometer when using heated humidifiers. The thermometer should be as close to the patient wye as possible.

  5. Warm, moist areas such as heated humidifiers are a breeding ground for microorganisms (especially *Pseudomonas*). The humidifier should be changed **every 24 hours**.

NOTE: Heated humidifiers are not as likely to deliver contaminated moisture to the patient because the small molecular water particles are not able to carry the organisms.

J. **Heat moisture exchanger** (artificial nose)

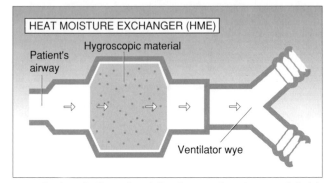

From Persing G. *Entry Level Respiratory Care Review*. Philadelphia: WB Saunders; 1992.

  1. This device is placed in-line between the patient and the patient wye of the ventilator circuit.

  2. As the patient exhales, gas at body humidity and body temperature enters the heat moisture exchanger heating the hygroscopic filter (made of felt, plastic foam, or cellulose sponge) and condensing water into it. During the next inspiration, gas passes through the heat moisture exchanger and is warmed and humidified.

  3. Under ideal conditions, the heat moisture exchanger can produce 70% to 90% body humidity.

NOTE: If the patient's secretions begin to thicken while using a heat moisture exchanger, a conventional humidifier should be substituted.

  4. Over a period of time, the heat moisture exchanger may cause a resistance to gas flow observed by increasing peak inspiratory pressures on the ventilator. If all pathologic reasons are ruled out as the cause of the increased pressures, **the heat moisture exchanger should be replaced with a new one**.

II. AEROSOL THERAPY

A. An aerosol is defined as water in particulate form or a mist. Nebulizers produce aerosols.

B. **Clinical uses for aerosol therapy**
1. To improve the mobilization of pulmonary secretions
2. To administer medications (via hand-held nebulizer or ultrasonic nebulizer)
3. To prevent dehydration
4. To prevent or relieve bronchospasm or inflammatory reaction following extubation
5. To hydrate the airways of a tracheostomy patient
6. To induce cough for sputum collection

C. **Hazards of aerosol therapy**
1. Bronchospasm—A bronchodilator may decrease the potential of this occurring
2. Overhydration
3. Overheating of inspired gas
4. Tubing condensation draining into the airway
5. Delivery of contaminated aerosol to the patient

D. **Characteristics of aerosol particles**
1. The ideal particle size for therapeutic use in respiratory care is 0.5 to 3 microns.
2. Numerous factors affect the penetration and deposition of aerosol particles:
   a. **Gravitational sedimentation**—the larger a particle is the more effect gravity has on it, and it will deposit sooner.
   b. **Brownian movement**—affects particles 0.1 microns or smaller in size. Particles in this size range will deposit too soon (possibly in aerosol tubing).
   c. **Inertial impaction**—larger particles have a greater inertia, which keeps them moving in a straight direction. They cannot make directional changes in the airway; therefore, they deposit sooner.
   d. **Hygroscopic properties**—aerosol particles are hygroscopic (retain moisture). As they travel down the airway, they may increase in size as they retain moisture, altering the time in which they deposit.
   e. **Ventilatory pattern**—in order to obtain optimal particle penetration, the patient should be instructed to take **slow, moderately deep breaths with 2- to 3-second breathholding at the end of each inspiration**.

E. **Types of nebulizers (pneumatic)**
1. **Mechanical nebulizer** (entrainment nebulizer)

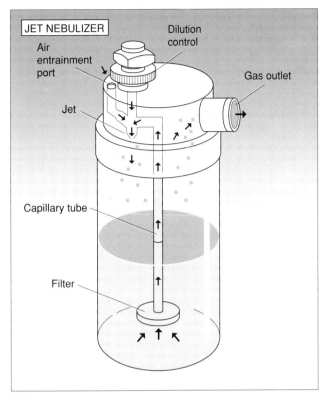

From Persing G. *Entry Level Respiratory Care Review*. Philadelphia: WB Saunders; 1992.

a. Uses the Bernoulli principle to draw water up the capillary tube into the gas stream to produce aerosol (mist)
b. Uses either a **Venturi** or **Pitot tube** for the entrainment of air for various oxygen percentages
   (1) **Venturi**—the objective is to allow air entrainment, increase flow, and restore postrestriction pressure to prerestriction pressure.

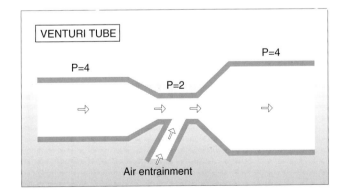

(2) **Pitot tube**—the objective is to maintain high forward velocity after air entrainment occurs, resulting in a high forward pressure, which is better able to counteract back pressure into the device, maintaining more stable oxygen percentages. (Postrestriction pressure is not restored to prerestriction levels.)

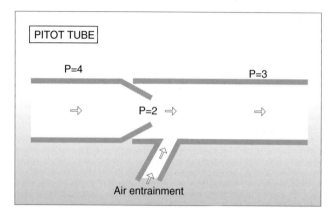

c. Mechanical nebulizers produce about **50%** of their particles in the **0.5 to 3 micron range**.

2. **Hydrosphere**

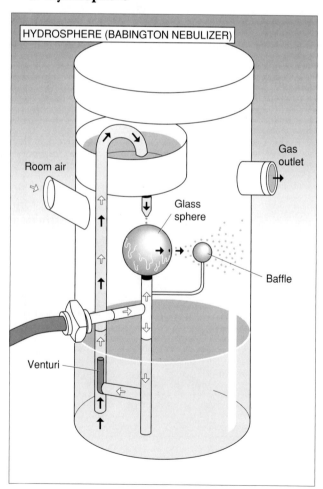

From Persing G. *Entry Level Respiratory Care Review*. Philadelphia: WB Saunders; 1992.

a. Water is pumped up into a reservoir above a glass sphere and drops out of the reservoir onto the sphere. The sphere has a small hole with high-velocity gas coming through it that decreases the pressure, pulling the water over the sphere. Water is then hit by high-velocity gas, producing an aerosol, and the particles hit a baffle, further reducing particle size.

b. Approximately 97% of the aerosol particles produced fall within the 1- to 10-micron range, with 50% smaller than 5 microns.

c. It is commonly used to deliver aerosol to an oxygen tent.

3. **Small-volume nebulizer**

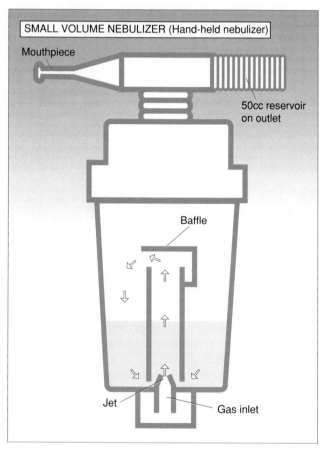

From Persing G. *Entry Level Respiratory Care Review*. Philadelphia: WB Saunders; 1992.

a. Used as a hand-held nebulizer or nebulizer on ventilator or intermittent positive pressure breathing (IPPB) circuit to deliver medications

b. Usually holds 3 to 6 ml of liquid medication

4. **Metered dose inhaler (MDI)**

a. This device delivers medication in aerosol form by squeezing the vial, in which the medication is stored, upward into the delivery port. This activates a small valve that allows the pressurized gas to nebulize the medication and deliver it to the patient.

b. MDIs have become a very popular method to deliver aerosolized drugs to the respiratory tract.

c. The particle size produced varies from 2 to 40 microns, with only about 10% of the dose actually reaching the lower respiratory tract.

d. It is essential that the patient be instructed thoroughly and **correctly on proper use of the MDI to assure optimal aerosol particle penetration.

e. The following points on the proper use of the MDI should be emphasized to the patient:

   (1) The patient should be instructed not to place the lips around the delivery port but to keep the mouth opened wide so that the teeth and lips will not obstruct the flow of aerosol.

   (2) The MDI should be held about 1 inch from the mouth, with the delivery port opening directed inside the mouth.

   (3) The patient should be instructed to inhale slowly and as deeply as possible. **The MDI should be activated just after the patient has started inhaling**.

   (4) Depending on the order, the patient may take two or three aerosol doses in one breath.

   (5) The patient should be instructed to hold the breath at peak inspiration for **5 to 10 seconds for optimal aerosol penetration.

   (6) MDIs are also used in patients breathing with a ventilator by placing the device directly into the inspiratory limb of the circuit; it is then activated by the respiratory care practitioner. Ideally, the aerosol should be delivered during a sigh breath with an inspiratory hold.

5. **Small-particle aerosol generator (Spag nebulizer)**

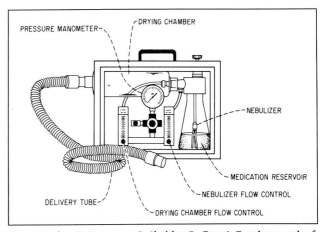

From Scanlon C, Spearman C, Sheldon R. *Egan's Fundamentals of Respiratory Care.* 5th ed. St. Louis: CV Mosby; 1990.

**a. This device is used to deliver the antiviral drug ribavirin (Virazole) to infant and pediatric patients with respiratory syncytial virus or bronchiolitis (discussed in further detail in Chapter 13).

b. The drug exits the nebulizer through a jet and then passes through a drying gas chamber that contains anhydrous (dry) gas. This further reduces the size of the particles, **the majority being smaller than 5 microns**.

F. **Electric nebulizers**

1. **Impeller nebulizer** (spinning disk or room humidifier)

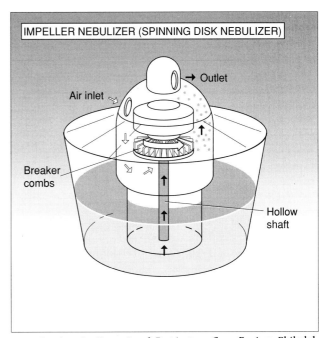

From Persing G. *Entry Level Respiratory Care Review.* Philadelphia: WB Saunders; 1992.

a. The disk rotates rapidly, drawing water up from the reservoir and throwing it through a slotted baffle, reducing the size of the particles.

b. They are popular for home use but clinically do not produce adequate aerosol output.

c. They are difficult to keep clean.

2. **Ultrasonic nebulizer**

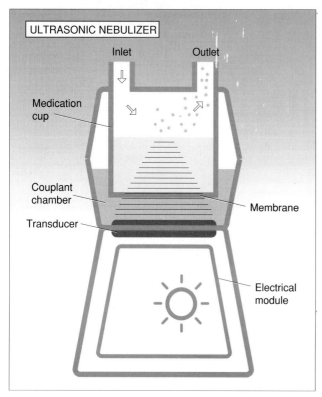

ULTRASONIC NEBULIZER

Inlet — Outlet

Medication cup

Couplant chamber

Transducer

Membrane

Electrical module

From Persing G. *Entry Level Respiratory Care Review.* Philadelphia: WB Saunders; 1992.

a. A piezoelectric transducer in the couplant chamber of the unit is electrically charged and produces high-frequency vibrations. These vibrations are focused on the diaphragm of the medication cup that sits in the couplant chamber. The vibrations break the medications in the cup into small particles, which are delivered to the patient.

b. **The frequency (which determines the particle size)** of the electric energy supplied to the transducer is approximately 1.35 megacycles (megacycle = 1 million cycles per second).

c. The couplant chamber contains **tap water** to help absorb mechanical heat and to act as a transfer medium for the sound waves to the medication cup.

d. **The amplitude control determines the volume of the aerosol output.** The volume

may be as high as **6 ml/min**, which is twice the output of pneumatic nebulizers.

e. A built-in blower delivers 20 to 30 L/min of air to the medication cup to aid in aerosol delivery and help evacuate heat.

** f. **90% of the aerosol particles produced fall within the 0.5- to 3-micron range**.

g. The temperature of the delivery aerosol is between 3 and 10°C above room temperature during normal operation.

h. **Hazards of ultrasonic therapy:**
   (1) Overhydration
   (2) Bronchospasm
   (3) Sudden mobilization of secretions
   (4) Electrical hazard
   (5) Water collection in the tubing
   (6) Swelling of secretions from the absorption of saline, obstructing the airway
   (7) Changes in drug dosage due to the drug reconcentrating as a result of the solvent in the medicine cup, leading to an increasingly stronger dose as the treatment continues

G. **Important points concerning nebulizers**

1. Of all respiratory equipment, heated nebulizers are the greatest source of delivery of contaminated moisture to the patient, *Pseudomonas* being the most common contaminant. They should be changed every 12 to 24 hours.

**2. Jets and capillary tubes must be clear of debris or buildup of minerals and must be cleaned after each use. If the nebulizer is not producing adequate mist, the cause could be a clogged capillary tube or jet.

3. All nebulizers have pressure pop-off valves that should be checked after the nebulizer is set up (usually set at 2 psi). The pop-off valve will be effective only if the nebulizer is on 100%.

4. Keep water drained out of the aerosol tubing, as water in the tubing will **increase the delivered oxygen percentage to the patient.

5. Keep the water level at the appropriate markings on the nebulizer to ensure optimal aerosol output.

6. Soap should not be used to clean the couplant chamber or medication cup of the ultrasonic nebulizer because residue interferes with the ultrasonic activity. Should this occur, a small amount of alcohol in the couplant chamber or medicine cup will help.

7. The filter at the end of the capillary tubes of pneumatic nebulizers must be decontaminated properly. A dirty or clogged filter will not allow the fluid to be drawn up the tube adequately, reducing aerosol output.

REFERENCES

1. Eubanks D, Bone R. *Comprehensive Respiratory Care.* 2nd ed. St. Louis: CV Mosby; 1990.
2. McPherson SP. *Respiratory Therapy Equipment.* 4th ed. St. Louis: CV Mosby; 1990.
3. McPherson, SP. *Respiratory Home Care Equipment.* Dubuque, IA: Kendall/Hunt Publishing; 1988.
4. Scanlan C, Spearman C. *Egan's Fundamentals of Respiratory Care.* 5th ed. St. Louis: CV Mosby; 1990.

PRETEST ANSWERS

1. B

2. A

3. C

4. E

5. E

6. D

Assessment of the Cardiopulmonary Patient

PRETEST QUESTIONS*

1. A patient coughs up yellow sputum following an intermittent positive pressure breathing (IPPB) treatment. Which one of the following statements is **true** in regard to this sputum production?

A. It is old and contains little water.
B. This production is termed hemoptysis.
C. It contains white blood cells (WBCs).
D. It is a normal color for sputum.
E. It contains large amounts of red blood cells (RBCs).

2. The term used to describe a condition in which a patient has difficulty breathing while in a supine position is which of the following?

A. Orthopnea
B. Hypoventilation
C. Paroxysmal nocturnal dyspnea
D. Kussmaul's respirations
E. Biot's respirations

3. Paradoxical respirations are seen in which of the following pulmonary conditions?

A. Pulmonary edema
B. Pneumonia
C. Flail chest
D. Pleural effusion
E. Asthma

4. Perfusion to the extremities may best be determined by which of the following methods?

A. Obtaining an arterial blood gas measurement and determining the PaO_2
B. Assessing the SaO_2 with a pulse oximeter
C. Assessing capillary refill
D. Palpating a brachial pulse
E. Checking for cool and clammy hands

5. While palpating the chest you determine that there are decreased vibrations over the right lower lobe. This may be the result of which of the following?

I. Pneumothorax
II. Atelectasis
III. Pneumonia

A. I only
B. II only
C. I and II only
D. II and III only
E. I, II, and III

6. A chest x-ray study following endotracheal intubation shows the tip of the endotracheal tube is resting at the fourth rib. Which of the following actions should be taken?

A. The tube should be advanced 2 cm.
B. The tube should be advanced until equal breath sounds are heard.
C. The tube should remain at this level.
D. The tube should be withdrawn 3 cm.
E. The tube should be replaced with a shorter tube.

---

*See answers at the end of the chapter.

Assessment of the Cardiopulmonary Patient

I. PATIENT HISTORY

A. Information to obtain from the patient:
  1. Chief complaint
  2. Symptomatology—what symptoms the patient is exhibiting and when they started
  3. Past medical problems
  4. Occupation
  5. Medications currently prescribed
  6. Allergies
  7. Patient's exercise tolerance and daily activities

II. ASSESSMENT OF SYMPTOMS

A. **Common symptoms in patients with pulmonary dysfunction:**
  1. **Cough**—aids in clearing the airway of secretions
    a. Nonproductive cough—caused by the following:
      (1) Irritation of the airway
      (2) Acute inflammation of the respiratory mucosal membrane
      (3) Presence of a growth
      (4) Irritation of the pleura
      (5) Irritation of the tympanic membrane
    b. Productive cough—monitor color of sputum
      (1) White and translucent—normal
      (2) Yellow—indicates infection and presence of WBCs—termed **purulent
      (3) Green—old, retained secretions
      **(4) Green and foul smelling—*Pseudomonas* infection
      (5) Brown—old blood
      (6) Red—fresh blood

NOTE: Foul-smelling sputum that often settles into several layers is characteristic of bronchiectasis (see Chapter 12).

    c. When cough is productive, it is important to record the amount, consistency, odor, and color of sputum, as changes over a 24-hour period may be important in diagnosing pulmonary disease.
    d. Sputum collection and laboratory analysis is an important part of the pulmonary assessment. Factors important to sputum collection:
      (1) The patient should understand the intent of collecting the sample.
      (2) Good oral hygiene should be maintained to prevent the collection from being contaminated by oral secretions.
      (3) Sputum collected must be from a deep cough.

NOTE: If patient cannot cough adequately, nasotracheal suctioning to obtain the sample may be necessary. To collect the sputum, a sputum trap or a Lukens' tube catheter is necessary.

    e. Characteristics of a cough
      (1) Barklike cough usually indicates croup.
      (2) Harsh, dry cough with inspiratory stridor usually indicates upper airway problems.
      (3) Wheezing-type coughs usually indicate a lower airway pathologic condition.
      (4) Chronic productive coughs are indicative of chronic bronchitis.
      (5) Frequent hacking cough and throat clearing may be the result of smoking or sinus or viral infection.
  2. **Dyspnea**—difficult or labored breathing
    a. It is a subjective symptom that is influenced by the patient's reactions and emotional state.

b. Causes of dyspnea
   (1) Increased airway resistance
   (2) Upper airway obstruction
   (3) Asthma and other chronic lung diseases
   (4) Decreased lung compliance
   (5) Pulmonary fibrosis
   (6) Pneumothorax
   (7) Pleural effusion
   (8) Abnormal chest wall
   (9) Anxiety state—no pathologic problem to explain it
c. Types of dyspnea:
   (1) **Orthopnea—dyspnea that occurs while patient is lying down; usually seen in patients with heart failure due to increased congestion of the lungs while in a supine position.
   (2) **Paroxysmal nocturnal dyspnea—sudden onset of shortness of breath after being in bed several hours; seen in cardiac patients and results in acute pulmonary edema, which usually subsides quickly
   (3) **Exertional dyspnea**—patients with cardiopulmonary disease often manifest this condition. The severity is determined by the amount of exertion.
3. **Hemoptysis**—the coughing up of blood from the respiratory tract
   a. Blood-tinged or blood-streaked sputum is not termed hemoptysis.
   b. Hemoptysis is determined by the coughing up of certain volumes of blood. The amount of bleeding indicates the severity of the hemoptysis.
   c. Causes of hemoptysis:
      (1) Pneumonia
      (2) Tuberculosis
      (3) Bronchiectasis
      (4) Lung abscess
      (5) Fungal lung infection—histoplasmosis
      (6) Neoplasms—bronchogenic carcinoma
      (7) Pulmonary embolism
      (8) Valvular heart disease
      (9) Mitral valve stenosis
   d. The patient may report "coughing up blood" when actually the blood is from the stomach or elsewhere. The site of the bleeding's origin must be determined.
4. **Chest pain**
   a. The thoracic wall is the most common source of chest pain.
   b. The pain may be from nerves, muscles, the skin, or bones of the thoracic wall.
   c. The lung parenchyma is not sensitive to pain.
   d. The parietal pleura (membrane lining the interior chest wall) is very sensitive to pain and is usually responsible for the pain associated with pneumonia, pleurisy, and other inflammatory processes.
   e. Chest pain may be associated with **pulmonary hypertension caused by the increased tension on the walls of the vessels and increased workload on the right side of the heart.
   f. Chest pain may originate from the heart because of inadequate blood supply. This pain is called **angina pectoris.
   g. Chest pain can also be associated with a ruptured aorta, myocardial infarction, and esophageal problems.

III. OTHER PHYSICAL ASSESSMENTS

A. **Breathing patterns**
   1. **Eupnea**—normal rate and depth of respirations; normal rate is 10 to 20 breaths/min
   2. **Bradypnea**—less than normal respiratory rate; may be seen with respiratory center depression due to head trauma or drug overdose
   3. **Apnea**—absence of breathing for a specific period (usually at least 10 seconds); seen with respiratory arrest due to asphyxia, severe drug overdose, central and obstructive sleep apnea, and other central respiratory center disorders
   4. **Tachypnea**—above-normal respiratory rate with a normal depth of breathing; may indicate decreased lung compliance and is associated with restrictive diseases, pneumonia, and pulmonary edema
   5. **Hypopnea**—shallow respirations (about one half of normal depth) with slower-than-normal respiratory rate; normal in well-conditioned athletes and accompanied by a slow pulse rate; may be seen with damage to the brainstem accompanied by a weak, rapid pulse
   6. **Hyperpnea**—deep, rapid, and labored breathing; associated with conditions in which there is an inadequate oxygen supply, as in cardiac and respiratory diseases; usually refers to hyperventilation
   7. **Kussmaul's respiration—increased rate and depth of breathing; usually seen in patients with severe metabolic acidosis (diabetic ketoacidosis)
   8. **Biot's respiration**—irregular depth of breathing with periods of apnea; breathing may be slow and deep or rapid and shallow; associated with elevated intracranial pressure or meningitis

**9. Cheyne-Stokes respiration—deep, rapid breathing followed by an apneic period; the breaths begin slow and shallow and gradually increase to a greater-than-normal volume and rate then gradually diminish in volume and rate followed by apnea, which may last 10 to 20 seconds before the cycle is repeated; seen with respiratory center depression from stroke or head injury, pneumonia in elderly individuals, or drug overdose

B. **Chest inspection**—should be performed with the patient seated and clothing removed above the waist. If patient is not able to sit in a chair, he/she should be placed in bed in the Fowler position (head of bed elevated 45°). **Inspection should include**:
1. The rate, depth, and regularity of breathing compared with the normal rates for the patient's age and activity level
2. Skin color, temperature, and condition, for example, bruises or scars—is skin diaphoretic (perspiring)?
3. Chest symmetry—comparison of one side of the chest to the other
   a. Observe chest excursion while standing in front of the patient to determine if both sides are expanding equally.
   **b. Unequal expansion may indicate:
   **(1) Atelectasis
   **(2) Pneumothorax
   (3) Chest deformities
   (4) Flail chest—may observe **"paradoxical"** respirations in which chest moves in on inspiration and out on expiration.
4. Shape and size of chest—compared with normal individuals
   a. Observe the anterior-posterior (A-P) diameter.
   b. An increased A-P diameter is called a **barrel chest and is indicative of chronic lung disease.
5. Work of breathing
   a. Should be evaluated to determine the level of breathing difficulty
   b. While observing the patient's breathing process, determine the following factors:
   (1) Is the chest movement symmetric?
   (2) Are the accessory muscles being used?
   (3) What is the shape of the chest?
   (4) What is the respiratory rate?
   (5) Is the breathing pattern regular or irregular?
   (6) Are there any bony deformities of the ribs, spine, or chest?
   (7) Is the patient's tidal volume normal in relation to size and age?

(8) Is expiration prolonged, shorter than inspiration, or equal to inspiration?
(9) Are substernal, suprasternal, or intercostal retractions or nasal flaring observed?

C. **Inspection of the extremities**
   1. **Digital clubbing**

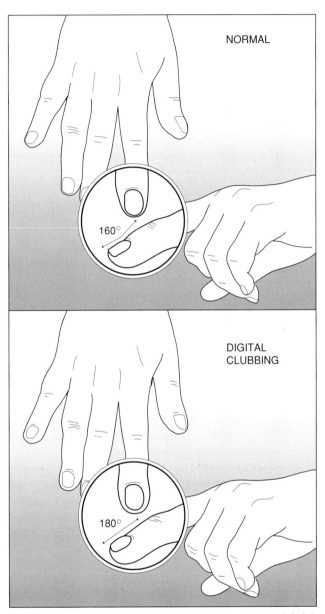

From Persing G. *Entry Level Respiratory Care Review*. Philadelphia: WB Saunders; 1992.

   a. Digital clubbing is indicative of longstanding pulmonary disease (75% to 85% of all clubbing is the result of pulmonary disease).
   b. It is an enlargement of the distal phalanges of the fingers, and less commonly of the toes. There is a loss of the angle between the nail and the dorsum of the terminal phalanx.
   c. It is the result of **chronic hypoxemia.

2. **Pedal edema**
   a. This refers to an accumulation of fluid in the subcutaneous tissues of the ankles.
   b. This symptom is commonly observed in patients with chronic pulmonary disease. The chronic hypoxemic state results in pulmonary vasoconstriction.
   c. This results in an increased workload on the right side of the heart, right ventricular hypertrophy, and, eventually, right-sided heart failure (cor pulmonale).
   d. Venous blood flow returning to the heart is diminished, and the peripheral blood vessels become engorged. The ankles are most affected because of gravity dependency.

3. **Cyanosis**
   a. This term refers to the bluish discoloration of the skin and nailbeds resulting from a 5 g/dl decrease in oxygenated hemoglobin.
   b. Cyanosis may indicate decreased oxygenation or reduced peripheral circulation.
   c. Patients with decreased hemoglobin levels (anemia) may not exhibit cyanosis even if tissue hypoxia is present. An anemic patient has a low oxygen-carrying capacity, which may result in tissue hypoxia, but will not be cyanotic unless 5 g/dl of unsaturated hemoglobin is present, which may not be the case.
   d. Conversely, a patient with an increased level of hemoglobin (polycythemia) has an increased capacity for carrying oxygen. This patient may have 5 g/dl of unsaturated hemoglobin, and therefore be cyanotic, yet have enough saturated hemoglobin to adequately oxygenate the tissues.

4. **Capillary refill**
   a. Perfusion to the extremities may be determined by assessing capillary refill.
   b. This is determined by compressing the patient's fingernail for a short time and then releasing it and observing the time it takes for blood flow to return to the nailbed.
   c. Normal refill time is less than 3 seconds.
   d. Patients with decreased cardiac output and poor digital perfusion will have a longer refill time.

D. **Chest deformities**

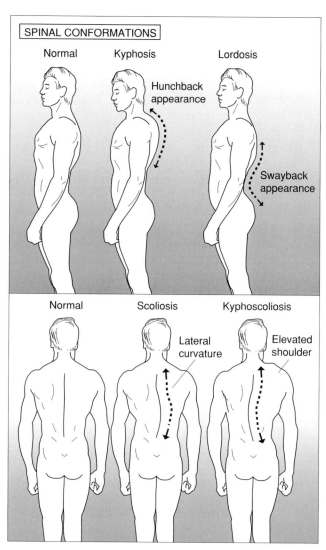

From Persing G. *Entry Level Respiratory Care Review.* Philadelphia: WB Saunders; 1992.

1. **Kyphosis**
   a. Backward curvature of the spine resulting in "hunchback" appearance
   b. Caused by degenerative bone disease or age or may be associated with chronic obstructive pulmonary disease (COPD)
2. **Lordosis**
   a. Backward curvature of the lumbar spine resulting in a "swayback" appearance
   b. Usually not responsible for respiratory difficulties
3. **Scoliosis**
   a. Lateral curvature of the thoracic spine, resulting in the chest protruding posteriorly and the anterior ribs flattening out
   b. Depending on severity, it may result in impaired lung movement

4. **Kyphoscoliosis**
   a. Combination of kyphosis and scoliosis
   b. May be most adequately observed by noticing differing heights of the shoulders
   c. Cardiopulmonary problems do not normally present until the patient reaches the age of 40 or 50 years.
   d. Pulmonary signs and symptoms of kyphoscoliosis:
   **(1) Dyspnea
   (2) Hypoxemia
   (3) Hypercapnia
   (4) Progressive respiratory insufficiency
   (5) Eventual cardiac failure
   (6) Decreased lung capacities evidenced by pulmonary function tests **(restrictive disease)
   (7) Frequent pulmonary infections
   (8) Uneven ventilation: perfusion ratio

5. **Pectus carinatum**

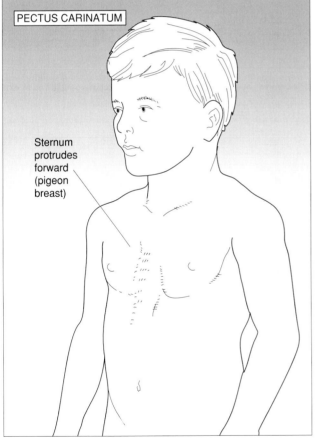

From Persing G. *Entry Level Respiratory Care Review.* Philadelphia: WB Saunders; 1992.

   a. Also called pigeon breast; results in the xiphoid process and lower sternum projecting forward
   b. Usually a congenital condition

   c. May cause dyspnea on exercise and more frequent respiratory infections because of interference with heart and lung movement
   d. In severe cases, surgical correction may be indicated.

6. **Pectus excavatum**

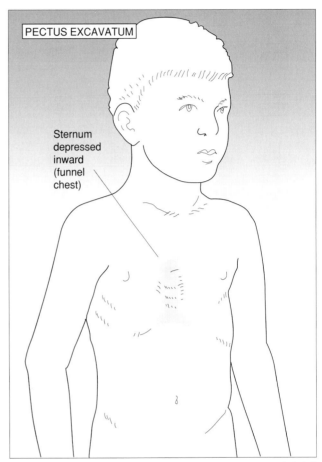

From Persing G. *Entry Level Respiratory Care Review.* Philadelphia: WB Saunders; 1992.

   a. Also called funnel chest; results in a funnel-shaped depression over the lower sternum
   b. Usually a congenital condition
   c. May lead to dyspnea on exertion and more frequent respiratory infections
   d. Reduces the ability to eat a full meal; therefore, many patients are underweight

7. **Barrel chest**

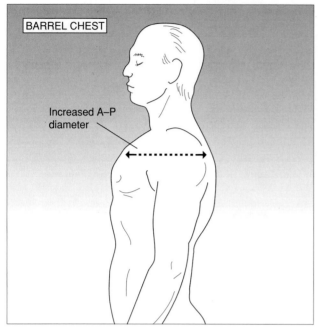

From Persing G. *Entry Level Respiratory Care Review*. Philadelphia: WB Saunders; 1992.

**a. Results from the premature closure of the airways, resulting in air-trapping and hyperinflated lungs, giving the chest a barrel appearance
   b. Also contributing is the increased musculature from the accessory muscles that are used during normal breathing in COPD patients
**c. Seen almost exclusively in patients with chronic lung disease
**d. This hyperinflated state of the lungs pushes down on the diaphragm, restricting its movement. This decreases alveolar ventilation and chest excursion, resulting in an increased work of breathing.
e. The muscles normally used for ventilation are the **diaphragm and external intercostal muscles, but since the diaphragm of COPD patients is flattened, the accessory muscles are used during normal ventilation.

E. **Palpation of the chest**
  1. The sense of touch is used on the chest wall to assess physical signs.
  2. Hands are placed on the chest to assess chest movement and vibration.
  3. Tactile fremitus
     a. Fremitus means vibration.
     b. With hands on the patient's chest, the patient is asked to say certain words such as "ninety-nine" and the practitioner feels over different areas of the chest.

**c. Vibrations are decreased over areas of atelectasis, fluid, pneumothorax, or masses.
   d. Increased vibrations are felt with pneumonia.

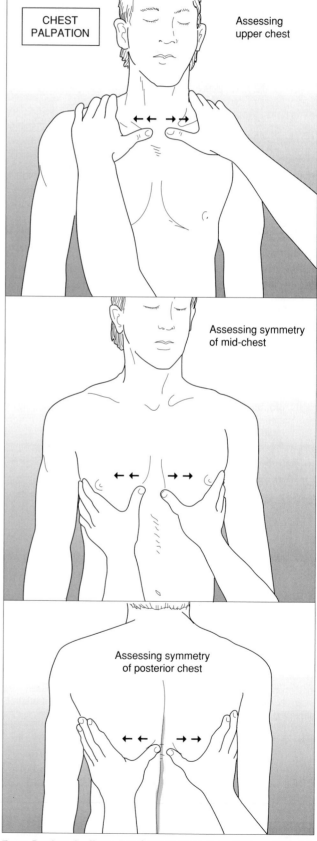

From Persing G. *Entry Level Respiratory Care Review*. Philadelphia: WB Saunders; 1992.

4. Position of the trachea

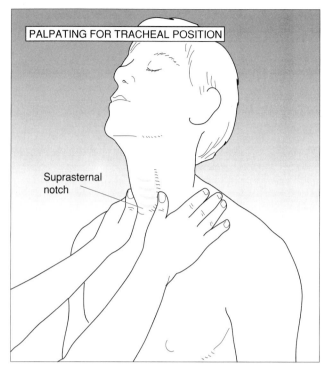

PALPATING FOR TRACHEAL POSITION

Suprasternal notch

From Persing G. *Entry Level Respiratory Care Review.* Philadelphia: WB Saunders; 1992.

a. This is assessed by placing both thumbs on each side of the suprasternal notch and gently pressing inward. One should feel soft tissue only. If the trachea is felt, this indicates it has shifted and is no longer positioned in the midline as it should be.
**b. A shift of the trachea may be the result of a pneumothorax or atelectasis.
  (1) Pneumothorax—trachea shifted to the unaffected side (opposite side of pneumothorax)**
  (2) Atelectasis—trachea shifted toward the affected side (same side as atelectasis)**
F. **Percussion of the chest wall**
  1. Tapping on the chest directly with one finger or indirectly by placing one finger on the chest area and tapping on that finger over different areas of the chest
  2. There are five different sounds heard from percussion:
    a. **Hyperresonance**
      (1) Recognized by a loud, low-pitched sound of long duration produced over areas that have a greater proportion of air than tissue
      (2) Examples: air-filled stomach, emphysema (air-trapping), pneumothorax
    b. **Resonance**
      (1) Recognized by a low-pitched sound of

long duration produced over areas with equal distribution of air and tissue
      (2) Example: normal lung tissue
    c. **Dullness**
      (1) Recognized by a sound of medium intensity and pitch with a short duration produced over areas containing a higher proportion of tissue or fluid than air
      (2) Examples: atelectasis, consolidation, pleural effusion, pleural thickening, pulmonary edema
    d. **Flatness**
      (1) Recognized by a sound of low amplitude and pitch produced over areas containing a higher proportion of tissue than air
      (2) Examples: massive pleural effusion, massive atelectasis, pneumonectomy
    e. **Tympany**
      (1) recognized by a "drumlike" sound
      (2) Example: tension pneumothorax
G. **Auscultation of breath sounds**
  1. **Normal breath sounds**
    a. **Vesicular**
      (1) Gentle rustling sound heard over the entire chest wall except the right supraclavicular area
      (2) Inspiration is longer than expiration with no pause between the two.
    b. **Bronchial**
      (1) Loud and generally high-pitched sound heard over the upper portion of the sternum, trachea, and main-stem bronchi
      (2) Expiration is longer than inspiration with a short pause between the two.
      (3) If heard in other lung areas, it is indicative of atelectasis or consolidation.
    c. **Bronchovesicular**
      (1) Combination of bronchial and vesicular breath sounds normally heard over the sternum, between the scapulae, and over the right apex of the lung
      (2) Inspiration and expiration are of equal duration with no pause between the two.
    d. **Tracheal**
      (1) Harsh and high-pitched sound heard over the trachea
      (2) Expiration is slightly longer than inspiration.
  2. **Adventitious breath sounds**
    a. **Rales (crackles)**
      (1) Bubbling or crackling sound heard primarily on inspiration produced by air flowing through fluid in the alveoli or small airways

(2) **Fine rales** are high-pitched and are heard on end inspiration. They are caused by pulmonary edema, pneumonia, atelectasis, or fibrosis.

(3) **Medium rales** are wetter and louder than fine rales, are heard during any part of inspiration, and are produced by air moving through fluid in the bronchioles. They are caused by emphysema, bronchitis, pneumonia, or pulmonary edema.

(4) **Coarse rales** are loud, low-pitched bubbling sounds heard on inspiration or expiration in larger airways as air moves through fluid. They are caused by emphysema, bronchitis, pneumonia, or pulmonary edema.

b. **Rhonchi**

(1) Sounds that are produced in airways filled with secretions or fluids. They have a typical rumbling sound and are heard on expiration.

(2) Heard primarily in larger airways

(3) **Sibilant rhonchi** are "squeaky-type" sounds heard in lower airway.

(4) **Sonorous rhonchi** are "snoring-type" sounds heard in the upper airway.

(5) Caused by asthma, emphysema, mucus plugs, or stenosis

NOTE: A distinguishing feature between rales and rhonchi is that rhonchi will generally clear after coughing, whereas rales usually will not.

c. **Wheezes**

(1) Often considered a rhonchi with a musical quality produced by air flow through constricted airways

(2) May be heard on both inspiration and expiration

**(3) Wheezes are heard characteristically with asthma due to bronchoconstriction

d. **Pleural friction rub**

(1) A clicking or grating sound caused by friction produced as the parietal and visceral pleura rub against each other during the breathing process

(2) Most commonly associated with pleurisy, it is very painful.

H. **Auscultation of heart sounds**—Heart sounds are thought to be produced as a result of sudden changes in blood flow through the heart that cause a vibration of the valves and chambers inside the heart. The normal heart sound is a "lub-dub" sound.

1. **Normal heart sounds**

a. The first heart sound ("lub") represents the closing of the atrioventricular (AV) valves.

(1) The AV valves are the mitral valve (between the left atrium and left ventricle) and the tricuspid valve (between the right atrium and right ventricle).

(2) The first heart sound is designated S_1.

b. The second heart sound ("dub") represents the closing of the semilunar valves.

(1) The semilunar valves consist of the pulmonic valve (between the right ventricle and the pulmonary artery) and the aortic valve (between the left ventricle and aorta).

(2) The second heart sound is designated S_2.

c. A third and fourth heart sound (S_3 and S_4) may be heard but are more difficult to hear than S_1 and S_2. They are more easily heard in children.

(1) S_3 is thought to result from blood rushing into the ventricles during early ventricular diastole.

(2) S_4 is thought to result from atrial contraction.

2. **Abnormal heart sounds (murmurs)**

a. Murmurs usually occur when blood flows in a turbulent fashion through heart structures that have a decreased cross-sectional area.

b. Murmurs are described in relation to the location of the sound, at what part of the cardiac cycle they occur, and the intensity of the sound.

**c. Conditions resulting in heart murmurs:

(1) Aortic valve disease (stenosis, regurgitation, and so on)

(2) Mitral valve disease (stenosis, regurgitation, and so on)

(3) Pulmonic valve stenosis

(4) Tricuspid valve insufficiency

I. **Chest x-ray interpretation**

1. Terms that are useful when interpreting chest x-ray films

a. **Anterior-posterior (A-P)**—chest x-ray view taken from front to back

b. **Consolidation**—well-defined, solid-appearing lung; appears light on x-ray film; **caused by pneumonia**

c. **Radiodensity**—this term is descriptive of white areas on the x-ray film. Fluids and solids appear white. **Radiodensity is caused by pneumonia, bony areas, and pleural effusion**

d. **Infiltrates**—descriptive term for scattered or patchy white areas on x-ray film** due to inflammatory processes. **They are caused by atelectasis or disease processes.**

e. **Radiolucency—appears dark on x-ray film. Air is dark on x-ray film. Hyperlucency is characteristic of emphysema, asthma, or subcutaneous emphysema**.
2. Respiratory care practitioners most commonly observe chest x-ray studies for the following findings:
   a. **Atelectasis**
      (1) Appears lighter than normal lung tissue
      (2) May observe elevated diaphragm, mediastinal shift (toward area of atelectasis), increased density, and decreased volume of a lung area
   b. **Pneumonia**
      (1) Appears white on x-ray film
      (2) Consolidation of entire lobe or more, causing **mediastinal shift toward the consolidation
   c. **Pneumothorax**
      (1) Air found in the pleural cavity, appearing dark with no vascular markings in the involved areas
      (2) **Tension pneumothorax may result in mediastinal shift and observance of the trachea **shifting away from the side of the pneumothorax.**
   d. **Endotracheal tube placement**
      **(1) Tube should rest about 2 to 7 cm above the carina
      (2) Carina is located on x-ray film at the level of the fourth rib or fourth thoracic vertebra
      (3) If endotracheal tube is inserted too far, it has a greater tendency to enter the **right main-stem bronchus
      (4) If the right main-stem bronchus is inadvertently intubated, diminished breath sounds will be heard on the left, as will possible asymmetric chest movement.
   e. **Heart shadow**
      (1) Should appear white in the middle of the chest with the left-sided heart border easily determined
      (2) A normal heart should be less than one half of the width of the chest. Increased heart size may indicate congestive heart failure.
   f. **Diaphragm**
      (1) Should be rounded or dome-shaped
      (2) Appears white on x-ray film at the level of the sixth rib
      **(3) Patient with hyperinflated lungs (COPD) will have flattened diaphragm
      (4) Both hemidiaphragms should be assessed for height and angle to the chest wall.
      (5) The dome of the right hemidiaphragm

is normally 1 to 2 cm higher than the left because of the liver.
      (6) Elevation of one hemidiaphragm may be the result of gas in stomach or lung collapse.
J. **Pulse**
   1. Pulse is a direct indicator of the heart's action.
   2. Normal heart rate in adult: 60 to 90 beats/min
   3. Normal heart rate in child: 90 to 120 beats/min
   4. An abnormally low heart rate is called **bradycardia**. It is caused by infection, hypothermia, and heart abnormalities.
   5. An abnormally high heart rate is called **tachycardia**. It is caused by hypoxemia, fever, loss of blood volume, heart abnormalities, and anxiety.
   6. **Peripheral edema and venous engorgement indicate inadequate pumping action of the heart resulting from right-sided heart failure (cor pulmonale) or left-sided heart failure (congestive heart failure).
K. **Blood pressure**—measured with a **sphygmomanometer**
   1. A measurement of the pressure within the arterial system
   2. Normal range for adults: 100 to 140/60 to 90 torr
   3. Normal range for child: varies depending on age
   4. Normal range for neonates: 60 to 90/30 to 60 torr
   5. Systolic (first number) pressure is the pressure measured during ventricular contraction.
   6. Diastolic (second number) pressure is measured while the ventricles are at rest.
   7. The diastolic pressure is the most critical measurement, as it is the lowest pressure that the heart and arterial system will be subjected to.
   8. An abnormally low blood pressure is called **hypotension**. It is caused by shock, volume loss, positioning, and depressant drugs.
   9. An abnormally high blood pressure is called **hypertension**. It is caused by cardiovascular imbalances, stimulant drugs, stress, and fluid retention caused by renal failure.
   10. Many factors affect blood pressure:
       a. Blood volume
       b. Blood viscosity
       c. Heart's pumping action
       d. Elasticity of the blood vessels
       e. Resistance to blood flow through the vessels
L. **Body temperature**
   1. Normal body temperature is 98.6°F (37°C)
   2. Slightly higher temperature in children because of higher metabolic rate
   3. An abnormally low body temperature is called

hypothermia and is caused by sweating (diaphoresis), blood loss, exposure, and increased heat loss.

4. An abnormally high body temperature is called **hyperthermia** and is caused by decreased heat loss, infection, or increased environmental temperature.

5. The term used for normal body temperature is **afebrile**.

M. **Assessing mental status**

1. **Level of consciousness**

a. Alert—patient is awake and responds to stimuli.

b. Obtunded and confused—patient is awake but responds slowly to commands; may be disoriented.

c. Lethargic—patient seems unconscious but when stimulated will awaken.

d. Coma—patient is unconscious and when stimulated will not awaken.

2. **Orientation to time and place**

a. Ask patients the date.

b. Ask patients if they know where they are.

3. **Ability to cooperate**

a. Ask patient to follow simple commands.

b. Must have patient cooperation for effective therapy such as incentive spirometry or IPPB

4. **Emotional state**

a. Ask patient to describe his/her feelings.

b. Note patient's response while asking questions.

IV. ASSESSMENT OF LABORATORY VALUES

A. **Serum electrolytes**

1. **Sodium** (Na^+)

**a. Normal value—135 to 145 mEq/L

b. Sodium is the major cation in the extracellular fluid, and its concentration is controlled by the kidneys through regulation of the amount of water in the body.

c. Causes of **hyponatremia (Na^+ level <135 mEq/L)

(1) Renal failure

(2) Congestive heart failure

(3) Excessive fever or sweating

(4) Long-term diuretic administration

(5) Inadequate sodium intake

(6) Excessive water ingestion

(7) Severe burns

(8) Gastrointestinal losses (vomiting, diarrhea)

d. **Clinical symptoms of hyponatremia**

(1) Muscle weakness—making ventilator weaning difficult**

(2) Confusion

(3) Muscle twitching progressing to convulsions

(4) Anxiety

(5) Alterations in level of consciousness

e. Causes of **hypernatremia** (Na^+ level >145 mEq/L)

(1) Excessive water loss (sweating, diarrhea)

(2) Renal failure

(3) Inadequate water intake

(4) Mannitol diuresis

(5) Steroid administration

f. **Clinical symptoms of hypernatremia**

(1) Confusion

(2) Central nervous system dysfunction

(3) Seizure activity

(4) Coma

2. **Potassium** (K^+)

**a. Normal value—3.5 to 5 mEq/L

b. Potassium is the major intracellular cation.

c. Causes of **hypokalemia** (K^+ level <3.5 mEq/L)

(1) Diuretics

(2) Adrenal steroids

(3) Vomiting, diarrhea

(4) Burns

(5) Severe trauma

d. **Clinical symptoms of hypokalemia**

**(1) Muscle weakness leading to paralysis, respiratory failure, and hypotension

**(2) Cardiac arrhythmias

(a) Premature atrial and ventricular contractions

(b) Atrial and ventricular tachycardia

(c) Asystole

(3) S-T segment depression on electrocardiogram

(4) Decreased gastrointestinal tract motility, resulting in abdominal distention

e. Causes of **hyperkalemia** (K^+ level >5 mEq/L)

(1) Acidosis

(2) Renal insufficiency

(3) Tissue necrosis

(4) Hemorrhage

f. **Clinical symptoms of hyperkalemia**

(1) Paralysis

**(2) Electrocardiographic abnormalities

(a) Shortened Q-T interval

(b) Widened QRS complex

(c) Prolonged P-R interval

(d) Lack of P wave

**(3) Cardiac arrhythmias

(a) Ventricular arrhythmias

(b) Nodal arrhythmias

3. **Chloride (Cl⁻)**

**a. Normal value—95 to 105 mEq/L

b. Chloride is the major anion in the body, of which two thirds is found in extracellular compartments. Since chloride is generally excreted with potassium as potassium chloride by the kidney, decreased levels of one will result in decreased levels of the other.

c. Causes of **hypochloremia** (Cl⁻ levels <95 mEq/L)

 (1) Vomiting, diarrhea

 (2) Furosemide (Lasix) diuresis

NOTE: Hypochloremia may result in metabolic alkalosis.

d. **Clinical symptoms of hypochloremia**

 (1) Muscle spasm

 (2) Coma (severe hypochloremia)

e. Causes of **hyperchloremia** (Cl⁻ levels >105 mEq/L)

 (1) Respiratory alkalosis

 (2) Metabolic acidosis

 (3) Dehydration

 (4) Administering excessive amounts of sodium chloride and potassium

f. **Clinical symptoms of hyperchloremia**

 (1) Headache

 (2) Malaise

 (3) Weakness

 (4) Unconsciousness

 (5) Coma

4. **Calcium (Ca)**

**a. Normal value—4.25 to 5.25 mEq/L

b. Most of the body's calcium is contained in the bones. It plays a major role in neuromuscular function and cellular enzyme reactions.

c. Causes of **hypocalcemia** (Ca level <4.25 mEq/L)

 (1) Severe trauma

 (2) Renal failure

 (3) Severe pancreatitis

 (4) Vitamin D deficiency

 (5) Parathyroid hormone deficiency

d. **Clinical symptoms of hypocalcemia**

 (1) Muscle spasm

 (2) Abdominal cramping

 (3) Convulsions (rare)

 (4) Prolonged Q-T interval on electrocardiogram

e. Causes of **hypercalcemia** (Ca level >5.25 mEq/L)

 (1) Hyperthyroidism

 (2) Vitamin A or D intoxication

 (3) Hyperparathyroidism

 (4) Sarcoidosis

 (5) Cancer metastasis to the bone

f. **Clinical symptoms of hypercalcemia**

(1) Muscle weakness—making ventilator weaning difficult**

 (2) Fatigue

 (3) Mental depression

 (4) Anorexia

 (5) Nausea, vomiting

 (6) Coma (severe cases)

5. Bicarbonate (HCO_3^-)—detailed in Chapter 10

B. **Blood urea nitrogen**

1. Urea is a substance produced in the liver and carried in the blood to the kidneys, where it is excreted in the urine.

2. If the kidneys fail to remove urea from the blood adequately, the blood urea concentration increases.

**3. The normal BUN value is 7 to 20 mg/dl.

4. **An elevated blood urea nitrogen (BUN) value is indicative of renal failure.

C. **Glucose**

**1. Normal serum level—70 to 105 mg/dl

**2. Elevated levels observed in diabetic ketoacidosis, with patient compensating through alveolar hyperventilation (Kussmaul's respirations, as mentioned earlier in this chapter)

D. **Hematology tests**

1. **Red blood cells**

a. RBCs determine the adequacy of oxygen transport and are also referred to as **erythrocytes**.

**b. Normal value—4 million to 6 million/mm³ of blood

**c. A decreased RBC count (anemia) indicates an inadequate oxygen-carrying capacity in the blood. Blood should be administered to the patient.

2. **Hemoglobin**

a. Hemoglobin is the portion of the RBC that carries oxygen, so it is an indicator of the oxygen-carrying capacity of the blood.

**b. Normal value—13.5 to 18 g/dl in males; 12 to 16 g/dl in females

c. A decreased hemoglobin level indicates inadequate oxygen-carrying capacity in the blood. Blood should be given to the patient.

3. **Hematocrit**

a. The percentage of the volume of RBCs in the total blood volume

b. Normal value—43% to 50% in males; 37% to 43% in females

c. A decreased hematocrit level indicates inadequate oxygen-carrying capacity of the blood. The patient should be given blood.

4. **White blood cells**

a. WBC count determines the presence of infection.

**b. Normal value—5000 to 10,000/mm³

**c. An elevated WBC count indicates the presence of infection. The respiratory care practitioner should recommend a chest x-ray study or sputum culture to determine lung involvement.

  d. WBCs are also referred to as **leukocytes**.

V. REVIEWING THE PATIENT CHART

A. Once the patient has been admitted and requires some type of respiratory care, the chart should be reviewed for the following:
   1. Patient history
   2. Physical examination on admission
   3. Current vital signs
      a. Heart rate
      b. Respiratory rate—if the rate remains elevated or there is little or no change in the patient's respiratory distress, the respiratory care practitioner should recommend modifications in the prescribed oxygen therapy (increasing the FIO_2, placement on continuous positive airway pressure, or institution of mechanical ventilation—see Chapter 11, "Ventilator Management").
      c. Blood pressure—a decrease in blood pressure may indicate excessive positive end-expiratory pressure (PEEP) levels, requiring a decrease in the prescribed level of PEEP (see Chapter 11, "Ventilator Management").
   4. Current respiratory care orders
      a. Oxygen delivery device
      b. Percentage or liter flow of oxygen
      c. Type of ventilator and prescribed parameters
      d. Frequency and duration of prescribed treatments
      e. Medications ordered with the treatment
   5. Patient progress notes
   6. **Arterial blood gas values**—abnormal values in PaO_2 and/or $PaCO_2$ indicate that changes in oxygen therapy or ventilatory parameters are necessary (see Chapter 10, "ABG Interpretation" and Chapter 11, "Ventilator Management").
   7. Pulmonary function results
      a. To determine severity of lung dysfunction
      b. To determine obstructive or restrictive abnormalities
      c. Recommendation of before-and-after bronchodilator studies to determine responsiveness to therapy

REFERENCES

1. Eubanks D, Bone R. *Comprehensive Respiratory Care.* 2nd ed. St. Louis: CV Mosby; 1990.
2. Farzan S. *A Concise Handbook of Respiratory Diseases.* 2nd ed. Reston, VA: Prentice-Hall; 1985.
3. Levitzky M. *Introduction to Respiratory Care.* Philadelphia: WB Saunders; 1990.
4. Scanlan C, Spearman C. *Egan's Fundamentals of Respiratory Care.* 5th ed. St. Louis: CV Mosby; 1990.

PRETEST ANSWERS

1. C

2. A

3. C

4. C

5. C

6. D

CHAPTER 4

Management of the Airway

PRETEST QUESTIONS*

1. Which of the following are hazards of an esophageal obturator airway (EOA)?

I. Tracheal intubation
II. Rupture of esophagus
III. Vomiting upon removal of the EOA

A. I only
B. II only
C. I and II only
D. I and III only
E. I, II, and III

2. Opening the patient's airway using an oropharyngeal airway will be most beneficial when the obstruction is caused by which of the following?

A. Secretions
B. Foreign body
C. Edema
D. Tongue
E. Laryngospasm

3. McGill's forceps are used during which of the following procedures?

A. Nasotracheal intubation
B. Oral intubation
C. Tracheotomy
D. Insertion of an EOA
E. Insertion of a nasopharyngeal airway

4. The physician wants to begin weaning a patient from a tracheostomy tube. How may this best be accomplished?

A. Deflate the cuff every 2 hours.
B. Change to a fenestrated tracheostomy tube.
C. Keep the cuff inflated and remove the inner cannula.
D. Change to a tracheostomy tube with a foam cuff.
E. Deflate the cuff and place a plug over the tracheostomy stoma.

5. You are called to a patient's room because of a ventilator alarm sounding. You hear an audible leak around the patient's endotracheal (E-T) tube during a ventilator breath and notice the exhaled volume reading is 150 ml less than the set tidal volume. You check the cuff pressure and find it is 12 torr. The appropriate measure to take at this time is which of the following?

A. Maintain the current cuff pressure and increase the patient's tidal volume to compensate for the leak.
B. Instill enough air to maintain a cuff pressure of 30 torr.
C. While listening with a stethoscope at the larynx, instill air into the cuff until a slight leak is heard on inspiration.
D. Instill air until only a slight audible leak is heard.
E. Instill air until the audible leak is no longer heard.

6. You want to attempt to pass a suction catheter into the patient's left lung to obtain a sputum specimen. What would be the most appropriate method to achieve this?

A. Have the patient turn the head to the left.
B. Have the patient turn the head to the right.
C. Use a Yankauer suction device.
D. Use a catheter one half of the internal diameter of the patient's airway.
E. Use a coudé suction catheter.

---

*See answers at the end of the chapter.

Management of the Airway

I. UPPER AIRWAY OBSTRUCTION

A. **Main causes of upper airway obstruction**
   1. Tongue falling back against the posterior wall of the pharynx because of unconsciousness or central nervous system abnormality
   2. Edema—postextubation inflammation and swelling of glottic area
   3. Bleeding
   4. Secretions
   5. Foreign substances
      a. Foreign bodies
      b. False teeth
      c. Vomitus
   6. Laryngospasm
B. **Signs of partial upper airway obstruction**
   1. Crowing, gasping sounds on inspiration
   2. Patient not able to cough (with slight obstruction, patient may be able to cough)
   3. Increasing respiratory difficulty
   4. Good to poor air exchange (depending on severity of obstruction)
   5. Exaggerated chest and abdominal movement without comparable air movement

6. Cyanosis (depending on severity of obstruction)
C. **Signs of complete upper airway obstruction**
   1. Inability to talk
   2. Increased respiratory difficulty with no air movement
   3. Cyanosis
   4. Sternal, intercostal, and epigastric retractions
   5. Use of accessory muscles of the neck
   6. Extreme panic
   7. Patient becomes unconscious and suffers respiratory arrest if obstruction not relieved
D. **Treatment of airway obstruction**
   1. If the patient is conscious with a partial airway obstruction, he/she should be allowed to try to relieve the obstruction without assistance.
   2. If the patient is conscious with a complete airway obstruction caused by food or other foreign object, abdominal thrusts must be performed until the object is dislodged (see Chapter 6).
   3. If the patient is unconscious with a partial or complete airway obstruction that is most likely caused by the tongue, the head tilt/chin lift maneuver will help relieve the obstruction by moving the tongue forward.

II. ARTIFICIAL AIRWAYS

A. Oropharyngeal airway

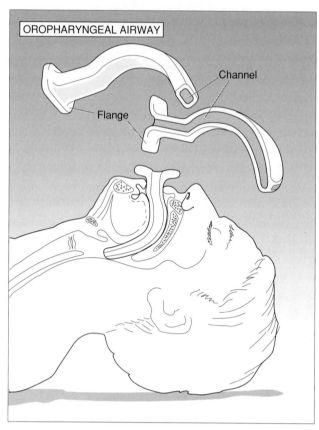

From Persing G. *Entry Level Respiratory Care Review.* Philadelphia: WB Saunders; 1992.

1. Maintains a patent airway by lying between the base of the tongue and the posterior wall of the pharynx, preventing the tongue from falling back and occluding the airway

**2. Must be used only on the *unconscious patient*, as a conscious patient would gag on the airway, leading to the potential of aspiration

3. This airway should **never be taped in place; if patient becomes conscious the airway must be easily removable to prevent vomiting and aspiration.

4. Proper insertion of the oropharyngeal airway:

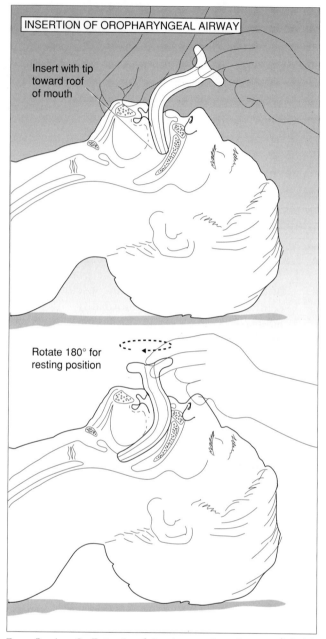

From Persing G. *Entry Level Respiratory Care Review.* Philadelphia: WB Saunders; 1992.

a. Measure the airway from the corner of the lip to the angle of the jaw to ensure proper length.
b. Remove foreign substances from the mouth.
c. Hyperextend the neck.
d. Using the cross-finger technique, open the patient's mouth and insert the airway with the tip pointing toward the roof of the mouth.
e. Observe the airway passing the uvula and rotate 180°.

5. **Hazards of oropharyngeal airways**
   a. Gagging or fighting the airway—remove immediately
   b. Base of tongue pushed into the back of the throat, obstructing the airway
   c. The epiglottis is pushed into the laryngeal area by an airway that is too large.
   d. The airway is aspirated or is not effective in relieving obstruction because it is too small.
6. **Important points concerning oropharyngeal airways**
   ** a. Oropharyngeal airways may be used in the unconscious, orally intubated patient to prevent the patient from biting the tube.
   b. Berman's airways are made of hard plastic and have a groove down either side to guide a suction catheter to the glottic area.
   c. Guedel's airways are made of a soft, more pliable material that has an opening through the middle to allow the passage of a suction catheter into the glottic area.

B. **Nasopharyngeal airway**

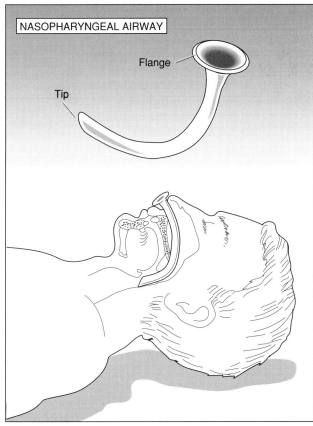

From Persing G. *Entry Level Respiratory Care Review.* Philadelphia: WB Saunders; 1992.

1. Maintains a patent airway by lying between the base of the tongue and the posterior wall of the pharynx
2. It is constructed of soft, pliable rubber and is inserted as follows:

a. Select the proper size airway by measuring the airway from the tip of the nose to the tragus of the ear. The outside diameter of the airway should be equal to the inside diameter of the patient's internal nares.
b. Lubricate the airway with a water-soluble gel and insert into the patient's nostril.
c. The flanged end should rest against the nose, and the distal tip should rest behind the uvula.
d. Place tape around the flanged end to secure it in place. (Safety pin may be inserted through the flange and pin taped to the face.)
3. This airway is tolerated by the conscious patient.
4. It may be used as a means to facilitate nasotracheal suctioning.
5. **Hazards of nasopharyngeal airways**
   a. Aspiration of an airway that is too small
   b. Nasal irritation—alternate nostrils daily

C. **Esophageal obturator airway**

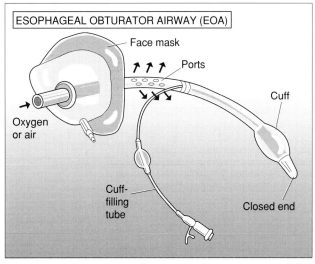

From Persing G. *Entry Level Respiratory Care Review.* Philadelphia: WB Saunders; 1992.

1. Developed in 1973 as an alternative to tracheal intubation, especially for those not skilled in that procedure
2. The tube is placed in the esophagus to prevent air from entering the stomach during manual ventilation. A resuscitator bag is attached to the proximal end of the tube and gas exits small holes in the tube in the laryngeal area. Since the stomach is sealed off with a cuff, gas enters the lungs only.
** 3. Used in emergency situations for **unconscious, apneic victims**
4. The tube is 30 to 37 cm long with a closed distal end and a 30-cc cuff just above the end of the tube.

5. Steps for proper insertion of the EOA:
   a. Check the cuff and lubricate the end of the tube with a water-soluble gel.
   b. Attach the mask and lock in place.
   c. Place the victim's head in a neutral position.
   d. Grasp the victim's jaw with the thumb along the tongue and lift up.
   e. Insert the tube along the right side of the mouth.
   f. Seal the mask on the victim's face and blow through the tube to observe the chest rise.
   g. Auscultate with a stethoscope to observe for equal breath sounds and listen over the stomach to make sure no air is entering it.
   h. Inflate the cuff with no more than 30 cc of air.

NOTE: The cuff of the EOA must be passed below the level of the carina before it is inflated. If it is not, the cuff could compress the trachea, resulting in an obstructed airway.

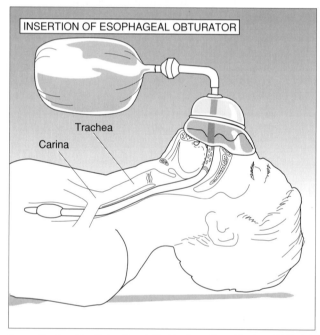

From Persing G. *Entry Level Respiratory Care Review.* Philadelphia: WB Saunders; 1992.

6. Removal of the EOA:
   a. Once the patient becomes conscious or begins breathing, or personnel trained in endotracheal intubation become available, the tube should be removed.
   b. Deflate the cuff and **turn the patient's head to the side as the tube is withdrawn. Vomiting is very common upon removal, and this helps prevent the aspiration of stomach contents. **Placement of a nasogastric tube to decompress the stomach prior to removal of the EOA will reduce the risk of aspiration also.**

**c. Intubating the patient's trachea prior to the removal of the EOA is the best method for preventing aspiration, especially if the patient will be requiring an E-T tube once the EOA is removed.
**d. Suctioning equipment must be readily available when removing an EOA.

7. **Contraindications to use of the EOA**
   a. Conscious or semiconscious victims
   b. Children younger than 16 years of age (tubes available in adult sizes only)
   c. Patients who can rapidly be brought out of a coma (drug overdose, hypoglycemic coma)
   d. Tube should not be in the esophagus more than 2 hours
   e. Patients with known esophageal trauma

8. **Hazards of the EOA**
   a. Esophageal perforation
   b. Rupture of the esophagus due to vomiting with the airway in place and the cuff inflated—recognized by chest pain, subcutaneous emphysema, and pneumomediastinum
   c. Inadvertent tracheal intubation—recognized by lack of breath sounds and no chest excursion
   d. Vomiting upon removal of the EOA

9. **Problems associated with the EOA**
   a. Failure to seal the mask adequately while ventilating the patient
   b. Inability to insert the EOA
   c. The EOA interferes with the placement of an E-T tube.

D. **E-T tubes**
   1. **Indications for E-T tubes**
      a. Relief of upper airway obstruction—resulting from laryngospasm, epiglottitis, or glottic edema
      b. Protection of the airway—the airway has four protective reflexes:
         (1) Pharyngeal reflex—gag and swallowing
         (2) Laryngeal reflex—laryngospasm
         (3) Tracheal reflex—coughing when trachea is irritated
         (4) Carinal reflex—coughing when carina is irritated

**NOTE: When these reflexes are obtunded or knocked out, the airway must be protected with an E-T tube. These reflexes may be obtunded by paralysis, drugs, loss of consciousness, or neuromuscular disease.

**NOTE: As these reflexes become obtunded, they are lost in progression from the pharyngeal to the carinal. As they recover, they do so in progression from the carinal to the pharyngeal.

      c. To facilitate tracheal suctioning

d. To assist manual or mechanical ventilation
2. **Hazards of E-T tubes**
   a. Contamination of the tracheobronchial tree
   b. Cough mechanism reduced
   c. Damage to the vocal cords
   d. Laryngeal or tracheal edema
   e. Mucosal damage leading to tracheal stenosis
   f. Tube occluded with inspissated secretions
   g. Loss of patient's dignity
   h. Loss of patient's ability to talk
3. Steps to perform endotracheal intubation

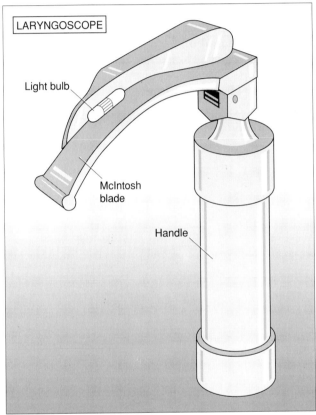

From Persing G. *Entry Level Respiratory Care Review.* Philadelphia: WB Saunders; 1992.

a. Select a laryngoscope with a **Miller (straight) blade or a McIntosh (curved) blade.** Make sure the light bulb is tight, as it will not light if it is loose.

b. Place the patient in the "sniffing position."

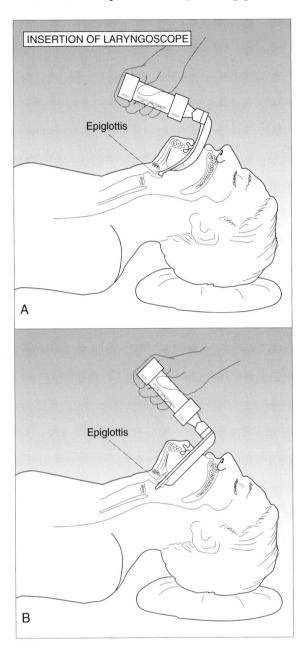

c. Select the proper size E-T tube, instill air into the cuff to make sure it holds it, and then deflate the cuff.
d. Insert a stylet to make the tube more rigid for easier insertion. Make sure the stylet does not extend past the end of the tube.
e. Insert the laryngoscope blade into the right side of the mouth (if laryngoscope is in left hand) and move tongue to the left.
f. Advance the blade forward.
   (1) The curved blade (McIntosh) should be inserted between the epiglottis and the base of the tongue (valecula); with a forward and upward motion, the epi-

glottis is raised to expose the glottis and vocal cords.

(2) The straight blade (Miller) should be placed under the epiglottis and lifted upward and forward to expose the cords.

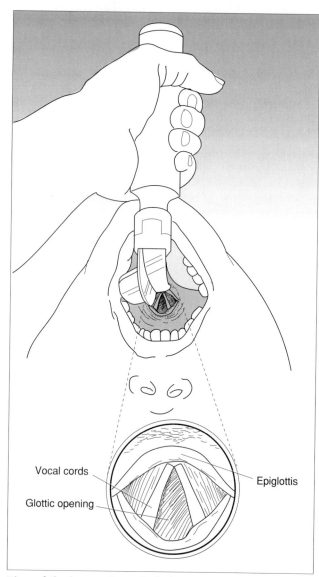

View of the larynx through the laryngoscope

From Persing G. *Entry Level Respiratory Care Review.* Philadelphia: WB Saunders; 1992.

NOTE: Never exceed 15 to 20 seconds per intubation attempt. The blade and tube in the back of the throat may stimulate the **vagus nerve, leading to bradycardia.** Remove the blade and tube and ventilate patient with a bag and mask.

    g. As the cords are observed, advance the E-T tube **approximately 5 cm past the cords.**
NOTE: If the tube is inserted too far, it will enter the right main-stem bronchus.

    **h. Inflate the cuff and listen for equal and bilateral breath sounds. If louder sounds are

heard on the right than on the left, the tube probably is in the right main-stem bronchus. Deflate the cuff and withdraw the tube until equal breath sounds are heard.

NOTE: The average distance from the teeth to the carina is 27 cm. Note that the E-T tube has markings in centimeters indicating the distance to the end of the tube from that point. Therefore, **taping the tube at the 23- to 25-cm mark** at the teeth will most likely place the tube between the clavicles and the carina.

    ** i. Obtain an immediate chest x-ray film for tube placement. The end of the tube should rest 2 to 7 cm above the carina. **The carina is located on x-ray film at the fourth rib or fourth thoracic vertebra.**

    j. Tape the tube securely.

4. **Parts of the E-T tube**

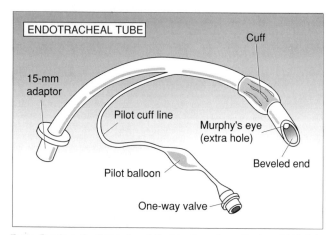

From Persing G. *Entry Level Respiratory Care Review.* Philadelphia: WB Saunders; 1992.

5. **E-T tube markings**

    a. IT—implantation tested; indicates that the material in the tube is nontoxic and is free from tissue reaction when implanted in rabbit tissue

**NOTE: Polyvinylchoride is the most common material used in E-T tubes.

    b. Z-79—The Z-79 Committee for Anesthesia Equipment for the American National Standards Institute; this committee ensures that the tube manufacturer is using material that is nontoxic to tissues

    c. ID—internal diameter of the tube in millimeters; this is how the tubes are designated by size

    d. OD—outside diameter of the tube in millimeters; also measured in French units, which is one third of a millimeter

    e. Numbers and marks indicating the distance in centimeters from that mark to the distal end of the tube

6. **Complications of oral E-T tubes**
   a. Poorly tolerated by conscious or semiconscious patients
   b. Difficult to stabilize because of the movement of the tube
   c. Stimulation of oral secretions
   d. Gagging resulting from tube irritation
   e. More difficult to pass suction catheter because of the curvature of the tube and poor stabilization
   f. Harder for patient to communicate
   g. Harder to attach equipment to a poorly stabilized E-T tube
   h. Patient may bite the tube, occluding air flow and setting off the ventilator high-pressure alarm, ending inspiration prematurely
7. **Nasotracheal tubes**
   a. These are considered nonemergency tubes.
   b. **Nasotracheal intubation**
      (1) Nose should be anesthetized with lidocaine or cocaine spray. A vasoconstrictor, such as phenylephrine hydrochloride (Neo-Synephrine drops), is used to shrink nasal mucosal blood vessels for easier tube insertion.
      (2) The tube is lubricated with water-soluble gel and inserted through a patent nostril.
      (3) If the patient is alert and breathing spontaneously, one should try advancing the tube as patient is taking a deep breath or coughing. This is called blind nasal intubation.
      (4) If the patient is not cooperative or is unconscious, the tube is visualized in the mouth and grasped by **McGill's forceps** and guided through the vocal cords via direct visualization with a laryngoscope.
      (5) The tube is taped in place when proper placement is assured.
   c. **Advantages of nasotracheal tubes (versus oral tubes)**
      (1) Easier to stabilize
      (2) Better tolerated by the patient because gagging is not likely
      (3) Less potential for inadvertent extubation
      (4) Equipment attaches more easily
      (5) Easier to pass suction catheter
      (6) Easier for patient to eat or drink
   d. **Complications of nasotracheal tubes**
      (1) Pressure necrosis of the nasal tissue
      (2) Sinus obstruction leading to sinusitis
      (3) Obstruction of eustachian tube, resulting in middle ear infections
      (4) Septal deviation

(5) Bleeding—during intubation or extubation

E. **Tracheostomy tubes**

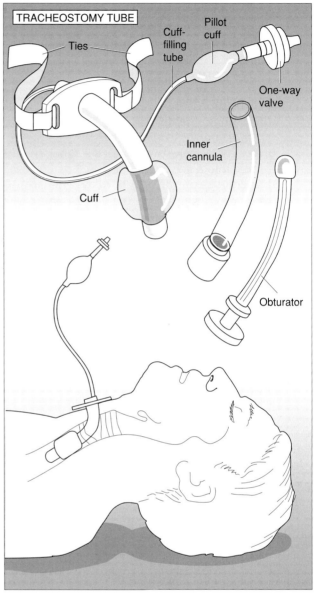

From Persing G. *Entry Level Respiratory Care Review.* Philadelphia: WB Saunders; 1992.

1. Tracheostomy tubes are inserted through an incision (stoma) made between the second and third tracheal rings.
2. The obturator should always be inserted into the outer cannula when the tube is being advanced into the stoma.
3. Once the tube is properly positioned, the obturator should be removed and the inner cannula inserted.
4. The cuff is then inflated and tracheostomy ties are used to secure the tube.
5. Some tubes use a foam cuff (Mikity-Wilson

Fome Cuff and Kamen Fome Cuff), which is deflated during insertion; when the tube is in place, the cuff is allowed to resume its normal foam shape, which provides an effective seal against the tracheal wall (exerts low pressure—20 torr).

6. **Indications for tracheostomies**
   a. To bypass upper airway obstruction
   b. To reduce anatomic deadspace (by 50%)
   c. To prevent problems posed by oral or nasal E-T tubes
   d. To allow patient to swallow and receive nourishment
   e. For long-term airway care (E-T tubes should be left in place no longer than 3 to 4 weeks)

7. **Immediate complications of tracheostomy tubes** (occurring within the first 24 hours; are associated with the tracheotomy procedure itself)
   a. Pneumothorax
   b. Bleeding
   c. Air embolism—tearing of pleural vein
   d. Subcutaneous emphysema

8. **Late complications of tracheostomy tubes** (occurring more than 1 to 2 days after the tracheotomy)
   a. Hemorrhage
   b. Infection
   c. Airway obstruction
   d. Tracheoesophageal fistula
   e. Interference with swallowing
   f. Rupture of innominate artery
   g. Stomal stenosis
   h. Tracheitis

**NOTE: Changing a tracheostomy tube within 48 hours of the tracheotomy is not advisable and should be done only by a surgeon if at all. The reason for this is that the tracheal rings may recede when the tube is removed, making reintubation difficult.

9. Special tracheostomy tubes

a. **Fenestrated tracheostomy tube**

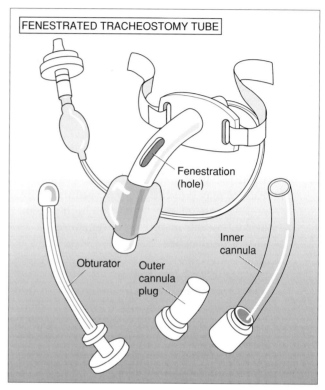

From Persing G. *Entry Level Respiratory Care Review*. Philadelphia: WB Saunders; 1992.

(1) This tube is used to aid in weaning the patient from a tracheostomy tube and to allow the patient to talk.

(2) With the inner cannula removed, air may pass through the hole (fenestration) in the outer cannula, allowing weaning from the tracheostomy tube, as well as talking.

(3) The outer cannula may be plugged with the cap on the proximal end of the tube. With the cuff deflated, all air flow will be through the patient's natural airway, but a passage for suctioning still exists.

(4) If ventilation should be necessary, the inner cannula may be reinserted and the cuff reinflated.

b. **Tracheostomy button**

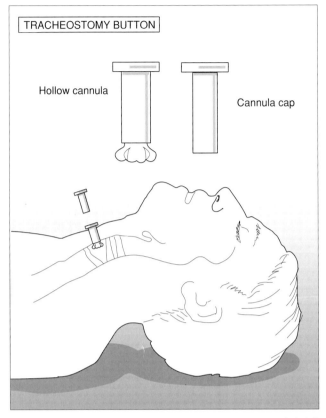

From Persing G. *Entry Level Respiratory Care Review.* Philadelphia: WB Saunders; 1992.

(1) This tube is used to wean the patient from the tracheostomy tube and yet maintain a patent stoma.
(2) Consists of a short, hollow tube that is used to replace the tracheostomy tube and still maintain a patent stoma if problems should arise.
(3) The patient has complete use of the upper airway.

c. **Kistner's tracheostomy tube**

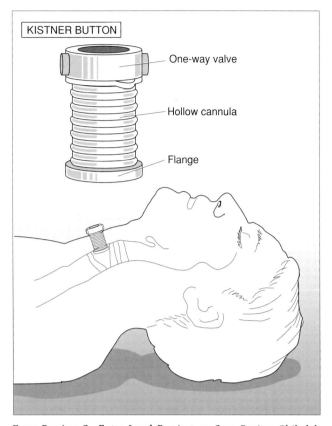

From Persing G. *Entry Level Respiratory Care Review.* Philadelphia: WB Saunders; 1992.

(1) This tube is also used to wean patients from tracheostomy tubes and yet maintain a patent stoma.
(2) Kistner's tubes are much like tracheostomy buttons, except they have a one-way valve on the proximal end of the tube.
(3) Air enters through the one-way valve and the tube during inspiration. As the patient exhales, the valve closes and the air flows up through the vocal cords and out the nose and mouth.

d. **Speaking tracheostomy tubes**

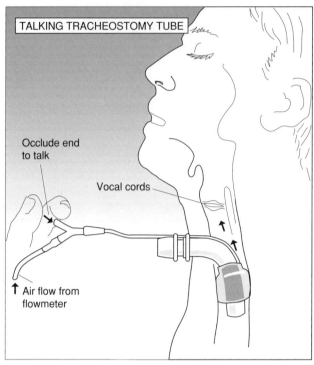

TALKING TRACHEOSTOMY TUBE

Occlude end
to talk

Vocal cords

↑ Air flow from
flowmeter

From Persing G. *Entry Level Respiratory Care Review.* Philadelphia: WB Saunders; 1992.

(1) A constant gas flow is available above the cuff and around the vocal cords to allow speech.
(2) The cuff remains inflated.

III. MAINTENANCE OF ARTIFICIAL AIRWAYS

A. **Cuff care**
1. Tubes should employ **high-volume, low pressure cuffs only.** They cause less occlusion to tracheal blood flow because they apply less pressure. They are also called floppy cuffs. It is important to note that if excessive air is placed in the cuff, it will act as a **high-pressure cuff.**
2. In order to ensure that the cuff is exerting the least amount of pressure on the tracheal wall and still providing an adequate seal, **the minimal leak technique or minimal occluding volume technique** should be employed.
   a. With the stethoscope beside the larynx, listen for air flow as the cuff is inflated. Inflate the cuff until no air flow is heard, then withdraw air slowly until a slight leak is heard. **This is the minimal leak technique.** (This is often performed on a sigh breath from the ventilator.)

b. **The minimal occluding volume technique** is accomplished the same way as the minimal leak technique, except you slowly inflate the cuff, just to the point at which no leak is heard.
** c. **Cuff pressures should be kept at less than 20 torr if at all possible.**
d. If the cuff is inflated to greater than 20 torr and a leak is still heard, continue inflating the cuff using the minimal leak or occluding volume technique. It may be that the E-T tube is too small and it is taking more air in the cuff to adequately seal the airway. In this case, the cuff pressure does not relate to the pressure on the tracheal wall. **To be safe, the E-T tube should be replaced with a larger one.
   e. **Effects of cuff pressure on the tracheal wall:**
Greater than 30 torr → obstructs arterial flow → ischemia
Greater than 20 torr → obstructs venous flow → congestion
Greater than 5 torr → obstructs lymphatic flow → edema
B. **Suctioning the airway**
   1. **Technique of suctioning**
      a. Preoxygenate the patient and instruct to breathe deeply. Hyperoxygenation is preferred to help prevent hypoxemia, which may lead to cardiac arrhythmias.
      b. Instill 3 to 5 ml of normal saline to help thin secretions (0.3 to 0.5 ml in infants).
      c. Insert the catheter without applying suction and advance until an obstruction (carina) is met. Do not jab catheter, as this may cause bradycardia (vagal stimulation).
      d. Withdraw the catheter approximately 1 to 2 cm and **apply intermittent suction** while rotating the catheter between the thumb and finger. **(This decreases mucosal damage.)**
      e. Once the catheter has been withdrawn into the E-T tube, continuous suction may be applied.
      f. Never leave the catheter in the airway for longer than **15 seconds.**
      g. Upon removal of the catheter, reoxygenate the patient and instruct him/her to breathe deeply and wait 30 seconds to 1 minute before entering the airway again.
NOTE: Monitor electrocardiogram and stop procedure if complications occur; hyperoxygenate and ventilate (if on ventilator).
      h. Repeat steps until secretions are aspirated and airway sounds clear.
      i. Suctioning the nasopharynx and oropharynx

may now be done, remembering **never** to reenter the E-T tube with this catheter.

2. **Proper suctioning levels**
   Adult: −80 to −120 torr
   Child: −60 to −80 torr
   Infant: −40 to −60 torr

NOTE: When nasotracheal suctioning is performed, the preceding steps should be followed and the following techniques added:

a. Lubricate catheter with water-soluble gel.

b. Instruct patient to take a deep breath or cough as the catheter advances to the oropharynx. This aids in inserting the catheter through the glottic opening.

3. **Selecting the proper sized catheter**

a. The suction catheter should not occupy more than **one half to two thirds of the internal diameter of the tube.

b. Suction catheters are sized by the French unit, **which is equal to 0.33 mm;** therefore, multiply the catheter size by 0.33 to determine its diameter in millimeters, which is how E-T tubes are sized. To determine the percentage of space the catheter occupies inside the E-T tube, divide the catheter size (mm) by the E-T tube size (mm).

EXAMPLE: How much of the internal diameter of an 8-mm E-T tube is occupied by a 14 French suction catheter?

14 French catheter = 4.62 mm (14 × 0.33)

$$\frac{4.62 \text{ mm}}{8 \text{ mm}} = 0.58 \times 100 = \textbf{58\%}$$

To calculate the maximum sized catheter to be used (when using one half as the maximum size):

$$\frac{\text{ET tube size} \times 3}{2} = \text{maximum catheter size}$$

4. Yankauer's suction (tonsil) — used to suction the oropharynx

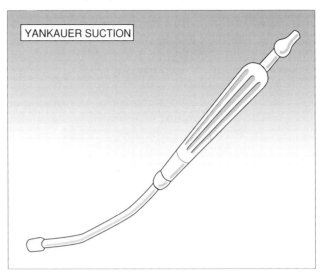

From Persing G. *Entry Level Respiratory Care Review.* Philadelphia: WB Saunders; 1992.

5. **Coudé suction catheter — angle-tipped catheter used to suction the left lung

6. **Indications for tracheal suctioning**
   a. Retained secretions patient cannot mobilize
   b. To maintain patency of artificial airways
   c. To obtain sputum for culture and sensitivity

7. **Hazards of tracheal suctioning**
   a. Hypoxemia — **increase FIO$_2$ prior to suctioning!**
   b. Arrhythmias — due to hypoxemia and vagal nerve stimulation; **vagus nerve is stimulated as catheter irritates the oronasal mucosa, tracheal mucosa, and carina, causing bradycardia**
   c. Hypotension — caused by bradycardia and prolonged coughing episode
   d. Atelectasis — caused by using a suction catheter that is too large or excessive suction pressure
   e. Tissue trauma — caused by jabbing catheter during insertion, improper lubrication while performing nasal suctioning, and not applying **intermittent** suction

---

IV. ENDOTRACHEAL EXTUBATION

A. Procedure of extubation
   1. Explain procedure to the patient.
   2. Increase the FIO$_2$ level.
   3. Suction down the E-T tube.

4. Suction the mouth and back of throat.
5. Untape the E-T tube, deflate the cuff, and instruct the patient to take a deep breath. **At peak inspiration, withdraw the tube.**

NOTE: It is permissible to withdraw the tube while suctioning, as this clears the airway while extubating.

B. **Complications of extubation**
1. **Laryngospasm**
   a. Spasm of the vocal cords due to irritation of the tube, resulting in airway obstruction; this is observed as respiratory difficulty immediately following extubation
   b. If laryngospasm occurs, administer high FIO_2 concentration, and if it persists for more than 1 to 2 minutes, administer a bronchodilator via a hand-held nebulizer.
2. **Glottic edema** (see further on)

NOTE: **Intubation equipment should be readily available at the bedside during extubation if reintubation becomes necessary.**

V. LARYNGEAL AND TRACHEAL COMPLICATIONS OF E-T TUBES

A. **Sore throat and hoarseness**
1. Common occurrence from tube irritation
2. Usually subsides within 2 to 3 days
3. Treat with cool mist.

B. **Glottic edema**
1. **Inspiratory stridor is the major clinical sign.
2. Caused by:
   a. Traumatic intubation
   b. Insertion of oversized E-T tube
   c. Poor E-T tube maintenance
   d. Allergic response to material in E-T tube
3. Should be treated with:
   **a. Cool aerosol to decrease swelling
   **b. Vasoconstrictor—racemic epinephrine via hand-held nebulizer
   **c. Steroids—Dexamethasone (Decadron) occasionally used to reduce swelling

C. **Subglottic edema**
1. Edema that occurs below the glottis at the level of the cricoid cartilage
**2. A serious complication following extubation that may lead to reintubation
3. If postextubation distress cannot be relieved, subglottic edema must be suspected.

D. **Vocal cord ulceration**
1. Suspected if hoarseness continues for more than 1 week
2. Caused by:
   a. Traumatic intubation
   b. Tight-fitting tube
   c. Allergic reaction to material in tube
   d. Excessive movement of the tube

E. **Tracheal mucosal ulceration**
1. Common occurrence following extubation
2. Occurs at the area of the cuff site

F. **Vocal cord paralysis**
1. Caused by damage to the recurrent laryngeal nerve
2. Usually occurs secondary to upper chest or neck surgery

G. **Laryngotracheal web**
1. Caused by necrotic tissue at the glottic or subglottic level, which leads to fibrin formation that combines with secretions and cellular debris to form a membrane or web
2. Stridor and acute airway obstruction generally occur.
3. The web should be suctioned from the airway immediately.
4. Often occurs several days after extubation

H. **Tracheal stenosis**
1. A lesion found at the cuff site or the level of the cricoid membrane
2. As the lesion heals it constricts, leading to a narrowing of the airway.
3. A narrowing of less than 50% of the diameter of the airway will not be symptomatic.
4. To help prevent tracheal stenosis, maintain cuff pressure by use of the **minimal leak technique.**

I. **Tracheal malacia**
1. Loss of the cartilaginous support of the trachea
2. Following extubation, the trachea collapses, leading to respiratory distress.

REFERENCES

1. Eubanks D, Bone R. *Comprehensive Respiratory Care.* 2nd ed. St. Louis: CV Mosby; 1990.
2. McPherson SP. *Respiratory Therapy Equipment.* 4th ed. St. Louis: CV Mosby; 1990.
3. Scanlan C, Spearman C. *Egan's Fundamentals of Respiratory Care.* 5th ed. St. Louis: CV Mosby; 1990.
4. Shapiro BA: *Clinical Application of Respiratory Care.* 4th ed. St. Louis: Mosby-Year Book Publishers; 1990.

PRETEST ANSWERS

1. E
2. D
3. A
4. B
5. C
6. E

Special Respiratory Care Procedures

PRETEST QUESTIONS*

1. Which of the following are complications associated with bronchoscopy?

   I. Pulmonary hemorrhage
   II. Pneumothorax
   III. Hypoxemia

   A. I only
   B. II only
   C. I and III only
   D. II and III only
   E. I, II, and III

2. While assisting on a bronchoscopy, it is noted that the physician is having difficulty entering the trachea. This may be the result of which of the following?

   A. Pneumothorax
   B. Hypoxemia
   C. Laryngospasm
   D. Pulmonary hemorrhage
   E. Atelectasis

3. Following a bronchoscopy, it is noted by the respiratory therapist that it is taking more ventilator pressure to ventilate the patient than before the procedure. This could be caused by which of the following?

   I. Bronchospasm
   II. Pneumothorax
   III. Hypoxemia
   IV. Pulmonary hemorrhage

   A. I and II only
   B. II and III only
   C. I, II, and IV only
   D. II, III, and IV only
   E. I, II, III, and IV

4. During a thoracentesis, the patient suddenly complains of chest pain and becomes dyspneic. This is most likely the result of which of the following?

A. Atelectasis
B. Myocardial infarction
C. Empyema
D. Pneumothorax
E. Pulmonary edema

5. To aid in the evacuation of air from the pleural space, a chest tube should be inserted at what level?

A. Supraclavicular space
B. Second intercostal space
C. Fourth intercostal space
D. Sixth intercostal space
E. Eighth intercostal space

6. The respiratory therapist notices that on a patient's chest tube drainage system there is fluctuation of the water level in the water seal chamber with each breath and that air bubbles are seen only in the vacuum control chamber, which has been filled to 15 cm of water. The most appropriate action to take is which of the following?

A. Clamp the chest tube and check for leaks.
B. Insert the chest tube farther until bubbling stops in the vacuum chamber.
C. Withdraw the chest tube until bubbling starts in the water seal chamber.
D. Decrease the vacuum pressure.
E. Recommend a chest x-ray study to determine if the pneumothorax has resolved.

7. The respiratory therapist observes that during a patient's breathing cycle there is no fluctuation in the water seal chamber of the pleural drainage system. The most appropriate action is which of the following?

A. Withdraw the tube until fluctuation is seen.
B. "Strip" the chest tube to clear a possible obstruction.
C. Increase the vacuum pressure.
D. Clamp the chest tube and observe for leaks.
E. No action is necessary, as this is a normal observation.

---

*See answers at the end of the chapter.

Special Respiratory Care Procedures

I. BRONCHOSCOPY

A. Bronchoscopy is a technique that uses an instrument called a bronchoscope. It is used for both therapeutic and diagnostic purposes.

B. **Types of bronchoscopes**

1. Rigid bronchoscope

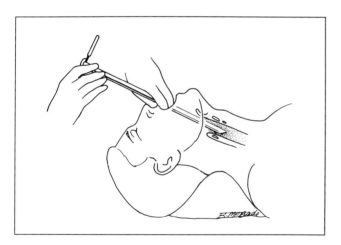

a. It consists of a hollow metal tube with a light on its distal end.

b. The tube is inserted orally and then passed through the vocal cords into the trachea.

c. It is useful for removing aspirated foreign bodies and thick secretions from the lungs.

2. Fiberoptic bronchoscope

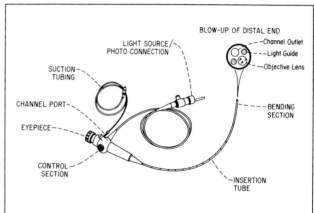

a. It consists of a collection of thin, threadlike glass strands called fiberoptic filaments and a light bulb on its distal end for visualization.

b. Because of its more flexible nature, it is better tolerated by patients and therefore more commonly used.

c. The tube may be inserted orally, nasally, or through the endotracheal tube. The tube should be lubricated with a water-soluble jelly for easier nasal insertion. Often lidocaine jelly is used both as a lubricant and for its numbing effects.

d. Because of its flexibility, it can be advanced farther into the airway than a rigid bronchoscope, thereby allowing greater visualization of the conducting airways.

e. Biopsy forceps and brushes may be inserted through this bronchoscope to obtain tissue samples.

C. **Indications for bronchoscopy**

1. Removal of foreign bodies

2. Removal of mucus plugs and thick secretions

a. Normally performed if secretions cannot be removed by routine suctioning techniques

b. Once the site of the secretions is visualized, the area should be lavaged with saline prior to suctioning.
3. Atelectasis affecting a lobe or entire lung
4. Pulmonary hemorrhage
   a. To locate the area of bleeding
   b. To control bleeding by instillation of epinephrine or iced saline lavage at the bleeding site
5. Difficult tracheal intubation as a result of upper airway trauma, obesity, tumors, or spinal deformity
   a. The endotracheal tube (E-T tube) is slipped over the fiberoptic bronchoscope with the scope protruding well past the end of the E-T tube.
   b. The vocal cords are visualized and the scope is advanced through the cords to the midtracheal level, where the E-T tube is then advanced over the scope to the proper position. The scope is then withdrawn.
6. Biopsy of suspected tumors
7. Obtaining sputum for culture and sensitivity studies

D. **Complications of bronchoscopy**
1. Hypoxemia
   a. Monitor oxygen saturation during procedure.
   b. Increase oxygen percentage during procedure.
2. Laryngospasm
   a. Makes advancing the tube more difficult
   b. A bronchodilator should be readily available.
3. Bronchospasm
   a. Result of irritation to the airway
   b. A bronchodilator should be readily available.
4. Arrhythmias
   a. Resulting from vagal stimulation
   b. Monitor electrocardiogram and remove bronchoscope until the patient's cardiac status is stabilized.
5. Hemorrhage
   a. May occur during insertion of the tube
   b. Also may occur following biopsy
6. Respiratory depression
   a. Resulting from sedatives given during the procedure
   b. Monitor respiratory status closely.
7. Hypotension
   a. Resulting from vagal nerve stimulation
   b. May result from sedatives given during the procedure
8. Pneumothorax
   a. Resulting from inadvertent puncture of the lung
   b. Monitor respiratory status closely.

E. **Respiratory care practitioner's responsibilities during bronchoscopy**
NOTE: Responsibilities of the respiratory care practitioner vary according to region. The following are among the most common responsibilities:
1. Prepare the patient and explain the procedure.
2. Administer aerosolized local anesthetic to the patient's upper airway.
3. Conduct patient monitoring throughout the procedure.
   a. Pulse
   b. Respiratory rate
   c. Electrocardiogram
   d. Oxygen saturation
4. Collect sputum and tissue samples that the physician has obtained and prepare them for laboratory analysis.
5. Clean the bronchoscope properly following the procedure.

II. THORACENTESIS

A. Thoracentesis is a procedure in which a needle is inserted into the chest wall to obtain material from the lung or drain fluid from the pleural space (pleural effusion or empyema).
B. **Technique of thoracentesis**
1. A local anesthetic is injected into the skin at the area where the fluid has been detected.
2. A local anesthetic is then injected into the periosteum of the rib with a 22-gauge needle.
3. With the patient in a sitting position, a needle (usually 22-gauge or larger) is inserted into the pleural space, and the fluid is removed.
C. After the fluid is removed it is analyzed for:
1. Odor
2. Color
3. Red blood cell count
4. White blood cell count
5. Characteristics on gram staining
6. Identification of the infecting organism by culture and sensitivity testing
NOTE: Pus in the pleural space (empyema) should be drained prior to chest physical therapy.
D. Thoracentesis may be performed in cases of pneumonia in which consolidation has occurred. The needle may be inserted into the affected area of the lung and the secretions withdrawn so that culture and sensitivity testing may be performed to identify the infecting organism.
E. Complications of thoracentesis
1. Pneumothorax
2. Bacterial infection
3. Subcutaneous emphysema

III. TRANSTRACHEAL ASPIRATION

A. Obtaining sputum for culture and sensitivity testing via nasotracheal suctioning may not accurately identify the organisms within the trachea and lower airway because the sample is contaminated by "normal bacterial flora" located in the naso- and oropharynx.

B. In order to avoid contamination of the lower respiratory tract with nasal and oral suctioning, transtracheal aspiration may be performed.

C. **Technique of transtracheal aspiration**
  1. This procedure is performed by introducing a thin polyethylene needle catheter into the trachea through the cricoid membrane under local anesthesia.
  2. The needle is removed while the catheter remains in place, and saline is instilled into the trachea through the catheter.
  3. This usually stimulates a strong cough and the catheter is aspirated with a syringe.
  4. Only a small amount of sputum is needed for analysis.

D. **Complications of transtracheal aspiration**
  1. Patient discomfort
  2. Subcutaneous emphysema
  3. Esophageal damage
  4. Damage to the nerves and blood vessels surrounding the area of entrance into the trachea

IV. CHEST TUBE INSERTION AND MONITORING

A. Chest tubes are used to drain substances that accumulate in the pleural space.

B. Substances that may accumulate in the pleural space and the appropriate medical names include:
  1. air—pneumothorax
  2. blood—hemothorax
  3. lymph—chylothorax
  4. serous fluid—pleural effusion
  5. pus—pyothorax or empyema

NOTE: The term **hydrothorax** is often used to refer to lymph, serum, or plasma in the pleural space.

C. To help evacuate air from the pleural space (pneumothorax), the chest tube is usually inserted in the second intercostal space. To remove fluids, the tube is placed lower, usually in the eighth intercostal space.

NOTE: Once the air is evacuated from the pleural space, spontaneous healing or sealing of the leak in the lung will usually occur.

D. **Chest tube drainage systems**
  1. **One-bottle system**

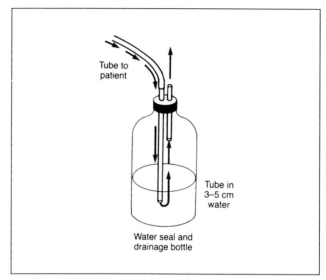

From O'Toole M, ed. *Miller-Keane Encyclopedia and Dictionary of Medicine, Nursing, and Allied Health.* 5th ed. Philadelphia: WB Saunders; 1992.

  a. Fluid or air drains from the pleural space through the chest tube and enters the drainage bottle through a glass tube that is submerged under water. This forms a seal, acting like a one-way valve to prevent air from entering the pleural cavity.
  b. Air entering the bottle is then vented out the short tube in the top of the bottle.
  c. The one-bottle setup is both a water seal container and a collection container.

  2. **Two-bottle system**

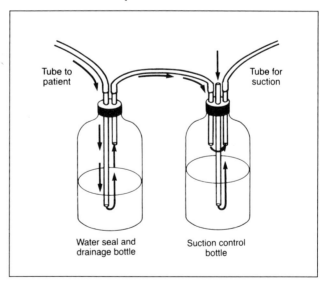

From O'Toole M, ed. *Miller-Keane Encyclopedia and Dictionary of Medicine, Nursing, and Allied Health.* 5th ed. Philadelphia: WB Saunders; 1992.

a. In this system, a second bottle is added to collect air exiting the pleural space. Liquid drains into the first bottle.

b. The purpose of this system is to better control the amount of suction applied. A suction source may be connected to the vent of the water seal bottle.

3. **Three-bottle system**

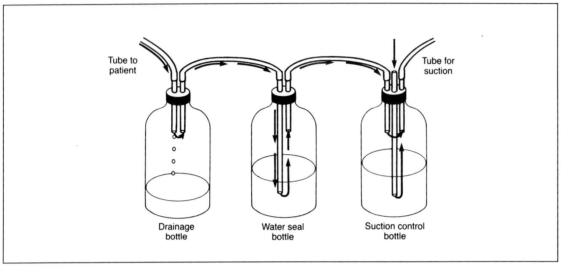

Tube to patient
Tube for suction

Drainage bottle
Water seal bottle
Suction control bottle

From O'Toole M, ed. *Miller-Keane Encyclopedia and Dictionary of Medicine, Nursing, and Allied Health.* 5th ed. Philadelphia: WB Saunders; 1992.

a. A third bottle may be added to determine the amount of subatmospheric pressure in the water seal bottle.

b. The amount of suction is determined by how far under the water the tube is submerged.

c. A suction source may be attached to the third bottle's vent to maintain a desired constant subatmospheric pressure.

E. **Important points concerning chest tube drainage**

** 1. The water level in the water seal bottle will fluctuate with changes in pleural pressure that occur with normal breathing. **If no fluctuation is occurring in the water seal bottle, obstruction of the tube must be suspected.**

2. Chest tubes may become obstructed as a result of blood clots or kinks in the tube itself. **Obstructed chest tubes may result in a tension pneumothorax.**

** 3. In order to assure adequate drainage and tube patency, the tube should be "stripped" or "milked" every 1 to 2 hours. This is accomplished by compressing and releasing the tubing, which creates a sudden gush of suction thereby keeping the tube clear of obstruction caused by a clot.

** 4. Occasional bubbling in the water seal bottle is normal as air enters from the pleural space.

Excessive or persistent bubbling may indicate air leaks in the system. The lack of bubbling indicates that no air is being removed from the pleural space, a sign of improvement.

** 5. If an air leak is suspected, the chest tube should be clamped to identify the source of the leak.

** 6. Clamping of the tube is required when changing drainage bottles but must be done with caution in patients with pleural air leaks, since a tension pneumothorax may result.

7. The drainage and collection bottles must be kept at a level below the chest to prevent backflow.

8. The drainage and collection system must be kept airtight with no leaks around the connections. The glass tube **must always** be kept submerged under the water.

9. If a suction source is connected to the vent tube in the suction bottle, a negative pressure not to exceed −15 cm of water is usually necessary.

10. After the lung reexpands, the chest tube should remain in place for another 1 to 2 days. After the tube is removed, the wound should be covered with a sterile petroleum jelly dressing to prevent air from entering the pleural space.

REFERENCES

1. Des Jardins T. *Clinical Manifestations of Respiratory Disease.* 2nd ed. Chicago: Year Book Medical Publishers; 1990.
2. Des Jardins T. *Cardiopulmonary Anatomy and Physiology—*

Essentials for Respiratory Care. Albany, NY: Delmar Publishers; 1988.
3. Kacmarek R, Stoller J. *Current Respiratory Care.* Philadelphia: B.C. Decker; 1988.
4. Levitzky M, Cairo J, Hall S. *Introduction to Respiratory Care.* Philadelphia: WB Saunders; 1990.
5. O'Toole M, ed. *Miller-Keane Encyclopedia and Dictionary of Medicine, Nursing, and Allied Health.* 5th ed. Philadelphia: WB Saunders; 1992.
6. Scanlan C, Spearman C. *Egan's Fundamentals of Respiratory Care.* 5th ed. St. Louis: CV Mosby; 1990.
7. Weinberger S. *Principles of Pulmonary Medicine.* 2nd ed. Philadelphia: WB Saunders; 1992.

PRETEST ANSWERS

1. E
2. C
3. C
4. D
5. B
6. E
7. B

CHAPTER 6

Cardiopulmonary Resuscitation Techniques

PRETEST QUESTIONS*

1. You enter a patient's room to give a treatment and observe that the patient is unconscious and not breathing. Your first action should be which of the following?

A. Deliver two breaths
B. Begin chest compressions
C. Perform abdominal thrusts
D. Place the patient in Fowler's position
E. Open the airway

2. Following 10 minutes of cardiopulmonary resuscitation (CPR), an infant's pulse returns, but no ventilatory effort is present. The respiratory care practitioner should do which of the following?

A. Continue compressions and rescue breathing at a ratio of 5 compressions to 1 breath.
B. Stop compressions and deliver one breath every 6 seconds.
C. Deliver five back blows until breathing resumes.
D. Stop compressions and deliver one breath every 3 seconds.
E. Continue compressions and rescue breathing at a ratio of 15 compressions to 2 breaths.

3. A patient has been intubated and CPR is being performed. The patient's electrocardiogram (EKG) strip indicates asystole, and the physician is unable to insert an intravenous line (IV). The respiratory therapist should recommend the immediate performance of which of the following?

A. Instill sodium bicarbonate directly down the endotracheal tube.
B. Continue to attempt to start an IV in a peripheral vein.

C. Instill epinephrine directly down the endotracheal tube.
D. Inject epinephrine directly into the myocardium.
E. Instill calcium chloride directly down the endotracheal tube.

4. Which of the following drugs is used to treat ventricular fibrillation during CPR?

  I. Epinephrine
 II. Lidocaine
III. Atropine sulfate

A. I only
B. II only
C. I and II only
D. II and III only
E. I, II, and III

5. During CPR, the patient's EKG indicates ventricular fibrillation. The patient has been defibrillated with 200 joule with no change in the EKG reading. The respiratory therapist should recommend which of the following?

A. Repeat defibrillation with 300 joule.
B. Repeat defibrillation with 450 joule.
C. Instill sodium bicarbonate directly down the endotracheal tube.
D. Continue two-rescuer CPR with a compression : ventilation ratio of 5 : 2.
E. Perform a precordial thump.

6. A patient's EKG indicates that atrial fibrillation and cardioversion should be attempted. The defibrillator should be set at what energy level to return the heart to normal function?

A. 50 joule
B. 150 joule
C. 250 joule
D. 400 joule
E. 500 joule

---

*See answers at the end of the chapter.

71

CHAPTER **6**

Cardiopulmonary Resuscitation Techniques

I. CARDIOPULMONARY RESUSCITATION

A. **Obstructed airway (conscious adult)**
1. Determine if airway obstruction is present by asking the victim if he/she is choking or if speech or coughing is possible.
2. Perform **abdominal thrusts** until the foreign body is expelled or the victim becomes unconscious.
3. If the victim becomes unconscious, place him/her on the back and call for help.
4. Use the tongue-jaw lift maneuver to open the mouth and perform a finger sweep with the victim's head turned to the side.
5. Open the airway by using the head-tilt/chin-lift method.
6. Give two breaths.
7. If the ventilation attempts fail (determined by observing the chest not rising or by difficulty in expelling air into the victim), reposition the airway and ventilate again. If there is still no air movement, straddle the victim's thighs and perform 6 to 10 abdominal thrusts.
8. Perform a finger sweep again and reattempt ventilations.
9. Repeat sequence until the airway is cleared.
B. **Obstructed airway (unconscious adult)**
1. Determine unresponsiveness.
2. Call for help.
3. Position the victim on the back.
4. Open the airway using the head-tilt/chin-lift method.
5. **Determine breathlessness** by placing ear over the victim's mouth, and **look, listen, and feel for air movement.**
6. Attempt to ventilate.

7. If there is no air movement, reposition the airway and reattempt to ventilate.
8. If there is still no air movement, straddle the victim's thighs and perform 6 to 10 abdominal thrusts.
9. Perform a finger sweep with the victim's head turned to the side.
10. Attempt ventilation.
11. Repeat the sequence until the airway is cleared.
C. **One-rescuer CPR (adult)**
1. Determine unresponsiveness.
2. Call for help.
3. Position victim on the back.
4. Open the airway using the head-tilt/chin-lift method.
5. Determine breathlessness by placing ear over the victim's mouth and look, listen, and feel for air movement.
6. Give two breaths while observing chest rise. (Allow lungs to deflate between breaths.)
7. Determine pulselessness by palpating the **carotid artery.** (Palpate **brachial artery** in the **infant.**)
8. Begin chest compressions at a rate of 80 to 100/min (15 compressions—2 breaths).
9. Continue until patient responds, help arrives, or you can no longer physically continue.
D. **Two-rescuer CPR (adult)**
1. When the second rescuer arrives, he/she should take over as the new compressor while the first rescuer gets into position to be the breather. Palpating for a spontaneous pulse should be performed at this time.
2. If no pulse is present, the breather delivers one breath and signals the compressor to resume CPR **(five compressions to one breath).**

3. The breather must make sure the breath is being delivered between compressions.
4. The patient should be intubated as soon as possible to provide a more effective airway and to prevent air from entering the stomach during ventilation.
5. As the compressor begins to tire, he/she may signal the breather to change positions by altering the pneumonic from "one, one thousand" to "change, one thousand." After the next 5:1 sequence, the compressor moves to the head to begin ventilations (first checking the pulse) while the breather gets into position to begin compressions.

II. ADULT, CHILD, AND INFANT CPR MODIFICATIONS

A. **Compression : ventilation ratios (one rescuer)**
1. Adult—15:2   80 to 100 compressions/min
2. Child—5:1   80 to 100 compressions/min
3. Infant—5:1   >100 compressions/min
B. **Compression : ventilation ratios (two rescuers)**
1. Adult—5:1
2. Child—5:1
3. Infant—5:1
C. **Rescue breathing—victim has pulse**
1. Adult—one breath every 5 seconds
2. Child—one breath every 4 seconds
3. Infant—one breath every 3 seconds
D. **Compression depth**
1. Adult—**1.5 to 2 inches** with two hands stacked and heel of one hand on lower half of the victim's sternum
2. Child—**1 to 1.5 inches** with one hand on the lower half of the victim's sternum
3. Infant—**0.5 to 1 inch** with two or three fingers one finger's width below the nipple line

III. CPR—SPECIAL CONSIDERATIONS

** A. **Do not** hyperextend the neck of an infant to open the airway, as this may close it off.
** B. If a manual resuscitator bag and mask is not available for rescue breathing, **a mask with a one-way valve should be used to prevent contamination from the patient's exhaled air.** Mouth-to-mouth ventilation is used only if no other means is available.

C. **Never** compress the chest of a victim who has even the weakest pulse.
1. A weak pulse more than likely delivers a higher cardiac output than do manual compressions.
2. Manual compressions achieve only approximately **25% to 35% of normal blood flow.**
D. Upon entering a room in which one-rescuer CPR is being performed, the first step to take before changing to two-rescuer CPR is to establish the presence or lack of a pulse.
E. The best way to determine adequate cerebral blood flow while performing chest compressions is by checking pupillary reaction.
F. Victims with suspected **neck injury** should have the airway opened by the **jaw thrust maneuver without head tilt.**
G. **Hazards of CPR**
1. Rib fracture (especially in infants and elderly individuals—may lead to pneumothorax or lacerated liver)
2. Fat embolism (microfractures of the ribs or sternum lead to the leaking of fat from bone marrow, which finds its way into the venous circulation)
3. Gastric distention (from air entering the stomach from rescue breathing—air should be removed because this interferes with lung expansion)

IV. MANUAL RESUSCITATORS

A. **Uses of manual resuscitators**
1. Rescue breathing
2. To hyperinflate the lungs prior to tracheal suctioning
3. Transporting patient who requires artificial ventilation

B. **The manual resuscitator**

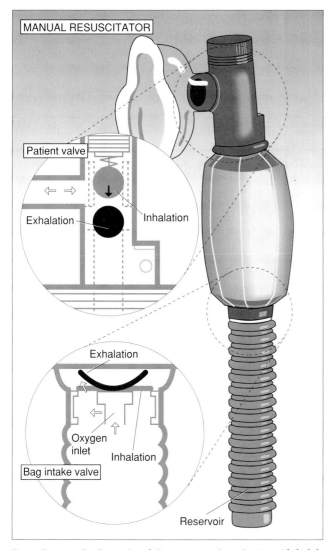

MANUAL RESUSCITATOR

Patient valve

⇐ ⇒

Exhalation — Inhalation

Exhalation

⇐ ⇑

Oxygen inlet — Inhalation

Bag intake valve

Reservoir

From Persing G. *Entry Level Respiratory Care Review*. Philadelphia: WB Saunders; 1992.

C. All resuscitators have basically the same design:
1. A patient valve with a standard universal adaptor consisting of a 22-mm outside diameter that fits standard resuscitation masks and a 15-mm internal diameter that connects to standard endotracheal or tracheostomy tubes
2. The patient valve also houses the exhalation valve and ports, which prevent the rebreathing of exhaled air.
3. The resuscitators use self-inflating bags by way of a bag intake valve.
**4. A reservoir attachment should be connected to the bag intake valve so that as the bag reinflates, it fills with supplemental oxygen instead of room air. This will ensure higher oxygen percentages (approaching 100%) being delivered to the patient.

5. Most resuscitator bags have pressure relief devices that open to the atmosphere at 40 cm of water pressure to prevent excessive pressures from being delivered to the patient's lungs.
6. Some resuscitators come equipped with positive end-expiratory pressure (PEEP) valves for "bagging" patients who are on PEEP on the ventilator. This is very beneficial, as it has been shown that patients taken off PEEP to be "bagged" will have drastic reductions in PaO_2 if ventilated with no PEEP.
**7. In order to achieve the highest delivered oxygen percentages possible, follow these criteria:
  **a. Always use a reservoir attachment if available.
  **b. Use the highest flowrate that will not cause the valves to jam (10 to 15 L/min).
  **c. Use the longest possible bag refill time, which means a slower ventilation rate. Allow the bag to fully refill before the next breath. A faster ventilation rate will decrease the delivered oxygen percentage.
  d. Do not use large stroke volumes (volume squeezed from the bag) if possible. Higher volumes delivered from the bag mean more room air entrained and thus lower oxygen percentages **(not that significant if a reservoir attachment is used).
D. **Hazards of using manual resuscitators**
1. Leaks during inspiration caused by improperly fitted face mask or inadequately filled endotracheal (E-T) tube cuff
2. Equipment malfunction due to sticking valves, missing parts, improper assembly, or dirty valve mechanisms
3. Poor ventilation technique

E. **Gas-powered resuscitators**

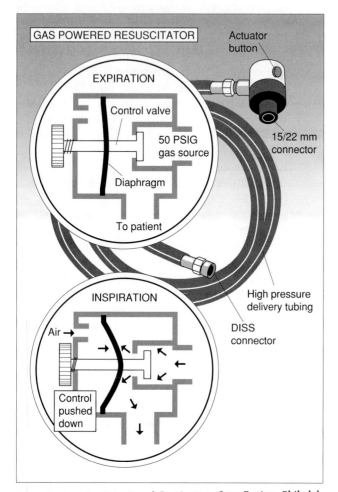

From Persing G. *Entry Level Respiratory Care Review*. Philadelphia: WB Saunders; 1992.

1. These are usually pressure-limited devices.
2. Some use demand valves, which open and deliver gas if a negative pressure is created.
3. They usually have manual control buttons to initiate inspiration if the patient is apneic.
4. They are able to deliver 100% oxygen.
5. Volume delivery will decrease if the pressure needed to ventilate the patient's lungs is higher than the capabilities of the unit.
6. The unit is powered from a 50-psig oxygen wall outlet. If the diaphragm in the unit breaks, the patient's airway could be exposed to this high pressure.
7. There are pressure relief devices that vent pressures greater than 50 cm of water.

V. PHARMACOLOGIC INTERVENTION DURING CPR

A. **Routes of administration**

1. Central venous line — ideal route if available
2. Peripheral IV line — best route if central venous line not available
3. **Endotracheal tube — drugs such as **lidocaine, epinephrine, and atropine** may be instilled directly into the tracheobronchial tree via the E-T tube for rapid absorption.
4. Intracardiac — epinephrine is the only drug that may be injected directly into the heart but only if the E-T tube or IV route is not available or failed to elicit a response.

B. **Drugs commonly administered during CPR**
1. **Epinephrine**
   a. Indications
      (1) Asystole
      (2) Sinus arrest
      (3) Ventricular fibrillation
   b. Route of administration
      (1) IV bolus
   **(2) E-T tube
      (3) Intracardiac
   c. Dosage — 0.1 ml/kg every 5 minutes (10 ml maximum) of a 0.1 mg/ml (1:10,000) preparation IV or 10 ml down E-T tube
   d. Pharmacologic actions
      (1) Increased heart rate
      (2) Increased force of contraction of the heart
      (3) Increased coronary perfusion pressure
      (4) Vasoconstriction
2. **Lidocaine**
   a. Indications
      (1) Ventricular fibrillation
      (2) Ventricular tachycardia
      (3) Premature ventricular contractions (PVCs)
   b. Route of administration
      (1) IV bolus
      (2) IV drip
   **(3) Endotracheal tube
   c. Dosage — 1 mg/kg IV bolus
   d. Pharmacologic actions
      (1) Decreases ventricular activity
3. **Atropine sulfate**
   a. Indications
      (1) Sinus bradycardia
      (2) Asystole
      (3) Nodal bradycardia
   b. Route of administration
      (1) IV bolus
   **(2) Endotracheal tube
   c. Dosage — 1 mg IV every 5 minutes for asystole or 0.5 mg every 5 minutes (2 mg maximum) for bradycardia
   d. Pharmacologic actions
      (1) Increased heart rate

(2) Increased force of contraction of the heart

4. **Procainamide**
   a. Indications
      (1) Ventricular tachycardia
      (2) Ventricular fibrillation
      (3) PVCs
   b. Route of administration
      (1) IV bolus
      (2) IV drip
   c. Dosage—50 mg bolus every 5 minutes or 1 to 4 mg/min IV drip of a 100 mg/ml preparation
   d. Pharmacologic actions
      (1) May cause hypotension
      (2) Increases electrical stimulation threshold
      (3) Decreases electrical activity of the ventricles

5. **Bretylium**
   a. Indications
      (1) Ventricular tachycardia
      (2) Ventricular fibrillation
      (3) PVCs
   b. Route of administration
      (1) IV bolus
   c. Dosage—5 mg/kg in 50 ml diluent over 5 to 10 minutes
   d. Pharmacologic actions
      (1) May cause hypotension
      (2) Increases electrical stimulation threshold
      (3) Decreases electrical activity of the ventricles

6. **Propranolol**
   a. Indications
      (1) Myocardial infarction
      (2) Angina pectoris
      (3) Supraventricular arrhythmias
      (4) Ventricular tachycardia
   b. Route of administration
      (1) IV bolus
   c. Dosage—1 to 5 mg (maximum 1 mg/min) of a 1 mg/ml preparation
   d. Pharmacologic actions
      (1) Decreased heart rate
      (2) Decreased stroke volume
      (3) Increased left ventricular end diastolic pressure

7. **Dobutamine**
   a. Indications
      (1) Depressed myocardial contractility
   b. Route of administration
      (1) IV drip
   c. Dosage—2.5 to 10 micrograms/kg/min
   d. Pharmacologic actions

(1) Increased cardiac output
(2) Enhanced atrioventricular conduction

8. **Isoproterenol**
   a. Indications
      (1) Bradycardia
      (2) Heart block
      (3) Hypotension
   b. Route of administration
      (1) IV drip
   c. Dosage—1 mg in 500 ml of 5% dextrose (2 micrograms/ml)
   d. Pharmacologic actions
      (1) Increased heart rate
      (2) Increased force of contraction of the heart

9. **Dopamine**
   a. Indications
      (1) Hypotension
   b. Route of administration
      (1) IV drip
   c. Dosage—2 to 30 micrograms/kg/min
   d. Pharmacologic actions
      (1) Increased cardiac output
      (2) Increased blood pressure

10. **Sodium nitroprusside (Nipride)**
    a. Indications
       (1) Hypertension
    b. Route of administration
       (1) IV drip
    c. Dosage—50 mg added to 250 ml of dextrose in water
    d. Pharmacologic actions
       (1) Peripheral vasodilation, decreased blood pressure

11. **Calcium chloride**
    a. Indications
       (1) Hypocalcemia
       (2) Hyperkalemia
    b. Route of administration
       (1) IV (should not be mixed with other medications)
    c. Dosage—0.2 ml/kg
    d. Pharmacologic actions
       (1) Increased force of contraction of the heart

**NOTE: Sodium bicarbonate is no longer recommended for use during CPR. It has been found to cause adverse effects, which include a shift of the oxyhemoglobin curve to the left (decreased release of oxygen by the hemoglobin), depression of cerebral and myocardial function, and the deactivation of catecholamines (isoproterenol, epinephrine) used during the resuscitative effort.

VI. DEFIBRILLATION AND CARDIOVERSION

A. **Defibrillation**
1. This is a nonsynchronized current of electricity delivered to the heart during ventricular fibrillation.
2. It is accomplished by the use of paddles placed on specific areas of the chest. After conducting gel is applied to the paddles, one paddle is placed below the clavicle and to the right of the upper part of the sternum. The other paddle is placed on the midaxillary line just to the left of the left nipple.
3. The initial electrical current delivered should be **200 joule (watt per second) for adults** and 2 joule/kg in infants and children. If this level is not effective in restoring normal ventricular activity, it may be increased to no more than 360 joule in adults or 4 joule/kg in infants and children.
4. This high charge of electricity delivered to the myocardium is intended to reverse life-threatening ventricular arrhythmias by causing complete depolarization of the cardiac muscle, thereby disrupting the electrical circuits in the heart that are causing the ventricular fibrillation.
5. Lidocaine and epinephrine should be administered because they improve the success of defibrillation.
6. It is essential that proper levels of electric current be used to help prevent myocardial damage and cardiac arrhythmias.

B. **Cardioversion**
1. This is a synchronized current of electricity delivered to the heart during ventricular depolarization (QRS complex).
2. Cardioversion is used to terminate the following arrhythmias:
   a. Atrial flutter
   b. Atrial fibrillation
   c. Ventricular tachycardia
   d. Paroxysmal supraventricular tachycardia
   e. Ventricular fibrillation (defibrillation usually indicated)
3. Cardioversion delivers a lower energy level than does defibrillation. The normal level for cardioversion is a charge between 25 and 100 joule to restore normal cardiac rhythm in adults and 0.2 to 1 joule/kg in infants and children.
4. A respiratory care practitioner's duties when assisting in this procedure should include the following:
   a. Monitor heart rate and respiratory rate
   b. Monitor oxygen saturation

   c. Have oxygen delivery device readily available
   d. Have manual resuscitator and intubation equipment readily available

NOTE: See Chapter 9 for further information on the EKG and identification of specific arrhythmias.

VII. TRANSPORTING THE CRITICALLY ILL PATIENT

A. Patients may be transported by either land or air.
B. Important points concerning the transport of patients by land or air:
1. Unstable patients must be transported with great care to avoid worsening of their condition.
2. The practitioner should hold the E-T tube with one hand while "bagging" with the other. This will better stabilize the tube and help avoid inadvertent extubation.
3. Sudden changes in speed or direction may cause a drop in the patient's blood pressure.
4. Special attention must be paid to monitoring lines that could become dislodged in transport.
5. The ventilators used should incorporate demand valves in their operation because this conserves gas.
6. Patients should be sedated adequately to help prevent anxiety and provide a safer transport.
**7. During transport in an unpressurized aircraft, rapid increases in altitude will result in decreased atmospheric pressure and PO_2. This may be managed by increasing the oxygen concentrations delivered.
8. Higher altitudes (lower atmospheric pressure) may increase the size of an untreated pneumothorax, as well as increase E-T tube cuff pressure, affecting capillary perfusion to the trachea.
9. Lightweight equipment (such as transport ventilators) is necessary for air transportation.
10. Patient monitoring is more difficult in aircraft, especially helicopters.
11. Heated humidity/aerosol for ventilators or masks during transport is not necessary for such short-term use.
C. Respiratory care equipment needed during transport:
   a. Oxygen system (tanks or liquid)
   b. Portable suction machine and catheters
   c. Portable ventilator

d. Portable EKG unit
e. Arterial pressure monitor
f. Pulse oximeter
g. Intubation equipment
h. Manual resuscitator

REFERENCES

1. Barnes T. *Respiratory Care Practice*. Chicago: Year Book Medical Publishers; 1988.
2. Eubanks D, Bone R. *Comprehensive Respiratory Care*. 2nd ed. St. Louis: CV Mosby; 1990.
3. Levitzky M. *Introduction to Respiratory Care*. Philadelphia: WB Saunders; 1990.
4. McPherson SP. *Respiratory Therapy Equipment*. 4th ed. St. Louis: CV Mosby; 1990.
5. O'Toole M, ed. *Miller-Keane Encyclopedia and Dictionary of Medicine, Nursing, and Allied Health*. 5th ed. Philadelphia: WB Saunders; 1992.
6. Scanlan C, Spearman C. *Egan's Fundamentals of Respiratory Care*. 5th ed. St. Louis: CV Mosby; 1990.

PRETEST ANSWERS

1. E

2. D

3. C

4. C

5. A

6. A

Intermittent Positive Pressure Breathing Therapy

PRETEST QUESTIONS

1. Which of the following will increase the delivered tidal volume (VT) to a patient having an intermittent positive pressure breathing (IPPB) treatment with the Bird Mark 7?

  I. Increasing flow
  II. Increasing inspiratory pressure
 III. Decreasing sensitivity
 IV. Decreasing flow

A. I and II only
B. I and III only
C. II and IV only
D. I, II, and III only
E. II, III, and IV only

2. During an IPPB treatment, the patient suddenly complains of chest pain and becomes short of breath. Upon assessing the patient, you auscultate decreased breath sounds on the left. These findings are consistent with which of the following?

A. Atelectasis
B. Left-sided pneumothorax
C. Pulmonary embolism
D. Pleural effusion
E. Right-sided pneumothorax

3. While administering IPPB, the patient complains of feeling lightheaded and dizzy. What should the respiratory therapist do to correct this?

A. Instruct the patient to pause longer between breaths.
B. Instruct the patient to take deeper breaths.
C. Increase the inspiratory pressure.
D. Decrease the inspiratory flow.
E. Decrease the sensitivity.

4. While administering IPPB, the patient begins coughing up large amounts of blood. The respiratory therapist should:

A. Continue the treatment and notify the physician that a chest x-ray study is needed.
B. Decrease the inspiratory pressure.
C. Stop the treatment briefly and resume when the patient is feeling better.
D. Continue the treatment but observe closely.
E. Stop the treatment and notify the physician.

5. Which of the following are hazards of IPPB therapy?

  I. Excessive ventilation
  II. Increased cardiac output
 III. Decreased intracranial pressure

A. I only
B. II only
C. I and III only
D. II and III only
E. I, II, and III

6. You have received an order to deliver IPPB to a patient with head trauma. What modifications in therapy might benefit this patient?

  I. Using a higher flowrate
  II. Using lower peak pressures
 III. Setting the sensitivity to -5 cm of water

A. I only
B. II only
C. I and II only
D. II and III only
E. I, II, and III

CHAPTER **7**

Intermittent Positive Pressure Breathing Therapy

I. INTRODUCTION TO IPPB THERAPY

A. IPPB is defined as a short-term (10 to 15 minutes) breathing treatment in which above atmospheric pressures are delivered to the patient's lung via a pressure-cycled ventilator.
B. Effective IPPB is dependent on four factors:
1. A respiratory care practitioner who has been well trained and exhibits a knowledge of the equipment, medications delivered, reasons for therapy, side effects of therapy, and goals of therapy
2. A relaxed, informed, and cooperative patient
3. A pressure-limited IPPB machine with a means of measuring V_T
4. Proper practitioner instruction on breathing patterns and cough techniques

II. PHYSIOLOGIC EFFECTS OF IPPB

A. **Increased mean airway pressure**
1. During normal spontaneous inspiration, airway pressure drops below atmospheric pressure (-2 cm of water), thereby setting up a pressure gradient between the atmosphere (at nose and mouth) and the airways. Air flows into the airways, gradually building back up to atmospheric pressure. Air flow stops and passive exhalation occurs because of the natural recoil properties of lung tissue. The lung is never subjected to significant positive pressure.
2. During an IPPB machine breath, positive pressure is applied to the airways to improve the ventilation status of the lung. This is what is meant by **increased mean airway pressure.** It

is the average (mean) pressure in the airways during one breathing cycle.
B. **Increased V_T**
1. IPPB should deliver V_Ts of 12 to 15 ml/kg of ideal body weight.
2. Delivered V_T is dependent upon the patient's lung status (compliance, airway resistance, and so on).
   a. Decreased compliance $\rightarrow$ decreased delivered V_T
   b. Increased compliance $\rightarrow$ increased delivered V_T
   c. Decreased airway resistance $\rightarrow$ increased delivered V_T
   d. Increased airway resistance $\rightarrow$ decreased delivered V_T
3. Delivered V_T may be measured with the use of a respirometer or gas collection bag on the exhalation port.
4. The inspiratory pressure control adjusts the delivered V_T.
   a. Increase pressure $\rightarrow$ increase delivered V_T
   b. Decrease pressure $\rightarrow$ decrease delivered V_T
C. **Decreased work of breathing**
1. A patient experiencing acute hypoventilation may avoid intubation and placement on mechanical ventilation by administration of frequent IPPB treatments (may be temporary).
2. The practitioner must encourage the patient to relax and allow the IPPB unit to do all the work in order for the patient's work of breathing to decrease.
3. IPPB may increase the patient's work of breathing if:
   a. The machine sensitivity is set too low, making it difficult for the patient to cycle the machine into inspiration. **The patient should pull no more than -2 cm of water pressure to initiate inspiration.**

b. The flowrate is inadequate to meet the patient's inspiratory flow demands. Increase the flowrate if inspiratory time is prolonged and you notice that the manometer needle is **rising slowly** to peak pressure.

c. The delivered VT is inadequate. Monitor VT and listen to basilar breath sounds to ensure that adequate volumes are being delivered.

d. Adequate time is not allowed for passive exhalation to occur. The machine **sensitivity** may be set **too high.**

D. **Alteration of the inspiratory and expiratory times**

1. By placing a patient with respiratory difficulties on IPPB, we should improve alveolar ventilation, thereby making the patient more comfortable, less "air hungry," and returning inspiration and expiration times and respiratory rate to normal.

2. Normal inspiration:expiration ratio for an adult is 1:2.

E. **Mechanical bronchodilation**

1. A patient with respiratory disease will experience an **increased resistance to air flow** as the diameter of the airways decreases **because of bronchospasm, secretions,** and so on.

2. When positive pressure is applied to constricted airways, dilation of these airways can occur to a greater degree than with spontaneous breathing.

NOTE: Some studies show that higher flowrates and pressures may cause a bronchoconstrictive reflex in the airways. This may be counteracted by the use of bronchodilators.

F. **Cerebral function**

1. A patient being administered IPPB may experience lightheadedness, dizziness, or faintness because of the reduced $PaCO_2$ levels and resultant alkalemia. **Decreased $PaCO_2$ levels result in cerebral vasoconstriction and thus decreased cerebral blood flow.**

2. In order to prevent reduced $PaCO_2$ levels, encourage the patient to breathe slowly and to pause between breaths.

3. A 50-ml flexible tube should be connected between the mouthpiece and manifold, which will allow for a slight rebreathing of carbon dioxide, preventing decreased PCO_2 levels.

III. INDICATIONS FOR IPPB THERAPY

A. Increased work of breathing
B. Hypoventilation
C. Inadequate cough
D. Increased airway resistance
E. Atelectasis—especially in sedated postoperative patients and patients recovering from chest or abdominal surgery who are reluctant to breathe deeply
F. Pulmonary edema
G. Aid in weaning from continuous mechanical ventilation
H. Placebo effect

IV. HAZARDS OF IPPB THERAPY

A. **Excessive ventilation**

1. Leads to decreased $PaCO_2$ levels, causing cerebral vasoconstriction resulting in dizziness (discussed earlier)

2. The patient should be instructed not to walk immediately following the treatment.

B. **Excessive oxygenation**

1. Patients with moderate to severe chronic obstructive pulmonary disease (COPD) breathe because of the "hypoxic drive" mechanism. If the IPPB treatment is given with oxygen, this may elevate the PaO_2 above the normal level (50 to 60 torr) knocking out the drive to breathe.

2. Hypoxic drive potential should be noted with the following arterial blood gas values:
pH   7.35 to 7.4 (compensated)
$PaCO_2$ >50 torr
PaO_2 <60 torr

C. **Decreased cardiac output**

1. Positive pressure applied to the airways will likewise be exerted on blood vessels returning blood to the heart. This restricts venous blood return to the heart, which, in turn, decreases cardiac output from the left ventricle.

2. Avoiding high inspiratory pressures and long inspiratory times will minimize this hazard.

3. If there is a decreased venous return during the therapy, the patient may experience **tachycardia** due to decreased left ventricular filling pressure, as well as a **drop in systemic blood pressure.**

D. **Increased intracranial pressure**

1. Blood flow from the head is restricted as positive pressure is exerted on the superior vena cava, returning blood to the heart. This keeps more blood in the cerebral vessels elevating intracranial pressure (ICP).

2. Normal ICP is <10 torr.

3. Using lower pressures and shorter inspiratory times (increased flows) and placing the patient

in the Fowler position or sitting on the edge of the bed will minimize this hazard.

4. This is not a common hazard except in patients with closed head injuries or central nervous system disease.

E. **Pneumothorax**
1. Most common in COPD patients with bullous disease or emphysema with bleb formation.
**2. A patient complaining of sudden chest pain, shortness of breath, or other breathing difficulties and tachycardia during IPPB must be suspected of having a pneumothorax.
3. Listen with stethoscope for bilateral breath sounds and observe for asymmetric chest movement.
**4. If pneumothorax is suspected, the treatment must be stopped immediately.

F. **Hemoptysis**
1. The coughing up of blood during or after IPPB may not be caused by IPPB itself but may be related to a strong cough accompanying the treatment.
2. The treatment must be stopped immediately, as air could be forced into a blood vessel, resulting in an air embolism.

G. **Gastric distention**
1. Caused by swallowing air during the treatment
2. May cause the patient to complain of nausea during or after the treatment

H. **Nosocomial infection**
1. Circuits should be changed every 24 hours.
2. Appropriate filters should be used on the IPPB unit to prevent machine contamination.
3. The practitioner should wash the hands before and after every treatment.

V. CONTRAINDICATIONS OF IPPB THERAPY

** A. **Untreated pneumothorax**
1. This is considered an **absolute contraindication.** IPPB should not be administered under any circumstances with this condition, as it will only worsen the problem.
2. IPPB is safe in patients with pneumothorax who have a chest tube in place.

** B. **Pulmonary hemorrhage**
1. This is considered an **absolute contraindication.**
2. If IPPB is administered in this situation, air may enter a blood vessel, resulting in an air embolism.

The following are **relative contraindications,** meaning under certain circumstances IPPB may be administered:

C. **Tuberculosis**
1. May lead to the spread of tuberculosis if patient is not receiving antituberculosis medications
2. IPPB is safe if patient is receiving antituberculosis drugs.

D. **Subcutaneous emphysema**
1. Indicates an air leak from the lung; further positive pressure would worsen the condition
2. Subcutaneous emphysema is not a danger in itself but may be an indication of greater severity such as a pneumothorax or pneumomediastinum.

E. **Hemoptysis**
1. This condition indicates an open pulmonary blood vessel, which could lead to an air embolism.
2. The origin of the bleeding must be determined.

F. **Closed head injury**
1. IPPB may increase ICP; therefore, it must be monitored closely in this type of patient.
2. To lessen the potential of increasing the ICP, use **higher flowrates (decreased inspiratory time) and lower peak pressures.

G. **Bullous disease
1. Patients with bullae or bleb formation, such as patients with COPD, are more prone to pneumothorax, as the weak areas of the lung may rupture.
2. The use of lower peak inspiratory pressures helps in alleviating this problem.
3. Rupturing of blebs or bullae may result from a strong coughing effort during the treatment. These patients must be monitored closely.

H. **Cardiac insufficiency**
1. Patients with decreased blood pressure, decreased cardiac output, or other such cardiac problems must be monitored closely for further cardiac embarrassment.
2. Further cardiac problems may result from the positive pressure, leading to decreased venous return, or from cardiac side effects from bronchodilator administration.

I. **COPD patient with air trapping**
1. IPPB may lead to an increase in air trapping in these patients, causing inadvertent positive end-expiratory pressure that may decrease cardiac output.
2. IPPB could lead to a further hyperinflated lung status, compromising adequate ventilation.

J. **Uncooperative patient**
1. The patient must be cooperative for treatment to be effective.
2. Alternate therapy should be considered.

VI. IPPB IN THE TREATMENT OF PULMONARY EDEMA

A. **IPPB aids in the treatment of pulmonary edema by:**
1. Decreasing venous return
2. Increasing tidal volume to improve ventilation and oxygenation, resulting in improved cardiac activity
3. Reducing the alveolar-capillary pressure gradient, thereby reducing the amount of fluid pouring into the airways from the capillaries
4. Delivering aerosolized ethanol (40% to 50%), which results in the dissipating of foamy edematous fluid

VII. PROPER ADMINISTRATION OF IPPB

A. Assemble all equipment and check machine for leaks.
B. Affirm physician order—if there is some question about the order, such as medication dosage, contact the physician for clarification.
C. Briefly review patient chart:
1. Last treatment given
2. Latest chest x-ray film interpretation
3. Latest arterial blood gas results
D. Wash hands.
E. Identify patient by wrist band and introduce yourself and explain the reasons for administering the treatment.
F. Connect the circuit to the IPPB unit and plug into gas source.
G. Place medications in nebulizer.
H. Auscultate breath sounds to locate problem areas (atelectasis, secretions, and so on).
I. Determine heart rate and respiratory rate.
J. Position patient upright, as this allows for better ventilation.
K. Place the mouthpiece in the patient's mouth and encourage the patient to keep the lips sealed tight and to breathe only through the mouth (use nose-clips if patient has difficulty).
L. Instruct the patient to "sip" on the mouthpiece and allow the machine to fill the lungs until it cycles off. **The patient then holds the breath for a count of three prior to exhalation** to better distribute medications and improve gas exchange and **pauses before the next breath.**
M. Set machine parameters.
**1. Inspiratory pressure (start lower than desired pressure and gradually increase as treatment

continues; increase flow likewise, as pressure is increased, to maintain same inspiratory time)
2. Flowrate
3. Nebulization
4. Sensitivity
N. Check vital signs halfway through the treatment. Allow a brief rest period.
NOTE: If the pulse rate increases more than 20 beats/min, stop treatment and notify the physician.
O. After 10 minutes or when the medications are completely nebulized, encourage the patient to cough.
P. Check vital signs again.
Q. Encourage the patient to cough periodically for the next 30 minutes to 2 hours, as the peak effect of the medications occurs then.
R. Wash hands.
S. Record vital signs, tolerance to treatment, cough effort, and sputum characteristics (color, amount, consistency) in the patient's chart.

VIII. CHARACTERISTICS OF SPECIFIC IPPB UNITS

A. **Bird Mark 7**

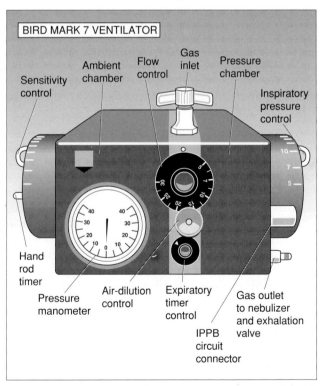

From Persing G. *Entry Level Respiratory Care Review.* Philadelphia: WB Saunders; 1992.

1. The Bird Mark 7 is a pneumatically powered and controlled ventilator. It is designed to operate with oxygen or air at a pressure of 50 psig. It is pressure-cycled and may be cycled on by the patient, by time, or manually.
2. **Gas flow through the Bird Mark 7**
   a. Gas enters the unit from the 50-psig wall outlet through a brass filter.
   b. The first control to which gas travels is the **flowrate control,** which is a simple needle valve.
   c. From the flowrate control, gas travels to the **ceramic switch,** which is positioned between the ambient chamber and the pressure chamber of the unit. Depending on the position of the ceramic switch, flow is either blocked or allowed through.
   d. In order for the patient to cycle the unit into inspiration, enough negative pressure must be created to separate a metal clutch plate from a magnet in the ambient chamber. This pulls the ceramic switch to the right, allowing gas flow to continue through the unit.
   e. As gas flows past the ceramic switch, it splits, with part of the flow supplying the expiratory drive line and nebulizer and the other part flowing into the ambient chamber through a Venturi that entrains ambient air. This increases flow and decreases the oxygen percentage.
   f. The "mixed" gas now travels through the Venturi gate and into the pressure chamber, where the patient circuit is connected, and flow continues on to the patient.
   g. Inspiration ends as gas in the patient's lungs builds up to a pressure that overcomes the magnetic force between another magnet and metal clutch plate located in the pressure chamber.
3. **Bird Mark 7 controls**
   a. **Flowrate control**
      (1) The scale simply consists of reference numbers and does not represent liters per minute.
      (2) Flows available are 0 to 80 L/min on air mix, 0 to 50 L/min on 100% oxygen
   **(3) Increase flow → decrease inspiration time
      Decrease flow → increase inspiration time
      (4) Flow wave patterns on Bird Mark 7:
         (a) Square wave (constant flow) on 100% oxygen
         (b) Tapered wave (decelerating flow) on air mix

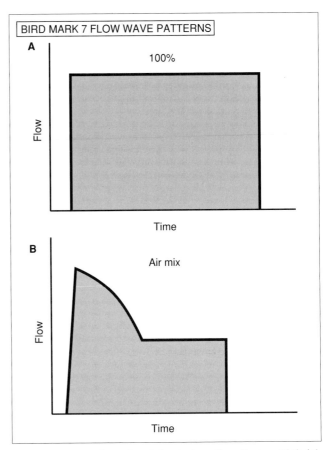

From Persing G. *Entry Level Respiratory Care Review.* Philadelphia: WB Saunders; 1992.

   b. **Air mix control**
      (1) When pulled out, allows flow into ambient chamber and then through a Venturi, resulting in air entrainment and an oxygen percentage of 40% to 90%
      (2) When pushed in, the flow is blocked to the ambient chamber, not allowing for air entrainment and therefore delivering 100% oxygen.
      (3) Air mix → higher flowrates
         100% oxygen → lower flowrates
   c. **Inspiratory pressure control**
      (1) Adjusts the position of the magnet in the pressure chamber closer to or farther away from the metal clutch plate
      (2) The closer the magnet is to the metal clutch plate, the higher the inspiratory pressure required to move the clutch plate (and *vice versa*)
      (3) Increase pressure → increase tidal volume
         Decrease pressure → decrease tidal volume
   d. **Sensitivity control**
      (1) Adjusts the position of the magnet in the

ambient chamber closer to or farther away from the metal clutch plate

(2) The closer the magnet is to the metal clutch plate, the more negative pressure is required by the patient to cycle the machine into inspiration (and *vice versa*).

(3) The position of the magnet should be such that the patient is required to generate no more than −2 cm of water pressure to initiate inspiration.

e. **Expiratory timing device**

(1) This is a needle valve that controls a leak from the expiratory timer cartridge and is used to automatically cycle the unit.

(2) Should always be turned off while administering IPPB or unit will self-cycle

f. **Hand timer rod**

(1) Located on the left side of the unit (ambient pressure side), it is used to manually cycle the unit off or on.

B. **Bennett PR-2 ventilator**

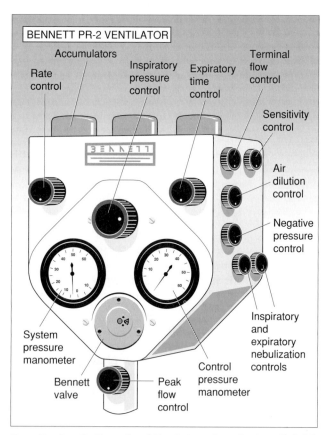

From Persing G. *Entry Level Respiratory Care Review.* Philadelphia: WB Saunders; 1992.

1. The PR-2 is a pneumatically powered, pressure-cycled ventilator that may be patient- or time-cycled and time-limited.

2. **Diluter regulator**

a. This is an adjustable reducing valve that con-trols the pressure generated in the patient circuit.

b. It is adjustable from 0 to 50 cm of water.

3. **Bennett valve**

a. This is the heart of the PR-2. Gas comes from the diluter regulator to this valve and rotates it to the opened position. Gas then travels on to the patient via the circuit. The valve also opens in response to patient's negative pressure.

b. As inspiratory pressure increases, the flow begins to decrease (due to decreased pressure gradient), and this rotates the Bennett valve to the closed position, stopping gas flow.

c. When inspiratory flow decreases to 1 to 4 L/min, the valve will rotate to the "off" position, stopping gas flow and ending inspiration.

4. **PR-2 controls**

a. **Inspiratory pressure control**

(1) Adjusts the peak inspiratory pressure

(2) Adjustable from approximately 0 to 50 cm of water

b. **Dilution control**

(1) When dilution control is pushed in, air entrainment is allowed and the oxygen delivered varies from 40% to 90%.

(2) When control is pulled out, no air entrainment is allowed, and 100% oxygen is delivered.

c. **Terminal flow control**

(1) Adds an additional 12 to 15 L/min of flow below the Bennett valve to help cycle the unit off in case leaks are present.

(2) This added flow goes to a Venturi, which decreases the oxygen percentage (especially important if patient is on 100% oxygen).

d. **Sensitivity control**

(1) Turning control counterclockwise increases the sensitivity, making it easier for the patient to cycle the unit into inspiration (and *vice versa*).

(2) When the sensitivity is turned off, it is "factory set" for the patient to initiate inspiration by generating −0.5 cm of water pressure.

e. **Peak flow control**

(1) In its full open position (all the way to the left), the flow is approximately 90 to 100 L/min with air dilution and 20 cm of water pressure.

(2) In the full closed position (all the way to the right), the flow is approximately 15 L/min.

f. **Nebulization control**
  (1) Separate controls for inspiratory or expiratory nebulization
  (2) Gas sent to the nebulizer is source gas (100% if plugged into oxygen outlet); therefore, percentage of oxygen increases when nebulizing medications.
g. **Rate control and expiratory time**
  (1) Used to automatically cycle the unit on
  (2) Turning rate control to the right sets the rate (adjustable from 0 to 50 breaths/min).
  (3) Expiratory time control lengthens expiratory time.
  (4) These controls should be turned off during the administration of IPPB, or the unit will self-cycle.

C. **Bennett AP-5**

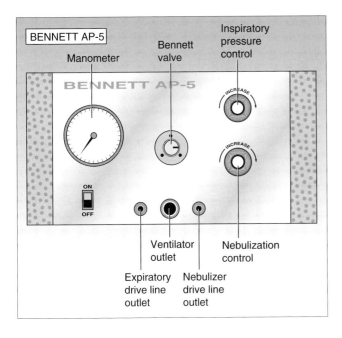

1. This IPPB unit is **electrically powered,** and inspiratory flow is powered by a compressor.
****2. Compressed gas is not necessary for the functioning of this IPPB machine; therefore, it is a popular model for use in the home setting.
3. It is pressure-limited and patient-cycled with a continuous flow for nebulization that comes from the compressor to the jet of the nebulizer.
4. Maximum peak pressure is approximately 30 cm of water.

IX. IMPORTANT FACTORS TO CONSIDER WHEN VENTILATING A PATIENT WITH A PRESSURE-LIMITED IPPB MACHINE

A. **Effects on delivered V_T**
  1. Increased airway resistance → decreased V_T
  2. Decreased airway resistance → increased V_T
  3. Increased lung compliance → increased V_T
  4. Decreased lung compliance → decreased V_T
  5. Increased inspiratory pressure → increased V_T
  6. Decreased inspiratory pressure → decreased V_T
  7. Increased flowrate → decreased V_T
  8. Decreased flowrate → increased V_T
B. **Effects on inspiratory time**
  1. Increased flowrate → decreased inspiratory time
  2. Decreased flowrate → increased inspiratory time
  3. Increased lung compliance → increased inspiratory time
  4. Decreased lung compliance → decreased inspiratory time
  5. Increased airway resistance → decreased inspiratory time
  6. Decreased airway resistance → increased inspiratory time

X. PROBLEMS ENCOUNTERED WHILE ADMINISTERING IPPB AND CORRECTIVE ACTIONS

A. The patient is having difficulty cycling the IPPB machine into the inspiratory phase. **Corrective actions:**
  1. Adjust the sensitivity so that the patient has to generate −0.5 to −2 cm of water pressure to start inspiration.
  2. Make sure machine is plugged into wall gas outlet.
  3. Ensure that machine tubing connections are all tight.
  4. Ensure that the patient has lips sealed tightly around the mouthpiece, or if a mask is used that there are no leaks around it.
  5. If the Bird Mark 7 is used, ensure that the flow control is turned on.
B. The patient complains of dizziness and tingling in the extremities during the treatment, with no appreciable increase in heart rate. **Corrective action:**
  1. Have the patient decrease the respiratory rate and pause longer between breaths.
C. Patient's heart rate increases more than 20 beats/min during the treatment. **Corrective action:**

1. Stop treatment immediately and notify the physician. This is most likely the result of the nebulized bronchodilator stimulating the heart.

D. The patient cannot cycle the IPPB machine off.
   Corrective actions:
   1. Tighten all tubing connections.
   2. Ensure that there are no leaks around the mouthpiece or mask.
   3. Ensure that the endotracheal tube or tracheostomy tube cuff is inflated adequately.
   4. If using the Bennett PR-2, check to make sure that the Bennett valve is not stuck.
   5. If using the Bennett PR-2, turn on the terminal flow control to help compensate for leaks.
   6. Check the expiratory valve function.

E. As the patient inhales, there is no nebulization of the medication occurring. **Corrective actions:**
   1. Ensure that the capillary tube of the nebulizer is connected.
   2. If using the Bennett PR-2, ensure that the nebulization control is turned on.
   3. Ensure that the nebulizer drive line is connected.
   4. Ensure that there is medication in the nebulizer.
   5. Ensure that the nebulizer is positioned in an upright position.

F. During inspiration, the manometer needle stays in the negative area for the first half of the breath and then rises to the positive area during the last half.
   Corrective action:
   1. Increase the machine flowrate.

G. The IPPB machine repeatedly cycles on shortly after the patient has begun the expiratory phase.
   Corrective actions:
   1. Decrease the machine sensitivity.

2. If using the Bird Mark 7, ensure that the expiratory time for apnea control is turned off.
3. If using the Bennett PR-2, ensure that the rate control is turned off.

REFERENCES

1. Eubanks D, Bone R. *Comprehensive Respiratory Care.* 2nd ed. St. Louis: CV Mosby; 1990.
2. McPherson SP. *Respiratory Therapy Equipment.* 4th ed. St. Louis: CV Mosby; 1990.
3. Shapiro BA. *Clinical Application of Respiratory Care.* 4th ed. Chicago: Mosby-Year Book Publishers; 1990.
4. Scanlan C, Spearman C. *Egan's Fundamentals of Respiratory Care.* 5th ed. St. Louis: CV Mosby; 1990.

PRETEST ANSWERS

1. C
2. B
3. A
4. E
5. A
6. C

CHAPTER 8

Chest Physiotherapy/
Incentive Spirometry

PRETEST QUESTIONS

1. Postural drainage and percussion **is not** indicated in which of the following conditions?

A. Bronchiectasis
B. Cystic fibrosis
C. Pulmonary edema
D. Pneumonia
E. Acute atelectasis

2. Which of the following is not necessary for incentive spirometry to be effective?

A. Respiratory rate <12 breaths/min
B. Cooperative patient
C. Forced vital capacity (FVC) >15 ml/kg of ideal body weight
D. Inspiratory capacity of >12 ml/kg of ideal body weight
E. Motivated patient

3. You receive an order for postural drainage to be performed on a patient in order to mobilize secretions from the anterior segment of the right upper lobe.

How should the patient be positioned in order to drain most effectively?

A. Patient lying supine with pillows under the knees
B. Patient lying on right side in the Trendelenburg position
C. Patient lying on stomach in the Trendelenburg position
D. Patient lying on the left side, rotated back 25° with the bed flat
E. Patient sitting up, legs straight out, with pillow behind the back with hands resting on knees

4. Which statement is **false** regarding incentive spirometry?

A. The patient should be positioned upright.
B. The initial goal should be twice the patient's tidal volume.
C. The patient's inspiratory time should be 3 to 5 seconds long.
D. The patient should be instructed to hold the breath at peak inspiration for 2 to 3 seconds.
E. Hyperventilation is a fairly common side effect.

CHAPTER 8
Chest Physiotherapy/ Incentive Spirometry

I. CHEST PHYSIOTHERAPY

A. Chest physiotherapy (CPT) consists of a variety of therapies aimed at the mobilization of pulmonary secretions and promoting a greater use of the respiratory muscles, resulting in an increase in the distribution of ventilation. Therapies included in CPT are:
1. Postural drainage
2. Chest percussion
3. Chest vibration
4. Coughing techniques
5. Breathing exercises (see Chapter 15)

B. **Goals of CPT**
1. Prevent the accumulation of pulmonary secretions
2. Improve the mobilization of retained secretions
3. Improve the distribution of ventilation
4. Decrease airway resistance

C. **Indications for CPT**
1. Lung conditions resulting in an increased difficulty in mobilizing pulmonary secretions:
    a. Bronchiectasis
    b. Cystic fibrosis
    c. Pneumonia
    d. Lung abscess
2. Acute respiratory failure with the presence of retained pulmonary secretions
3. Acute atelectasis
4. Ventilation/perfusion abnormalities resulting from retained pulmonary secretions
5. Patients with chronic obstructive pulmonary disease (COPD) and inefficient breathing patterns
6. Preventive use for postoperative respiratory complications

D. **Postural drainage positions**

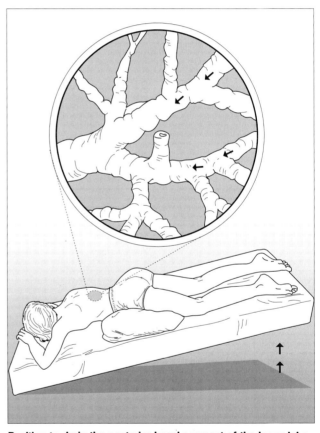

Position to drain the posterior basal segment of the lower lobe

From Persing G. *Entry Level Respiratory Care Review.* Philadelphia: WB Saunders; 1992.

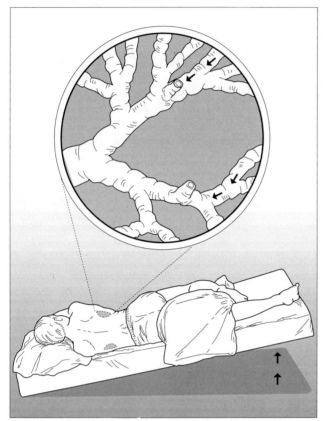

Position to drain the lateral basal segment of the lower lobe

From Persing G. *Entry Level Respiratory Care Review.* Philadelphia: WB Saunders; 1992.

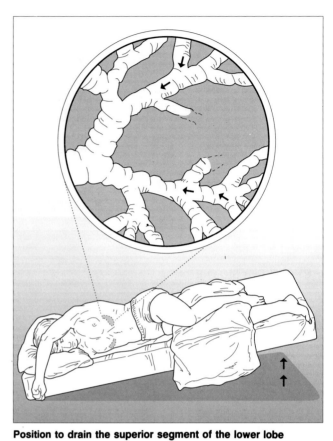

Position to drain the superior segment of the lower lobe

From Persing G. *Entry Level Respiratory Care Review.* Philadelphia: WB Saunders; 1992.

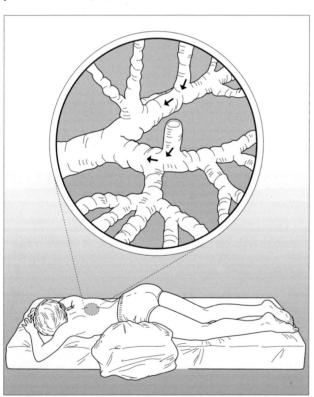

Position to drain the anterior basal segment of the lower lobe

From Persing G. *Entry Level Respiratory Care Review.* Philadelphia: WB Saunders; 1992.

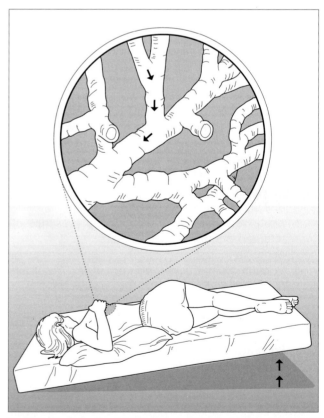

Position to drain the lateral and medial segments of the right middle lobe

From Persing G. *Entry Level Respiratory Care Review.* Philadelphia: WB Saunders; 1992.

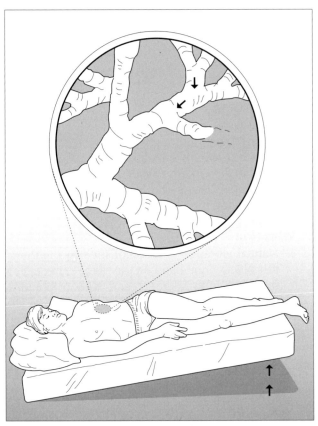

Position to drain the superior and inferior lingular segments of the left lung

From Persing G. *Entry Level Respiratory Care Review.* Philadelphia: WB Saunders; 1992.

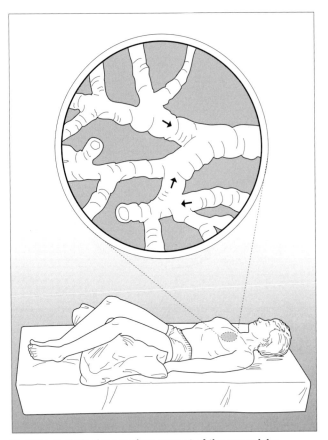

Position to drain the anterior segment of the upper lobe

From Persing G. *Entry Level Respiratory Care Review.* Philadelphia: WB Saunders; 1992.

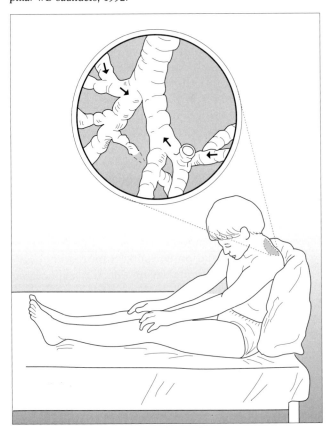

Position to drain the apical segment of the upper lobe

From Persing G. *Entry Level Respiratory Care Review.* Philadelphia: WB Saunders; 1992.

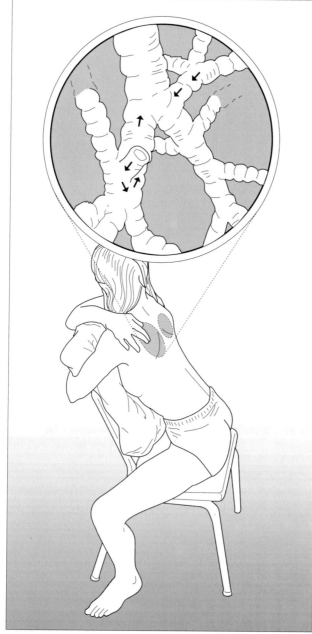

Position to drain the posterior segment of the upper lobe

From Persing G. *Entry Level Respiratory Care Review*. Philadelphia: WB Saunders; 1992.

E. **Percussion**
1. This is a means of improving the mobilization of pulmonary secretions by manually striking the chest wall with a cupped hand or placing a mechanical percussor on the chest wall. Both of these techniques are generally performed with the patient in postural drainage positions.
2. Mechanical percussors operate on either compressed air or electricity and are felt to be more effective than manual hand percussion.
3. Percussion should be performed over each specified area for 2 to 5 minutes.

4. Percussion should not be performed over the following areas:
   a. Spine
   b. Sternum
   c. Scapulae
   d. Clavicles
   e. Surgical sites
   f. Areas of trauma
   g. Bare skin (although some advocate manually percussing over bare skin, it has been shown that the energy wave produced by the air trapped under the hand is not significantly reduced by a light covering such as a hospital gown)

F. **Vibration**
1. Manual vibration is accomplished by the therapist placing one hand on top of the other over a specified lung segment and with a vibrating motion applying moderate pressure.
2. The patient should be instructed to take a deep breath, **with vibration applied during exhalation.
3. Mechanical vibrators may be used by placing the vibrator attachment over specified areas. The vibrator should not be applied to one area for more than 45 to 60 seconds at a time.
4. Vibration aids in the mobilization of retained pulmonary secretions.

G. **Complications of chest physiotherapy**
1. Hypoxemia
   a. Especially in individuals with COPD or in cardiac or obese patients
   b. Modification of drainage position will make the therapy more tolerable for these patients.
   c. May be minimized by the administration of a bronchodilator prior to CPT and the delivery of supplemental oxygen during the treatment
2. Rib fractures
   a. Caused from too vigorous percussion
   b. Most common in neonates and elderly patients
3. Increased airway resistance
   a. Patient should cough periodically throughout the treatment.
   b. Suction equipment should be readily available for patients having difficulty expectorating secretions.
4. Increased intracranial pressure
   a. Patients with head trauma should not be placed in the Trendelenburg (head down) position
   b. Increased intracranial pressure may result from prolonged coughing associated with CPT
5. Hemorrhage

6. Decreased cardiac output
   a. Often the result of positional hypotension
   b. Check heart rate periodically during the treatment.
7. Aspiration
   a. Caused by vomiting during the treatment
   b. CPT should be performed no sooner than 1 hour following a meal.

H. **Cough technique**
1. While sitting, the patient should be instructed to inhale deeply through the nose and hold the breath for 3 to 5 seconds.
2. The therapist should clasp the patient's arms across the abdomen and instruct him/her to produce two to three sharp coughs without taking a breath while the therapist presses the arms into the abdomen.
3. A pillow should be used to splint thoracic or abdominal incisions to decrease pain and improve the coughing effort.

II. INCENTIVE SPIROMETRY (SUSTAINED MAXIMAL INSPIRATORY THERAPY)

A. **Goals of incentive spirometry**
1. To treat atelectasis
2. To improve the cough mechanism
3. To maintain an airway during preoperative period
   a. Strengthens lung muscles prior to surgery
   b. Improves the mobilization of secretions
4. To prevent postoperative atelectasis

5. To provide early detection of lung disease
6. To provide psychologic support

B. **Hazards of incentive spirometry**
1. Hyperventilation
2. Pneumothorax (unlikely; there is a higher incidence in COPD patients)
3. Contaminated spirometer (except with disposables)
4. Increased intrapleural pressure and stimulation of the vagal reflex, causing bradycardia if the sustained maximal inspiratory pause is performed against a closed glottis (Valsalva maneuver)

C. **Guidelines for effective incentive spirometry**
1. Cooperative patient
2. Motivated patient
3. Patient's respiratory rate should be less than 25 breaths/min
4. Patient's forced vital capacity (FVC) should be greater than 15 ml/kg of body weight **(IPPB may be indicated if FVC is less than 15 ml/kg)**

D. **Important points concerning incentive spirometry**
1. The patient should be positioned upright in the Fowler or semi-Fowler position.
2. The initial inspiratory goal should be twice the patient's tidal volume.
3. The inspiratory time should be 5 to 15 seconds with a 2- to 3-second pause at the end of inspiration.
4. Incentive spirometry is an alternative to IPPB in treating atelectasis if the patient is able to achieve an FVC of greater than 15 ml/kg of body weight.

E. **Incentive spirometry devices**

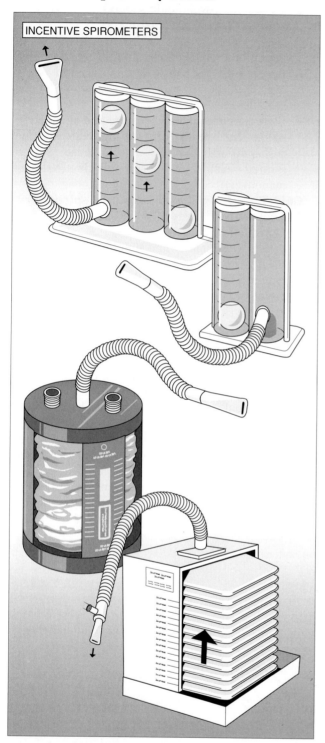

INCENTIVE SPIROMETERS

From Persing G. *Entry Level Respiratory Care Review*. Philadelphia: WB Saunders; 1992.

REFERENCES

1. Eubanks D, Bone R. *Comprehensive Respiratory Care*. 2nd ed. St. Louis: CV Mosby; 1990.
2. Shapiro BA. *Clinical Application of Respiratory Care*. 4th ed. St. Louis: CV Mosby; 1990.
3. Scanlan C, Spearman C. *Egan's Fundamentals of Respiratory Care*. 5th ed. St. Louis: CV Mosby; 1990.

PRETEST ANSWERS

1. C

2. A

3. A

4. C

Cardiac Monitoring

PRETEST QUESTIONS*

1. Which statement about the P wave on the electro-cardiogram (EKG) is **false**?

A. It represents atrial depolarization.
B. It is a positive wave on the graph.
C. Normal duration time is 0.06 to 0.10 second.
D. It represents ventricular repolarization.
E. It precedes the QRS complex.

2. Artifacts found on an EKG may be caused from which of the following?

I. Electric interference at the bedside
II. Poor electrode contact with the skin
III. Excessive movement of the patient

A. I only
B. II only
C. I and III only
D. II and III only
E. I, II, and III

3. In which of the following cardiac arrhythmias is the QRS complex abnormally shaped as well as wider than normal?

A. Sinus tachycardia
B. Premature ventricular contraction (PVC)
C. Atrial fibrillation
D. Premature atrial contraction (PAC)
E. Ventricular tachycardia

_____

*See answers at the end of the chapter.

4. A patient with a blood pressure of 110/50 and a pulse rate of 75 beats/min has a pulse pressure of which of the following?

A. 40 torr
B. 50 torr
C. 60 torr
D. 70 torr
E. 80 torr

5. A weak pulse is detected distal to the arterial catheter in a patient. This is indicative of which of the following?

A. Infection
B. Hemorrhage
C. Thrombosis
D. Tachycardia
E. Increased cardiac output

6. Which of the following conditions results in a decreased central venous pressure (CVP) reading?

I. Hypovolemia
II. Vasoconstriction
III. Air bubbles in the CVP line

A. I only
B. II only
C. I and II only
D. I and III only
E. II and III only

Cardiac Monitoring

I. ELECTROCARDIOGRAPHY

A. **Electrical conduction of the heart**
1. The sinoatrial node (SA node) is the pacemaker of the heart. It usually initiates about 75 impulses/min.
2. Once an impulse has been initiated by the SA node, the impulse travels down to the atrioventricular node (AV node).
3. From the AV node, the impulse travels down to the bundle of His, located in the interventricular septum.
4. The bundle of His divides into the right and left bundle branches, which deliver the impulses to the right and left sides of the heart.
5. The bundle branches divide even further into the Purkinje fibers, which send the impulse to individual muscle fibers of the ventricles, causing ventricular contraction.
6. Once the SA node sends an impulse, the conduction system depolarizes, sending the impulse through the conduction system to heart muscle, which depolarizes and contracts. After contraction, repolarization occurs; this is the heart in a resting state or **diastole. Systole** is the term used when the heart is contracting.

B. Through the use of various numbers of electrodes (leads) placed on the patient's body, the electrical activity of the heart can be monitored. The device to which the electrodes are attached is the **electrocardiograph.** The electrical activity of the heart recorded on graph paper is called the **electrocardiogram (EKG).**

C. **The standard 12-lead EKG** consists of three lead systems.
1. Standard limb leads (three leads)
   a. The leads are placed on the right arm, left arm, and left leg.
   b. Limb lead I measures the electrical potential between the right arm (−) and the left arm (+).
   c. Limb lead II measures the electrical poten-

tial between the right arm (−) and the left leg (+).
   d. Limb lead III measures the electrical potential between the left arm (−) and the left leg (+).
   e. A ground is placed on the right leg.
2. Augmented leads (three leads)
NOTE: The same leads are used for both the standard and augmented leads.
(+) indicates positive pole; (−) indicates negative pole
   a. Lead aVR—right arm (+); left arm and left leg taken together are zero
   b. Lead aVL—left arm (+); right arm and left leg taken together are zero
   c. Lead aVF—left leg (+); right arm and left arm taken together are zero
3. Precordial (chest) leads (six leads)
   a. Lead 1 (V_1)—positioned at the **fourth** intercostal space at the **right** border of the sternum
   b. Lead 2 (V_2)—positioned at the **fourth** intercostal space at the **left** border of the sternum
   c. Lead 3 (V_3)—positioned in a straight line between lead 2 and lead 4
   d. Lead 4 (V_4)—positioned at the midclavicular line and at the **fifth** intercostal space
   e. Lead 5 (V_5)—positioned at the anterior axillary line level with lead 4 horizontally
   f. Lead 6 (V_6)—positioned at the midaxillary line level with leads 4 and 5 horizontally

See diagram on next page.

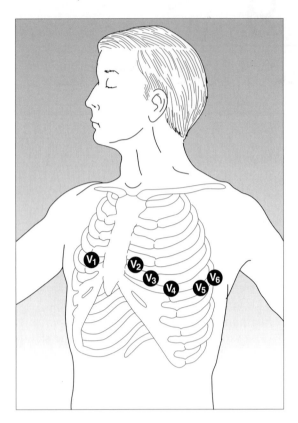

NOTE: The 12-lead EKG is not normally used for long-term EKG monitoring like that seen in the intensive care unit or the cardiac care unit.

D. **Long-term EKG monitoring**
  1. Lead placements (three leads)
    a. The first electrode is placed on the upper right side of the chest (−).
    b. The second electrode is placed on the lower left side of the chest (+).
    c. The third electrode is used as a ground and may be attached to any location that is convenient.
  2. In order to obtain a clear EKG reading, there must be good skin contact with the electrode. An electrode gel is used to improve conduction. Hair should be shaved from the chest if an electrode is to be attached in that area.

E. EKG graph paper

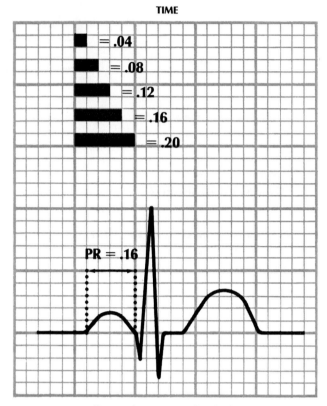

From Davis D. *Differential Diagnosis of Arrhythmias.* Philadelphia: WB Saunders; 1992.

  1. The EKG paper is made up of very small squares that represent 0.04 second horizontally (time) and 0.5 mV (millivolts) vertically (voltage).
  2. In order to make counting time easier, there is a darkened line at every fifth small square. In other words, from one darkened line to the next is 0.20 second (0.04 × 5).
  3. Most EKG paper will have short vertical lines at the top to designate 3-second intervals, making it easier to calculate the heart rate.

F. **Normal EKG pattern**

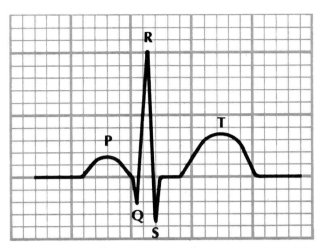

From Davis D. *Differential Diagnosis of Arrhythmias*. Philadelphia: WB Saunders; 1992.

1. The EKG strip shows a baseline, along with positive and negative deflections.
2. One cardiac cycle in made up of a series of waves represented by the letters P, Q, R, S, and T.
   a. P wave
      (1) positive wave
   **(2) Represents atrial depolarization
      (3) Duration time: 0.06 to 0.10 second
   b. Q wave
      (1) Negative wave that follows the P wave
      (2) May be lacking even in healthy individuals
   c. R wave—positive wave that follows the Q wave
   d. S wave—Negative wave that follows the R wave
   **e. QRS complex
      **(1) Represents ventricular depolarization

NOTE: Atrial repolarization occurs during the QRS and therefore is not seen on the EKG.
      (2) Duration time: 0.06 to 0.12 second
      (3) **Widened QRS seen in right bundle branch block**

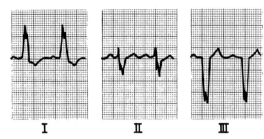

EKG tracing showing the widened QRS complex

From Levitsky MG, Cairo JN, Hall SM. *Introduction to Respiratory Care*. Philadelphia: WB Saunders; 1990.

   f. T wave
      (1) Positive wave
      (2) Represents ventricular repolarization
      (3) Inverted (negative wave) T waves indicate that coronary artery disease is present.
   g. P-R interval
      (1) Measured from the beginning of the P wave to the beginning of the Q wave
      (2) It represents the time it takes for the impulse to travel from the SA node through the AV node.
      (3) Duration time: 0.12 to 0.20 second
      (4) May be prolonged in first- and second-degree heart block

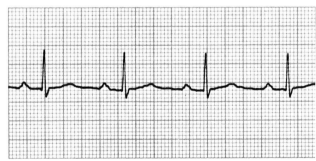

EKG tracing showing a prolonged P-R interval

From Davis D. *Differential Diagnosis of Arrhythmias*. Philadelphia: WB Saunders; 1992.

   h. S-T segment
      (1) Measured from the end of the S wave to the beginning of the T wave
      (2) This measures the time that is required for ventricular repolarization to begin.
      (3) The S-T segment may be elevated above the baseline or depressed below the baseline. This is an indication of **cardiac ischemia,** which is a deceased

amount of oxygenated blood reaching the left ventricle because of narrowed coronary arteries. If the blood supply is not restored, ventricular muscle may die and this is called **infarction.** ****Therefore, S-T segment elevation or depression is a sign of coronary artery disease.**

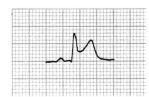

EKG tracing showing S-T segment elevation

From Davis D. *Differential Diagnosis of Arrhythmias*. Philadelphia: WB Saunders; 1992.

NOTE: Blood supply to the heart is supplied by two main arteries, **the right and left coronary arteries, which originate from the aorta. The right coronary artery extends down to feed the right ventricle and then separates into several branches. The left coronary artery divides into two major branches, the **circumflex branch,** which feeds the upper lateral wall of the left atrium and left ventricle, and the **left anterior descending branch** (anterior interventricular artery), which feeds the anterior portion of the heart.

G. **Normal heart rhythm**

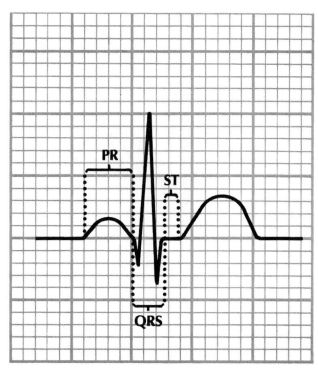

From Davis D. *Differential Diagnosis of Arrhythmias*. Philadelphia: WB Saunders; 1992.

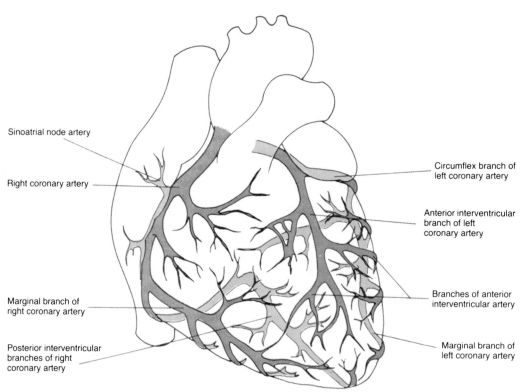

From O'Toole M, ed. *Miller-Keane Encyclopedia and Dictionary of Medicine, Nursing, and Allied Health*. 5th ed. Philadelphia: WB Saunders; 1992.

1. Atrial depolarization—represented on EKG as P wave
2. Cardiac impulse travels to the AV node, bundle of His, and the Purkinje fibers—represented on EKG as the P-R interval
3. Cardiac impulse reaches muscles in the ventricles, causing ventricular depolarization—represented on EKG as the QRS complex
4. Ventricular repolarization—represented on EKG as the S-T segment and T wave

H. **Basic steps to EKG interpretation**
   1. **Calculation of heart rate**
      a. As mentioned earlier in this chapter, most EKG paper will have 3-second intervals marked off at the top. **Count the number of R waves in a 6-second period and multiply by 10 to obtain the number of beats per minute.**
      *b. Normal rate: 60 to 100 beats/min
      * c. bradycardia: <60 beats/min
      *d. tachycardia: >100 beats/min
   2. **Determining regularity of the rhythm**
      a. Using calipers, measure the distance between a pair of R waves. Leave the calipers at that distance and measure the next pair of R waves and see if the distance is the same.
      b. Continue measuring the distance between successive pairs of R waves to see if they are constant. If they remain constant, the rhythm is termed regular.
   3. **Observation of P waves and the P-R interval**
      a. Make sure that there is a P wave before every QRS complex and that they are of the same shape.
      b. Using calipers, measure several P-R intervals to determine if they are consistent.
      c. As stated earlier in this chapter, the normal P-R interval is 0.12 to 0.20 second. If the P-R interval is longer than 0.20 second, first-degree heart block is present.
   4. **Determine the length of the QRS complex**
      a. Remember, the QRS complex represents the time it takes for ventricular depolarization to occur. With the normal QRS complex taking 0.06 to 0.12 second, any longer duration would indicate heart block.

NOTE: If all the preceding observations are within normal limits, the EKG is called <u>normal sinus rhythm</u>.

I. **Cardiac arrhythmias** (most often encountered by respiratory care practitioners)

1. Sinus bradycardia

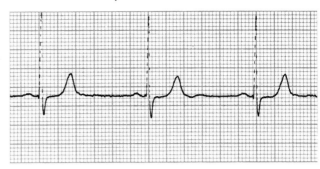

From Davis D. *Differential Diagnosis of Arrhythmias.* Philadelphia: WB Saunders; 1992.

   * a. Rate: less than 60 beats/min
   b. Rhythm: regular
   c. Wave pattern abnormalities: none
   d. Cause: increased vagal tone, hypothermia, increased intracranial pressure; may be normal in well-conditioned athletes
   e. Treatment: if accompanied by shortness of breath, hypotension, or abnormal beats, use atropine. A pacemaker may be indicated.

2. Sinus tachycardia

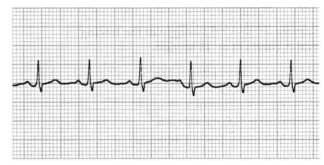

From Davis D. *Differential Diagnosis of Arrhythmias.* Philadelphia: WB Saunders; 1992.

   a. Rate: 100 to 160 beats/min
   b. Rhythm: regular
   c. Wave pattern abnormalities: none
   d. Cause: Hypoxemia, increased sympathetic nervous system stimulation (fear, anxiety, and so on), medication
   e. Treatment: stop underlying cause; digitalis, beta-blockers

3. Sinus arrhythmia

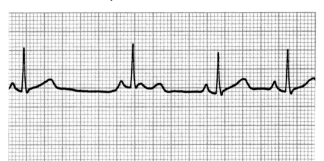

From Davis D. *Differential Diagnosis of Arrhythmias.* Philadelphia: WB Saunders; 1992.

    a. Rate: 60 to 100 beats/min
    b. Rhythm: irregular
    c. Wave pattern abnormalities: R to R cycles vary more than 0.16 seconds. **(Note how the distance between the R wave of the QRS complex varies and is inconsistent.)**
    d. Cause: none; it is normal in young, healthy individuals; heart rate may increase during inspiration and decrease during expiration
    e. Treatment: none necessary

4. Premature atrial contractions (PACs)

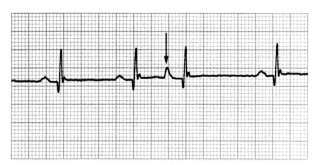

From Davis D. *Differential Diagnosis of Arrhythmias.* Philadelphia: WB Saunders; 1992.

    a. Rate: 60 to 100 beats/min; **if there are less than six PACs/min it is considered a minor arrhythmia, but more than six PACs/min is considered major.**
    b. Regular, except for PAC
    c. Wave pattern abnormalities: the premature P wave looks different from the sinus P wave; the PAC occurs sooner than the next beat would be expected
    d. Cause: atrial irritability due to organic heart disease, central nervous system disturbances, sympathomimetic drugs, tobacco, caffeine
    e. Treatment: if more than six PACs/min lidocaine may be used

5. PVCs

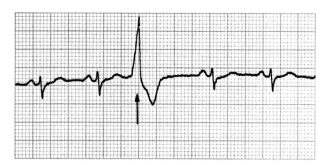

From Davis D. *Differential Diagnosis of Arrhythmias.* Philadelphia: WB Saunders; 1992.

    a. Rate: 60 to 100 beats/min; less than six PVCs/min is considered minor, with more than six PVCs/min considered major
    b. Rhythm: regular, except for PVCs

NOTE: When every other beat is a PVC, it is termed bigeminy, which is considered a dangerous arrhythmia.

    c. Wave pattern abnormalities: the shape of the QRS complex is abnormal and wider than 0.12 second
    d. Cause: ventricular irritability due to excessive digitalis, congestive heart failure, myocardial inflammation, coronary artery disease
    e. Treatment: intravenous (IV) lidocaine or other antiarrhythmia drugs such as procainamide or propranolol if more than six PVCs/min

6. Atrial fibrillation

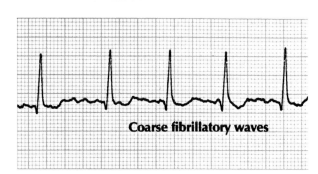

Coarse fibrillatory waves

From Davis D. *Differential Diagnosis of Arrhythmias.* Philadelphia: WB Saunders; 1992.

    a. Rate: variable; atrial rate greater than 350 beats/min
    b. Rhythm: irregular
    c. Wave pattern abnormalities: it is not possible to distinguish P waves and there is an uneven baseline; P-R interval is also indistinguishable
    d. Cause: arteriosclerotic heart disease, mitral stenosis, valvular heart disease

e. Treatment: cardioversion, propranolol, dig-italis

NOTE: This is considered a major arrhythmia whereby the atria fail to pump blood adequately to the ventricles.

7. Atrial flutter

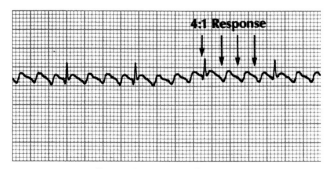

From Davis D. *Differential Diagnosis of Arrhythmias.* Philadelphia: WB Saunders; 1992.

    a. Rate: atrial—200 to 400 beats/min; ventricular—60 to 150 beats/min
    b. Rhythm: regular or irregular
    c. Wave pattern abnormalities: P waves have a characteristic sawtooth pattern and thus are often referred to as "F" waves.
    d. Cause: arteriosclerotic heart disease, myo-cardial infarction, rheumatic heart disease
    e. Treatment: cardioversion, carotid artery massage, procainamide, digitalis, tran-quilizers

NOTE: This arrhythmia results in blocking of atrial impulses in what is called a 2:1, 3:1, or 4:1 block. In a 2:1 block there are two atrial impulses for each ventricular beat and three or four impulses to each ventricular beat in a 3:1 or 4:1 block.

8. Ventricular tachycardia (lethal)

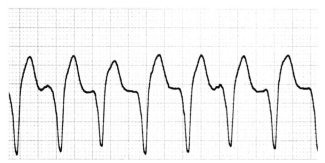

From Davis D. *Differential Diagnosis of Arrhythmias.* Philadelphia: WB Saunders; 1992.

    a. Rate: 140 to 200 beats/min
    b. Rhythm: regular
    c. Wave pattern abnormalities: P waves and P-R intervals are lacking or hidden in the QRS complex; each QRS interval is wider than normal and looks like a run of PVCs
    d. Cause: arteriosclerotic heart disease, cor-

onary heart disease, myocardial ische-mia, mitral valve prolapse
    **e. Treatment: lidocaine, defibrillation, car-diopulmonary resuscitation

9. Ventricular fibrillation (lethal)

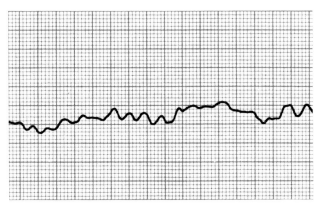

From Davis D. *Differential Diagnosis of Arrhythmias.* Philadelphia: WB Saunders; 1992.

    a. Rate: cannot be determined
    b. Rhythm: cannot be determined
    c. Wave pattern abnormalities: no distin-guishable waves
    d. Cause: acute myocardial infarction, digi-talis overdose
    **e. Treatment: defibrillation, cardiopulmo-nary resuscitation; if this arrhythmia is not reversed death will soon result because there is essentially no blood being pumped out of the heart

10. First-degree heart block

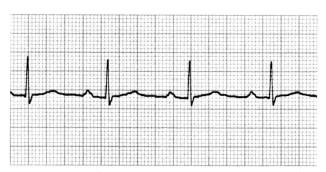

From Davis D. *Differential Diagnosis of Arrhythmias.* Philadelphia: WB Saunders; 1992.

    a. Rate: 60 to 100 beats/min
    b. Rhythm: regular
    c. Wave pattern abnormalities: P-R interval longer than 0.20 second
    d. Cause: excessive digitalis, ischemia of the AV node
    e. Treatment: atropine, isoproterenol

11. Second-degree heart block

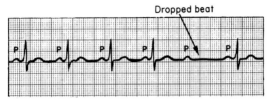

From Levitsky MG, Cairo JN, Hall SM: *Introduction to Respiratory Care*. Philadelphia: WB Saunders; 1990.

    a. Rate: 60 to 100 beats/min

    b. Rhythm: regular or irregular

    c. Wave pattern abnormalities: the QRS complex is normal but may be preceded by two to four P waves

    d. Cause: ischemia; may be a progression from first-degree block

    e. Treatment: isoproterenol, atropine, pacemaker

12. Third-degree heart block

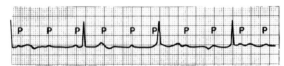

From Levitsky MG, Cairo JN, Hall SM. *Introduction to Respiratory Care*. Philadelphia: WB Saunders; 1990.

    a. Rate: atrial rate—normal; ventricular rate—less than 40 beats/min

    b. Rhythm: atrial and ventricular rhythms are regular but are independent of each other

    c. Wave pattern abnormalities: P-R interval not able to be determined; QRS complex may be normal or widened

    d. Cause: ischemia, AV node damage

    e. Treatment: pacemaker

II. HEMODYNAMIC MONITORING

A. Arterial catheter (arterial "line")

1. Systemic arterial blood pressure is most accurately measured by placing a catheter directly into a peripheral artery.

2. Peripheral arterial lines should be used in patients with unstable hemodynamic parameters. Along with the measurement of blood pressure, these lines provide a direct route for the frequent blood samples drawn from these patients.

3. The most common peripheral artery sites used are:

    **a. Radial—most common because of its easy access and good collateral circulation (with ulnar artery)

NOTE: An Allen's test to determine collateral circulation must be performed prior to puncture. (This procedure is described in Chapter 10.)

    b. Brachial

    c. Femoral

4. Using sterile technique, the 18- or 20-gauge catheter may be placed in the artery by either surgical cutdown or percutaneous puncture. The catheter is connected to a system that delivers a continuous flow of fluid from an IV bag to maintain patency of the system. The IV bag, which should contain normal saline and heparin, is pressurized by the use of a hand-bulb pressure pump.

5. The system is also equipped with stopcocks to allow for calibration with atmospheric pressure as well as for arterial sampling.

6. A **strain gauge pressure transducer (the most commonly used transducer) is connected to the system to provide a display of the pressure waveform as well as a digital reading of the arterial pressure in torr.

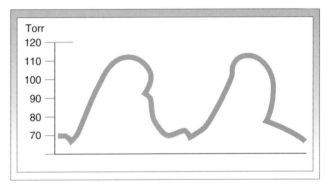

Normal arterial waveform

7. Pressures measured on the arterial waveform are

    a. **Systolic pressure**—equal to the peak of the waveform **(normally 90 to 140 torr).** Systole occurs as the heart contracts, forcing blood through the aorta (to the systemic circulation) and pulmonary arteries (to the lungs).

    b. **Diastolic pressure**—measured at the lowest point of the waveform **(normally 60 to 90 torr).** Diastole occurs between the contractions of the atria and ventricles (or while the heart is at rest) as these chambers begin refilling with blood.

    c. **Pulse pressure—the difference between the systolic and diastolic pressures **(normally about 40 torr)**

    d. Mean arterial pressure—represents the average pressure during the cardiac cycle **(normally 80 to 100 torr)**

8. **Complications of arterial catheters**
   a. Infection—may be reduced with removal of the catheter within 4 days
   b. Hemorrhage—make sure all connections in the system are tight
   c. Ischemia—note the color and temperature of the skin distal to the insertion site to determine distal perfusion
   d. Thrombosis and embolization—a weak pulse distal to the puncture site may indicate thrombosis; a continuous flush of saline and heparin through the system will help avoid this

NOTE: The catheter site and points distal to it should be assessed frequently by the respiratory care practitioner for signs of the preceding complications.

9. **Troubleshooting of problems in arterial lines**

NOTE: In many instances the respiratory care practitioner is responsible for the maintenance and troubleshooting of problems in arterial lines.

   a. "Damped" pressure tracing
   Causes:
   1. **Occlusion of the catheter tip by a clot**
      Correct by: aspirating the clot and flushing with heparinized saline
   2. **Catheter tip resting against the wall of the vessel**

Correct by: repositioning catheter while observing waveform
   3. **Clot in transducer or stopcock**
      Correct by: flushing system; if no improvement in the waveform tracing, change the stopcock and transducer
   4. **Air bubbles in the line**
      Correct by: disconnecting transducer and flushing out air bubbles
   b. Abnormally high or low pressure readings
   Causes:
   1. **Improper calibration**
      Correct by: recalibration of monitor and strain gauge
   2. **Improper transducer position**
      Correct by: ensuring the transducer is kept at the level of the patient's heart
   c. No pressure reading
   Causes:
   1. **Improper scale selection**
      Correct by: selecting appropriate scale
   2. **Transducer not open to catheter**
      Correct by: checking system and making sure the transducer is open to the catheter

B. **Use of the four-channel Swan-Ganz catheter**

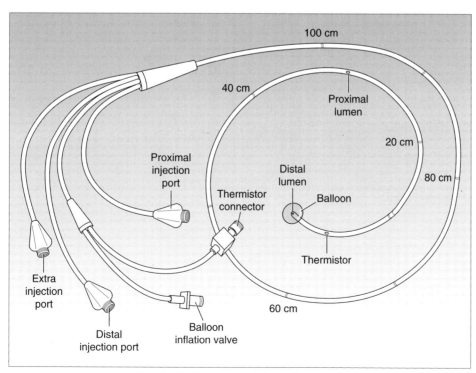

Quadruple (four)-channel Swan-Ganz catheter

1. The Swan-Ganz catheter is a balloon-tipped catheter made of polyvinyl chloride that is used to measure **CVP, pulmonary artery pressure (PAP),** and **pulmonary artery wedge pressure (PAWP),** sometimes referred to as pulmonary capillary wedge pressure.

2. The catheter also allows for the aspiration of blood from the pulmonary artery for **mixed venous blood gas sampling** as well as injection of fluids to determine cardiac output.

3. The distal channel (lumen) is used for the measurement of PAP as well as for obtaining mixed venous blood from the pulmonary artery.

4. The proximal channel (lumen) is used for the measurement of CVP or right atrial pressure as well as for the injection of fluids to determine cardiac output.

5. The balloon inflation channel controls the inflation and deflation of a small balloon located about 1 cm from the distal tip of the catheter and is used to measure PAWP.

6. The fourth channel is an extra port for the continuous infusion of fluid as may be necessary.

7. This catheter is also equipped with a computer connector in order to measure cardiac output using the thermodilution technique.

NOTE: Some catheters are equipped with only two channels, the distal channel and the balloon inflation channel.

8. **Insertion of the Swan-Ganz catheter:**

   a. The catheter is inserted through the brachial, femoral, subclavian, internal, or external jugular vein.

   b. Continuous monitoring of the catheter pressure and waveform is necessary as is EKG monitoring.

   c. Once the vein is entered, the catheter is advanced into the right atrium, at which time the balloon is inflated and the catheter flows through the right atrium and right ventricle and into the pulmonary artery where it "wedges" into a distal branch.

   d. Pressures and pressure waveform tracings are recorded as the catheter passes through the right side of the heart. Shown is a normal pressure waveform tracing of the right atrium, right ventricle, pulmonary artery, and PAWP.

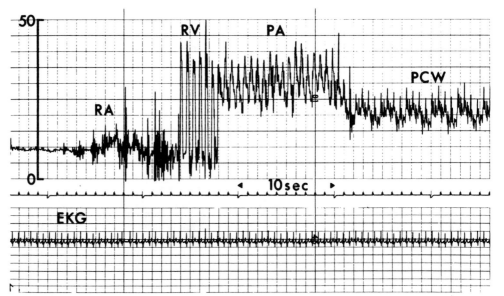

From Grossman W. Cardiac Catheterization and Angiography. 3rd ed. Philadelphia: Lea & Febiger; 1986. Used with permission.

e. Once the catheter "wedges" in a distal branch of the pulmonary artery, the PAWP may be measured, and the balloon should then be deflated. This allows for blood flow past the tip of the catheter. Since blood flow is stopped distal to the wedge position when the balloon is inflated, it should not be inflated any longer than **15 to 20 seconds or pulmonary infarction may occur.**

C. **Monitoring of CVP, PAP, and PAWP**

1. **CVP**

a. CVP may be monitored with a Swan-Ganz catheter as mentioned earlier or with a separate CVP catheter that is inserted through the subclavian, jugular, or brachial vein. The CVP catheter is connected to a water manometer that reflects the pressure in centimeters of water. Measuring the CVP with a Swan-Ganz catheter reflects the pressure in torr.

NOTE: When monitoring CVP with a water manometer, the manometer must be level with the heart while the patient is lying flat.

b. CVP is a measurement of right atrial pressure, which reflects systemic venous return and right ventricular preload. **The normal value is 5 to 15 cm of water or 4 to 10 torr.

**c. Conditions that increase CVP:

(1) Hypervolemia (volume overload)

(2) Pulmonary hypertension

(3) Right ventricular failure

(4) Pulmonary valve stenosis

(5) Tricuspid valve stenosis

(6) Pulmonary embolism

(7) Arterial vasodilation resulting in increased blood volume into the venous system

(8) Left-sided heart failure

(9) Improper transducer placement (transducer below the level of the right atrium)

(10) Positive pressure ventilator breath (measure CVP at end of expiration)

(11) Severe flail chest or pneumothorax—these conditions may compress the superior and inferior venae cavae, decreasing venous return while increasing CVP because of compression of the heart.

NOTE: To determine what effect positive end-expiratory pressure (PEEP) has on venous return and CVP, measure CVP while patient is on PEEP. To determine CVP without the effects of PEEP, some patients may be taken off PEEP for the measurement. It is important to remember though that patients with critical lung conditions who are receiving high levels of PEEP cannot tolerate being removed from PEEP; therefore, CVP must be measured while the patient remains on PEEP.

**d. Conditions that decrease CVP:

(1) Hypovolemia (inadequate circulating blood volume)

(2) Vasodilation (from decreased venous tone)

(3) Leaks or air bubbles in pressure line

(4) Improper transducer placement (transducer above the level of the right atrium)

2. **PAP**

a. PAP is a very important measurement in the care of critically ill patients with sepsis, adult respiratory distress syndrome, pulmonary edema, and myocardial infarction.

**b. It is especially important to monitor PAP and mixed venous blood ($P\bar{v}O_2$) values in patients who are on at least 10 cm of water of PEEP because high levels of PEEP may compromise the cardiac status of the patient by decreasing cardiac output and oxygen delivery to the tissues.

c. $P\bar{v}O_2$ sampling is achieved by obtaining blood from the pulmonary artery. **Normal $P\bar{v}O_2$ is 35 to 45 torr. $P\bar{v}O_2$ reflects tissue oxygenation, and should this value drop after the initiation of or increase in PEEP, it is an indication of a decrease in tissue oxygenation due to a drop in cardiac output resulting from the PEEP. PEEP should be decreased to maintain an adequate $P\bar{v}O_2$ (discussed further in Chapter 11).

d. **Normal systolic PAP is 20 to 30 torr

** **Normal diastolic PAP is 5 to 15 torr**

** **Normal mean PAP is 10 to 20 torr**

**e. Conditions that increase PAP:

(1) Pulmonary hypertension

(2) Mitral valve stenosis

(3) Left ventricular failure

** f. Conditions that decrease PAP:

(1) Decreased pulmonary vascular resistance (pulmonary vasodilation)

(2) Decreased blood volume

3. **PAWP**

a. When the balloon at the distal end of the catheter is inflated, it "wedges" in a branch of the pulmonary artery, blocking blood flow from the right side of the heart. The transducer measures the back pressure through the pulmonary circulation, which is a reflection of pressure in the **left atrium and the left ventricular end diastolic pressure.

**b. PAWP, therefore, is a measurement of left-sided heart pressures.

c. As stated previously, the balloon should not be inflated any longer than 15 to 20 seconds because blood flow obstructed for any longer may cause a pulmonary infarction.

**d. Normal PAWP value is 4 to 12 torr. PAWP of greater than 18 torr usually indicates impending pulmonary edema.

NOTE: PAWP is elevated with cardiogenic pulmonary edema and is normal with noncardiogenic pulmonary edema.

   **e. Conditions that increase PAWP:
   (1) Left ventricular failure
   (2) Mitral valve stenosis
   (3) Aortic valve stenosis
   (4) systemic hypertension
   ** f. Conditions that decrease PAWP:
   (1) Hypovolemia
   (2) Pulmonary embolus (PAWP may be normal)

D. **Complications from Swan-Ganz catheter insertion**
   1. Damage to tricuspid valve
   2. Damage to pulmonary valve
   3. Pulmonary infarction
   4. Pneumothorax
   5. Cardiac arrhythmias
   6. Air embolism
   7. Ruptured pulmonary artery

E. **Measurement of cardiac output**
   1. Cardiac output may be measured through the Swan-Ganz catheter using the **thermodilution technique.** A saline or dextrose solution at room temperature or 0°C is injected through the proximal port of the catheter. Heat loss occurs from the injection port to the distal tip of the catheter. The rate of blood flow determines the amount of heat loss and is measured on the cardiac output computer.
   2. Cardiac output may be calculated using the **Fick equation:

$$Q_T = \frac{V_{O_2}}{[CaO_2 - C\overline{V}O_2] \times 10}$$

Q_T = cardiac output (liters per minute)

V_{O_2} = oxygen consumption (milliliters per minute)

$[CaO_2 - C\overline{V}O_2]$ = arterial and mixed venous oxygen content difference of oxygen/100 ml of blood (also called vol %) (see section F further on)

NOTE: Grams of oxygen must be changed to milliliters of oxygen in order to express the cardiac output in liters per minute. This is accomplished by multiplying the oxygen content difference by the **factor 10.**

**NOTE: Normal output is 5 L/min.

EXAMPLE: Calculate a patient's cardiac output given the following information.

$$V_{O_2} = 250 \text{ ml/min}$$

$$CaO_2 - C\overline{V}O_2 = 5 \text{ vol \%}$$

$$Q_T = \frac{250 \text{ ml/min}}{[5] \times 10} = \textbf{5 L/min}$$

F. **Measurement of arterial and venous oxygen content**
   1. Oxygen content refers to the total amount of oxygen dissolved in the plasma and bound to hemoglobin in arterial or mixed venous blood.
   2. The difference between arterial and venous oxygen content is used to calculate cardiac output and cardiopulmonary shunting.
   3. Total oxygen content of arterial blood (CaO_2) is calculated by using the following formula:

$1.34 \times Hb \times SaO_2$ (represents milliliters of oxygen bound to hemoglobin)

$+ PaO_2 \times 0.003$ (represents milliliters of oxygen dissolved in plasma)

NOTE: 1.34 ml of oxygen is capable of binding with 1 g of hemoglobin, and 0.003 ml of oxygen is dissolved in the plasma for each torr of the PaO_2

EXAMPLE: Calculate the total arterial oxygen content given the following data:

Hb	15 g%
SaO_2	98%
PaO_2	86 torr

$1.34 \times 15 \times 0.98 = 19.7$ ml of oxygen (bound to hemoglobin)

$86 \times 0.003 = 0.26$ ml of oxygen (dissolved in the plasma)

$$CaO_2 = 19.7 \text{ ml} + 0.26 \text{ ml} = \textbf{19.96 ml}$$

   4. Total oxygen content of mixed venous blood ($P\overline{V}O_2$) is calculated by using the following formula:

$$(1.34 \times Hb \times S\overline{V}O_2) + (P\overline{V}O_2 \times 0.003)$$

EXAMPLE: Calculate the total venous oxygen content given the following data:

Hb   15 g%
S$\bar{v}O_2$ 75%
P$\bar{v}O_2$ 40 torr

$1.34 \times 15 \times 0.75 = 15$ ml of oxygen (bound to hemoglobin)

$40 \times 0.003 = 0.12$ ml of oxygen (dissolved in the plasma)

$C\bar{v}O_2 = 15$ ml $+ 0.12$ ml $= $ **15.12 ml**

G. **Intrapulmonary shunting**
  1. Intrapulmonary shunting is defined as the portion of the cardiac output that perfuses through the lungs without coming into contact with ventilated alveoli. This portion of the cardiac output, therefore, passes through the lungs and into the left side of the heart without being oxygenated.
  2. In the normal, healthy person, intrapulmonary shunting occurs. This results from blood flow through the bronchial, pleural, and thebesian veins. These veins return blood back to the left atrium, therefore bypassing the oxygenation process in the lungs (anatomic shunt). **Normally, intrapulmonary shunting is about 2% to 5% of the cardiac output and is primarily due to anatomic shunting.
  3. Physiologic shunting represents only a small portion of the normal shunt. Increased physiologic shunting results in a worsening cardiopulmonary status.
  4. Conditions that **increase physiologic shunting:
    a. Pneumonia
    b. Pneumothorax
    c. Pulmonary edema
    d. Atelectasis
  5. The amount of shunt may be determined using the clinical shunt formula:

$$\frac{Q_s}{Q_T} = \frac{(PAO_2 - PaO_2)\ (0.003)}{CaO_2 - C\bar{v}O_2 + (PAO_2 - PaO_2)\ (0.003)}$$

NOTE: This formula requires a 100% hemoglobin saturation of oxygenation in arterial blood.

Q_s = shunted blood
Q_T = total blood flow
0.003 = dissolved oxygen factor
PAO_2 = partial pressure of alveolar oxygen
PaO_2 = partial pressure of arterial oxygen

**6. If measurement of P$\bar{v}O_2$ is not available (via pulmonary artery catheter), the modified shunt equation may be used:

$$\frac{Q_s}{Q_T} = \frac{(PAO_2 - PaO_2)\ (0.003)}{(4.5\ vol\ \%) + (PAO_2 - PaO_2)\ (0.003)}$$

4.5 vol % represents a normal arterial/venous content difference ($CaO_2 - C\bar{v}O_2$)
Calculate a patient's percentage of shunt given the following data:

pH   7.37
$PaCO_2$ 45 torr
PaO_2 60 torr
FIO_2 0.40

Barometric pressure (P_B) 747 torr
$PAO_2 = (P_B - 47)\ (FIO_2) - (PaCO_2 \times 1.25)$
$(747 - 47)\ (0.4) - (45 \times 1.25)$
$280 - 56 = $ **224 torr**

$$\frac{Q_s}{Q_T} = \frac{(PAO_2 - PaO_2)\ (0.003)}{(4.5\ vol\ \%) + (PAO_2 - PaO_2)\ (0.003)}$$

$$= \frac{(224 - 60) \times 0.003}{4.5 + (224 - 85)\ (0.003)} = \frac{0.49}{4.5 + 0.49}$$

$$= \frac{0.49}{5} = 0.098$$

$$\frac{Q_s}{Q_T} = 0.098 \times 100 = \textbf{9.8\%}$$

This means that almost 10% of the patient's cardiac output is not being oxygenated in the lungs.
  7. **Interpreting calculated shunt values**
    a. $<10\%$ = normal
    b. 10% to 20% = abnormal intrapulmonary status, which is usually of no significance clinically
    c. 20% to 30% = significant intrapulmonary disease, which may be life-threatening and require cardiopulmonary support
    d. $>30\%$ = a serious life-threatening condition that requires aggressive cardiopulmonary support.

H. **Measuring cardiac index**
  1. Cardiac output varies according to the patient's body surface area (BSA). The cardiac index (CI) is a value that correlates the patient's cardiac output with the specific body surface area.

  2. $CI = \dfrac{cardiac\ output\ (L/min)}{body\ surface\ area\ (m^2)}$

3. Normal CI is 2.6 to 4.3 L/min/m²
4. Factors that **increase** cardiac index:
   a. Drugs that increase cardiac contractility (dopamine, epinephrine, digitalis)
   b. Hypervolemia
   c. Decreased vascular resistance
   d. Septic shock (early stages)
5. Factors that **decrease** cardiac index
   a. Drugs that decrease cardiac contractility (propanolol, metoprolol)
   b. Hypovolemia
   c. Congestive heart failure
   d. Increased vascular resistance
   e. Myocardial infarction
   f. Septic shock (late stages)
   g. Positive pressure ventilation
   h. PEEP, continuous positive airway pressure (CPAP)

I. **Measuring stroke volume**
   1. Stroke volume (SV) is the amount of blood ejected from the ventricle during ventricular contraction.

   $$2. \ SV = \frac{\text{cardiac output (ml/min)}}{\text{heart rate (beats/min)}}$$

   3. Normal stroke index is 50 to 80 ml/beat.

J. **Measuring systemic vascular resistance**
   1. Systemic vascular resistance (SVR) is a reflection of the resistance the left ventricle must overcome in order to eject its volume of blood. This is known as **afterload.**
   2. SVR is calculated using the following formula:

   $$SVR = \frac{\text{MSAP} - \text{CVP (torr)}}{Q_T \text{ (L/min)}}$$

   MSAP = mean systemic arterial pressure
   CVP = central venous pressure
   Q_T = cardiac output

NOTE: This resistance formula may be multiplied by 80 to convert to resistance units of dyne $\times$ sec $\times$ cm^{-5}.

   3. Normal SVR is 10 to 18 torr/L/min or 800 to 1440 dynes $\times$ sec $\times$ cm^{-5}
   4. Factors that **increase** SVR
      a. Vasoconstrictors (dopamine, epinephrine)
      b. Hypovolemia
      c. Hypocapnia
      d. Septic shock (late stages)
   5. Factors that **decrease** SVR
      a. Vasodilators (sodium nitroprusside, morphine, nitroglycerin)
      b. Hypercapnia
      c. Septic shock (early stages)

K. **Measuring pulmonary vascular resistance**
   1. Pulmonary vascular resistance (PVR) is a reflection of the afterload of the right ventricle.
   2. PVR is calculated using the following formula:

   $$PVR = \frac{\text{MPAP} - \text{PAWP (torr)}}{Q_T \text{ (L/min)}}$$

   MPAP = mean pulmonary artery pressure
   PAWP = pulmonary artery wedge pressure
   Q_T = cardiac output

NOTE: This resistance formula may be multiplied by 80 to convert to resistance units of dynes $\times$ sec $\times$ cm^{-5}.

   3. Normal PVR is 1.5 to 3 torr/L/min or 120 to 240 dynes $\times$ sec $\times$ cm^{-5}
   4. Factors that **increase** PVR
      a. Vasoconstrictors (dopamine, epinephrine)
      b. Hypercapnia
      c. Hypoxemia
      d. Acidemia
      e. Pulmonary embolism
      f. Pneumothorax
      g. Positive pressure ventilation
      h. PEEP, continuous positive airway pressure

L. **Measurement of oxygen consumption (VO_2)**
   1. Oxygen consumption is defined as the amount of oxygen (milliliters) extracted by the peripheral tissues in 1 minute. It is also a measurement of the oxygen uptake in the lung.
   2. VO_2 may be calculated using the following formula, which is based on the Fick equation:

   $$VO_2 = Q_T \left[C(a - v)O_2 \right] \times 10$$

   Q_T = cardiac output (L/min)
   $C(a - v)O_2$ = arterial/venous oxygen content difference
   10 = factor to convert $C(a - v)O_2$ to milliliters of oxygen per liter

EXAMPLE: Given the following data, calculate a patient's oxygen consumption (uptake).

   Q_T = 5 L/min
   CaO_2 = 20 vol %
   $C\overline{v}O_2$ = 14.5 vol %

   $VO_2 = 5 \times [20 - 14.5] \times 10$
   $VO_2 = 5 \times \quad 5.5 \quad \times 10$

   $VO_2 =$ **275 ml oxygen/min**

3. Normal oxygen consumption is **150 to 275 ml oxygen/min

4. Factors that **increase** V_{O_2}
   a. Hyperthermia
   b. Exercise
   c. Seizures
   d. Shivering
5. Factors that **decrease** V_{O_2}
   a. Hypothermia
   b. Cyanide poisoning
   c. Musculoskeletal relaxation

REFERENCES

1. Barnes T. *Respiratory Care Practice.* Chicago: Year Book Medical Publishers; 1988.
2. Davis D. *How to Quickly and Accurately Master ECG Interpretation.* Philadelphia: JB Lippincott; 1985.
3. Des Jardins T. *Cardiopulmonary Anatomy and Physiology.* Albany, NY: Delmar Publishers; 1988.
4. Levitzky M. *Introduction to Respiratory Care.* Philadelphia: WB Saunders; 1990.
5. Scanlan C, Spearman C. *Egan's Fundamentals of Respiratory Care.* 5th ed. St. Louis: CV Mosby; 1990.
6. Shapiro B. *Clinical Application of Respiratory Care.* 4th ed. St. Louis: Mosby-Yearbook; 1991.

PRETEST ANSWERS

1. D

2. E

3. B

4. C

5. C

6. D

CHAPTER **10**

Arterial Blood Gas Interpretation

PRETEST QUESTIONS*

1. Which of the following blood gas measurements determines how well a patient is ventilating?

A. pH
B. $PaCO_2$
C. PaO_2
D. HCO_3
E. $P\overline{v}O_2$

2. Which of the following blood gas measurements determines the level of tissue oxygenation?

A. pH
B. $PaCO_2$
C. PaO_2
D. HCO_3
E. $P\overline{v}O_2$

3. The following information has been obtained from a patient receiving 40% oxygen from an aerosol mask:

pH	7.42
$PaCO_2$	36 torr
HCO_3	26 mEq/L
PaO_2	122 torr

What is this patient's A-a gradient?
(barometric pressure = 747 torr)

A. 45 torr
B. 77 torr
C. 113 torr
D. 235 torr
E. 280 torr

4. Which of the following conditions shift the oxyhemoglobin dissociation curve to the right?

A. Hypercapnia
B. Hypothermia
C. Alkalosis
D. Hypocapnia
E. Decreased levels of 2,3-diphosphoglycerate (2,3-DPG)

5. A patient on a 2-L nasal cannula has the following arterial blood gas (ABG) results:

pH	7.51
$PaCO_2$	27 torr
HCO_3	23 mEq/L
PaO_2	62 torr

These blood gas measurements represent which of the following?

A. Uncompensated respiratory acidosis
B. Chronic respiratory alkalosis
C. Compensated metabolic alkalosis
D. Acute respiratory alkalosis
E. Partially compensated metabolic alkalosis

6. The respiratory therapist has received an order to obtain arterial blood from a patient for analysis, but upon performance of an Allen's test it is determined that collateral circulation is not present in the right wrist. At this time you would

A. Obtain blood from the right radial artery
B. Obtain blood from the right brachial artery
C. Wait for the physician to evaluate collateral circulation
D. Check collateral circulation in the left wrist
E. Obtain blood from the right femoral artery

---

*See answers at the end of the chapter.

Arterial Blood Gas Interpretation

I. ARTERIAL BLOOD GAS ANALYSIS

A. Blood gas analysis monitors the following physiologic parameters:
   1. Arterial oxygenation—PaO_2
   2. Alveolar ventilation—$PaCO_2$
   3. Acid-base status—pH
   4. Oxygen delivery to tissues—$P\bar{v}O_2$
B. Arterial samples are used because the values reflect the patient's total cardiopulmonary status.
C. Mixed venous blood, obtained from the pulmonary artery via a Swan-Ganz catheter, is used to determine oxygen delivery to the tissues (discussed in detail in Chapter 11).
D. Blood gas measurements are ordered to determine whether to change current therapy or maintain it.
E. Common sites to obtain arterial blood are the radial, brachial, femoral artery or the dorsal artery of the foot.
   1. The radial artery is the most common site because it has good collateral circulation and is easily accessible.
   2. A modified Allen's test is performed to determine collateral circulation.
      a. The patient is instructed to close hand tightly as practitioner occludes both the radial and ulnar arteries.
      b. The patient is instructed to open the hand as the practitioner releases the pressure on the ulnar artery while watching for hand color to return to normal.
      c. Color should be restored in 10 to 15 seconds. If not, the test is considered negative, meaning collateral circulation is not present. Blood **must not** be obtained from this wrist. Check the other wrist.

II. ARTERIAL OXYGENATION

A. **Partial pressure of arterial oxygen**
   1. The partial pressure of arterial oxygen (PaO_2) is the portion of oxygen that is dissolved in the plasma of the blood. It is what is left after the hemoglobin molecules have been saturated.
   2. For every **1 torr of PaO_2**, there is 0.003 ml of dissolved oxygen.
B. **Partial pressure of alveolar oxygen**
   1. The partial pressure of alveolar oxygen (PAO_2) is calculated by the following formula:

$$PAO_2 = [(PB - 47\ torr)(FIO_2)] - (PaCO_2 \times 1.25)$$

$$PAO_2 = (760 - 47\ torr)(0.21) - (40\ torr \times 1.25)$$

$$PAO_2 = (713 \times 0.21) - 50$$

$$PAO_2 = 150 - 50 = \textbf{100 torr}$$

2. This value is often compared with PaO_2 to determine P(A-a) gradient or the difference between alveolar oxygen tension and arterial oxygen tension (normal on room air is 4 to 12 torr**).

EXAMPLE: A patient breathing 50% oxygen through a Venturi mask has the following values:

pH	7.36
$PaCO_2$	45 torr
PaO_2	94 torr

What is this patient's A-a gradient? (PB = 747 torr)

$$PAO_2 = [(747 - 47)(0.5)] - 45 \times 1.25$$
$$350 \qquad - \quad 56 \ = \ 294$$

A-a gradient = $P_{A}O_2 - P_{a}O_2$

$$294 - 94 = 200 \text{ torr}$$

C. The majority of oxygen carried in the blood is bound to hemoglobin (see Chapter 1).

D. **Oxyhemoglobin dissociation curve**

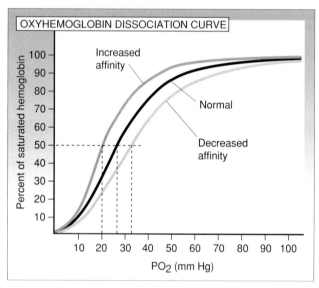

From Persing G. *Entry Level Respiratory Care Review.* Philadelphia: WB Saunders; 1992.

1. This curve plots the relationship between $P_{a}O_2$ and the arterial oxygenation saturation ($S_{a}O_2$) and the affinity that hemoglobin has for oxygen at various saturation levels.

2. This S-shaped curve indicates that at $P_{a}O_2$ levels of less than 60 torr, small increases in $P_{a}O_2$ result in fairly large increases in $S_{a}O_2$. As an example, 50% of the hemoglobin molecules would be carrying oxygen at a $P_{a}O_2$ of only 26 torr. As the $P_{a}O_2$ increases to 40 torr, the $S_{a}O_2$ increases substantially to about 75%. As the $P_{a}O_2$ continues to rise to 60 torr, the saturation increases to approximately 90%.

3. The flat portion of the curve indicates that at $P_{a}O_2$ levels greater than 60 torr, saturation rises slowly, with a $P_{a}O_2$ of 70 torr yielding an $S_{a}O_2$ of 93% and a $P_{a}O_2$ between 80 and 100 torr, resulting in $S_{a}O_2$ levels of 95% to 100%.

4. Various factors affect the affinity that hemoglobin has for oxygen. These factors shift the oxyhemoglobin dissociation curve to the right or to the left.

5. If the curve is **shifted to the right,** it indicates that **hemoglobin's affinity for oxygen has decreased** or that hemoglobin will release oxygen to the tissues more readily. **Factors that shift the curve to the right include:**

   a. Hypercapnia
   b. Acidosis
   c. Hyperthermia
   d. Increased levels of 2,3-DPG

6. If the curve is **shifted to the left,** it indicates that **hemoglobin's affinity for oxygen has increased** or that hemoglobin will not release oxygen to the tissues as readily. **Factors that shift the curve to the left include:**

   a. Hypocapnia
   b. Alkalosis
   c. Hypothermia
   d. Decreased levels of 2,3-DPG
   e. Carboxyhemoglobin

7. As oxygen diffuses from the alveoli to the blood (because of pressure gradient) it enters a red blood cell (RBC) where it combines with hemoglobin.

8. As oxygen combines with the hemoglobin, this enhances the release of carbon dioxide. This is called the **Haldane effect.**

9. As the RBC travels to the tissue, it releases the oxygen. This release of oxygen is due to the fact that elevated carbon dioxide levels, which are present around tissues, decrease hemoglobin's affinity for oxygen. This is known as the **Bohr effect.**

10. **Levels of hypoxemia**

60 to 70 torr	Mild hypoxemia
40 to 59 torr	Moderate hypoxemia
<40 torr	Severe hypoxemia

11. **Normal $P_{a}O_2$ levels**

Age	*$P_{a}O_2$ (torr)*
<60	80 to 100
60	80
65	75
70	70
75	65
80	60

NOTE: Subtract 1 torr from 80 torr for each year past 60 years to determine normal $P_{a}O_2$ by age.

12. **P-50**
   a. The P-50 represents the $P_{a}O_2$ when the hemoglobin is 50% saturated.
   b. Normal P-50 is 26.6 torr
   c. Used to describe hemoglobin's affinity to oxygen
      (1) Increased P-50 → decreased affinity
      (2) Decreased P-50 → increased affinity

13. **Arterial oxygen saturation**
   a. Arterial oxygen saturation ($S_{a}O_2$) refers to the quantity of oxygen being carried by the

hemoglobin compared with the maximum that may be carried.

    b. **Normal SaO_2 is 95% to 100%**

III. CARBON DIOXIDE TRANSPORT AND ALVEOLAR VENTILATION

A. Carbon dioxide makes up approximately 0.03% of inspired air.

B. Carbon dioxide is the by-product of cellular metabolism, and it is by this mechanism that it enters the blood.

C. After carbon dioxide enters the blood, it takes one of two routes:

    1. Five percent of the carbon dioxide dissolves in the plasma.

    2. The remaining 95% enters the RBC.

        a. Approximately 65% of the carbon dioxide entering the RBC is quickly converted to hydrogen and bicarbonate ions. (These ions are produced from carbonic acid, which is formed when water and carbon dioxide dissociate.)

        b. The remaining carbon dioxide entering the RBC combines with hemoglobin.

        c. Therefore, carbon dioxide is carried in the blood in three ways:

            (1) Dissolved in the plasma

            (2) Bound to hemoglobin

            (3) As bicarbonate (HCO_3)

D. **The adequacy of ventilation is determined by the $PaCO_2$ level.

    1. Normal $PaCO_2$ range is 35 to 45 torr

    2. **$PaCO_2$ < 35 torr** is termed **hypocapnia** and indicates excess carbon dioxide elimination or **hyperventilation.**

    3. **$PaCO_2$ > 45 torr** is termed **hypercapnia** and indicates that not enough carbon dioxide is being eliminated or **hypoventilation.**

** E. $PaCO_2$ increases when respiratory rate or tidal volume (minute volume) decreases or deadspace increases. $PaCO_2$ decreases when rate or tidal volume increases or deadspace decreases.

IV. ACID-BASE BALANCE (pH)

A. In simple terms, the pH level is determined by the amount of acid (carbonic acid; H_2Co_3) in the blood in relation to the amount of base (bicarbonate; HCO_3) in the blood

    1. The Henderson-Hasselbach equation states:

$$pH = pK + \log \frac{base}{acid}$$

$$pK = \text{dissociation constant} = 6.1$$

    2. Clinically we may state:

$$pH = pK + \log \frac{HCO_3}{PCO_2}$$

    3. The important ideas to remember from this equation are:

    a. **When bicarbonate increases and carbon dioxide remains unchanged, the **pH increases.**

    b. **When bicarbonate decreases and carbon dioxide remains unchanged, the **pH decreases.**

    ** c. **When carbon dioxide increases** and bicarbonate remains unchanged, the **pH decreases.**

    d. **When carbon dioxide decreases and bicarbonate remains unchanged, the **pH increases.**

B. The ratio of bicarbonate to carbonic acid is 20:1, which is a pH of 7.40.

C. The normal plasma pH range is **7.35 to 7.45.**

    1. A **pH < 7.35** is termed **acidemia.** It indicates a greater than normal hydrogen ion concentration. **Acidemia occurs as a result of:**

    ** a. Increased PCO_2 levels

    **b. Decreased bicarbonate levels

    2. A **pH > 7.45** is termed **alkalemia.** It indicates a less than normal hydrogen ion concentration. **Alkalemia occurs as a result of:**

    ** a. Decreased PCO_2 levels

    **b. Increased bicarbonate levels

D. **Respiratory versus metabolic components**

    1. When the initial pH change is the result of a PCO_2 change, this is a respiratory disturbance.

        a. An **increased PCO_2 (>45 torr) decreases the pH (<7.35).** This is termed **respiratory acidosis.**

The following values represent **respiratory acidosis,** and since the bicarbonate is still within normal limits, it is acute or uncompensated.

pH	7.25
$PaCO_2$	60 torr
HCO_3	25 mEq/L

(Normal HCO_3 level: 22 to 26 mEq/L)

        b. A **decreased PCO_2 (<35 torr) increases the pH (>7.45).** This is termed **respiratory alkalosis.**

The following values represent **respiratory alka-**

losis, and since the bicarbonate is still within normal limits, it is acute or uncompensated.

pH	7.53
$PaCO_2$	29 torr
HCO_3	23 mEq/L

2. When the initial pH change is the result of a bicarbonate change, this is a metabolic disturbance.

   a. A **decreased bicarbonate value (<22 mEq/L) decreases the pH (<7.35).** This is termed **metabolic acidosis.**

The following values represent **metabolic acidosis,** and since the $PaCO_2$ is within normal limits, it is acute or uncompensated.

pH	7.24
$PaCO_2$	38 torr
HCO_3	13 mEq/L

   b. An **increased bicarbonate value (>26 mEq/L) increases the pH (>7.45).** This is termed **metabolic alkalosis.**

The following values represent **metabolic alkalosis,** and since the $PaCO_2$ is within normal limits, it is acute or uncompensated.

pH	7.54
$PaCO_2$	41 torr
HCO_3	33 mEq/L

E. **pH compensation**
   1. The levels of bicarbonate and carbon dioxide will always change in order to keep the pH within the normal range. This is called **compensation.**
   2. If the $PaCO_2$ initially changes the pH, the bicarbonate will change accordingly to return the pH to normal.

(A) pH	7.27
$PaCO_2$	58 torr
HCO_3	31 mEq/L
(B) pH	7.37
$PaCO_2$	58 torr
HCO_3	35 mEq/L

The (A) example is a **partially compensated respiratory acidosis.** The elevated $PaCO_2$ caused the initial drop in pH. The bicarbonate is increasing to elevate the pH back to normal. Since the pH is approaching normal but is still low, this makes it **partially compensated.**

When the pH returns to normal (B), resulting from the continued increase in bicarbonate, this is called **chronic or compensated respiratory acidosis.**

(A) pH	7.53
$PaCO_2$	26 torr
HCO_3	16 mEq/L
(B) pH	7.43
$PaCO_2$	27 torr
HCO_3	12 mEq/L

The (A) example is a **partially compensated respiratory alkalosis.** The decreased $PaCO_2$ caused the initial increase in pH. The bicarbonate is decreasing to drop the pH back to normal. Since the pH is approaching normal but is still high, this makes it **partially compensated.**

When the pH returns to normal (B), resulting from the continuing decrease of bicarbonate, this is a **chronic or compensated respiratory alkalosis.**

3. If the bicarbonate initially changes the pH, the PCO_2 will change accordingly to return the pH to normal.

**(A) pH	7.21
$PaCO_2$	22 torr
HCO_3	12 mEq/L
(B) pH	7.36
$PaCO_2$	14 torr
HCO_3	13 mEq/L

The (A) example is a **partially compensated metabolic acidosis.** The decreased bicarbonate caused the initial drop in pH. The patient is hyperventilating (decreasing PCO_2 levels) to elevate the pH back to normal. Since the pH is approaching normal but is still low, it is **partially compensated.**

When the pH returns to normal (B), resulting from the continuing drop in PCO_2, it is a **compensated metabolic acidosis.**

(A) pH	7.50
$PaCO_2$	51 torr
HCO_3	31 mEq/L
(B) pH	7.44
$PaCO_2$	59 torr
HCO_3	31 mEq/L

The (A) example is a **partially compensated metabolic alkalosis.** The increased bicarbonate caused the initial increase in pH. The patient is hypoventilating (increasing PCO_2 levels) to drop the pH back to normal. Since the pH is approaching normal but is still high, it is **partially compensated.**

When the pH returns to normal (B), resulting from the continuing PCO_2 retention, it is a **compensated metabolic alkalosis.**

IMPORTANT NOTE: When interpreting compensated blood gas readings:

If the compensated pH is 7.35 to 7.4, the pH must be assumed to have been acidotic initially. Decide if the PCO_2 or bicarbonate caused the initial acidemia.

If the compensated pH is 7.4 to 7.45, the pH must be assumed to have been alkalotic initially. Decide if the PCO_2 or bicarbonate caused the initial alkalemia.

NOTE: Metabolic compensation takes several hours to occur, whereas respiratory compensation may occur in minutes.

F. **Mixed respiratory and metabolic component**
   1. When both the PCO_2 and the bicarbonate cause the pH to move in the same direction, it is called a mixed component.

pH	7.21
$PaCO_2$	55 torr
HCO_3	18 mEq/L

This is an example of **mixed respiratory and metabolic acidosis.** An elevated PCO_2 and decreased bicarbonate level both contribute to acidemia.

V. ABG INTERPRETATION

A. **ABG normal value chart summary**

pH	7.35–7.45
$PaCO_2$	35–45 torr
PaO_2	80–100 torr
HCO_3	22–26 mEq/L
B.E.	−2 to +2 (refers to the total base deficit or excess)

B. **Basic steps to ABG interpretation**
   1. Determine the acid-base status by observing the pH.
      a. Is the pH acidotic (<7.35)?
      b. Is the pH alkalotic (>7.45)?
   2. Determine if the pH change is the result of a PCO_2 change or a bicarbonate change.
   3. When this is determined, observe for signs of compensation. If the PCO_2 caused the initial pH

change, is the bicarbonate changing to return the pH back to normal?
   4. Determine oxygenation status by observing PO_2.
C. **ABG example problems**
   1.
pH	7.23
$PaCO_2$	57 torr
HCO_3	23 mEq/L
PaO_2	81 torr
B.E.	−1

   a. Acid-base status: **acidemia**
   b. Ventilatory status: **elevated $PaCO_2$ — hypoventilation resulting in decreased pH**
   c. Metabolic status: **normal bicarbonate level — no compensation occurring at this time**
   d. Oxygenation status: **normal PaO_2**

Interpretation: **uncompensated (acute) respiratory acidosis**

To correct: **institute mechanical ventilation to increase the patient's minute volume or increase the ventilator rate or tidal volume if patient is already on a ventilator.**

   2.
pH	7.57
$PaCO_2$	25 torr
HCO_3	25 mEq/L
PaO_2	98 torr
B.E.	0

   a. Acid-base status: **alkalemia**
   b. Ventilatory status: **decreased $PaCO_2$ — hyperventilation resulting in an increased pH**
   c. Metabolic status: **normal bicarbonate level — no compensation occurring at this time**
   d. Oxygenation status: **normal PaO_2**

Interpretation: **uncompensated (acute) respiratory alkalosis**

To correct: **decrease the ventilator rate or tidal volume or add mechanical deadspace.**

   3.
pH	7.45
$PaCO_2$	35 torr
HCO_3	26 mEq/L
PaO_2	53 torr
B.E.	+2

   a. Acid-base status: **normal pH**
   b. Ventilation status: **normal $PaCO_2$**
   c. Metabolic status: **normal bicarbonate**
   d. Oxygenation status: **moderate hypoxemia**

Interpretation: **normal acid-base status with moderate hypoxemia**

To correct: **if patient is receiving 60% or more oxygen through a mask, place on continuous positive airway pressure, or add positive end-expira-**

tory pressure on ventilator patient if on 60% oxygen or more.

4. pH   7.38
   PaCO₂   61 torr
   HCO₃   33 mEq/L
   PaO₂   54 torr
   B.E.   +9

   a. Acid-base status: **normal pH**
   b. Ventilatory status: **increased PaCO₂ — hypoventilation resulting in decreased pH**
   c. Metabolic status: **elevated bicarbonate level — compensating for initial acidemia**
   d. Oxygenation status: **moderate hypoxemia**

Interpretation: **compensated (chronic) respiratory acidosis**

Since the compensated pH is between 7.35 and 7.4, we must assume this was initially an acidemia caused by an elevated PaCO₂.

To correct: ****This is a classic example of "normal" ABG results in a patient with chronic lung disease; therefore, no change in present therapy is needed.**

5. pH   7.29
   PaCO₂   43 torr
   HCO₃   16 mEq/L
   PaO₂   87 torr
   B.E.   −7

   a. Acid-base status: **acidemia**
   b. Ventilatory status: **normal PaCO₂**
   c. Metabolic status: **decreased bicarbonate level resulting in decreased pH**
   d. Oxygenation status: **normal PaO₂**

Interpretation: **uncompensated metabolic acidosis**

No compensation is occurring because the PaCO₂ is normal.

To correct: **give sodium bicarbonate.** No ventilator parameter changes or oxygenation modifications are necessary at this time.

6. pH   7.20
   PaCO₂   22 torr
   HCO₃   15 mEq/L
   PaO₂   83 torr
   B.E.   −10

   a. Acid-base status: **acidemia**
   b. Ventilatory status: **decreased PaCO₂ — hyperventilation — compensating for initial acidemia**
   c. Metabolic status: **decreased bicarbonate level — resulting in decreased pH**
   d. Oxygenation status: **normal PaO₂**

Interpretation: **partially compensated metabolic acidosis**

This was an initial metabolic acidosis followed by hyperventilation. By removing more carbon dioxide, the pH is returning toward normal. It is not fully compensated, since the pH is not within normal limits at this time. **This is an example of a patient with diabetic acidosis (ketoacidosis).**

To correct: **may administer sodium bicarbonate**

VI. ARTERIAL BLOOD GAS INTERPRETATION CHART

N — Normal, I — Increased, D — Decreased

	pH	PCO₂	HCO₃
Normal	N	N	N
Uncompensated (acute)			
Respiratory acidosis	D	I	N
Respiratory alkalosis	I	D	N
Metabolic acidosis	D	N	D
Metabolic alkalosis	I	N	I
Partially compensated			
Respiratory acidosis	D	I	I
Respiratory alkalosis	I	D	D
Metabolic acidosis	D	D	D
Metabolic alkalosis	I	I	I
Fully compensated (chronic)			
Respiratory acidosis	N	I	I
Respiratory alkalosis	N	D	D
Metabolic acidosis	N	D	D
Metabolic alkalosis	N	I	I
Mixed respiratory and metabolic			
Acidosis	D	I	D
Alkalosis	I	D	I

VII. BLOOD GAS ANALYZERS

A. Current blood gas analyzers have the following capabilities:

1. Accurate measurement of pH, PCO_2, and PO_2
2. Self-calibration
3. Accurate measurement of base excess/deficit
4. Accurate measurement of plasma bicarbonate
5. Correction for temperature
6. Self-troubleshooting abilities
7. Automated blood gas interpretation
B. **Blood gas electrodes**
   1. **Sanz electrode — measures pH** by quantifying the acidity and alkalinity of a solution of blood. This is accomplished by the measurement of the potential difference across a pH-sensitive glass membrane.
   2. **Severinghaus electrode — measures PCO_2** by causing the carbon dioxide gas to produce hydrogen ions through a chemical reaction.
   3. **Clark electrode — measures PO_2** as a result of a chemical reaction whereby electron flow is measured.

REFERENCES

1. Barnes TA. *Respiratory Care Practice.* Chicago: Year Book Medical Publishers; 1988.
2. Eubanks D, Bone R. *Comprehensive Respiratory Care.* 2nd ed. St. Louis: CV Mosby; 1990.
3. Lane, EE. *Clinical Arterial Blood Gas Analysis.* St. Louis: CV Mosby, 1987.
4. Malley WJ. *Clinical Blood Gases: Application and Noninvasive Alternatives.* Philadelphia: WB Saunders; 1990.
5. McPherson SP. *Respiratory Therapy Equipment.* 4th ed. St. Louis: CV Mosby; 1990.
6. Shapiro BA. *Clinical Application of Blood Gases.* 4th ed. Chicago: Year Book Medical Publishers; 1989.

PRETEST ANSWERS

1. B
2. E
3. B
4. A
5. D
6. D

Ventilator Management

PRETEST QUESTIONS*

1. The following measurements have been obtained from a patient on a ventilator:
Peak inspiratory pressure—48 cm of water
Plateau pressure—27 cm of water
Tidal volume (V_T)—850 ml
Positive end-expiratory pressure (PEEP)—4 cm of water
Based on these data, the patient's static lung compliance is approximately which of the following?

A. 18 ml/cm of water
B. 20 ml/cm of water
C. 31 ml/cm of water
D. 37 ml/cm of water
E. 42 ml/cm of water

2. The Bear 2 is in the control mode and the inspiratory: expiratory (I:E) ratio alarm is sounding. Which control adjustment would correct this problem?

A. Decrease the flowrate.
B. Increase the V_T.
C. Increase the respiratory rate.
D. Increase the flowrate.
E. Decrease the sensitivity.

3. Mechanical ventilation can lead to which of the following complications?
 I. Increased renal output
 II. Barotrauma
III. Increased cardiac output

A. I only
B. II only
C. I and II only
D. II and III only
E. I, II, and III

4. Static lung compliance will decrease as a result of which of the following?

A. Bronchospasm
B. Mucosal edema
C. Atelectasis
D. Bronchial secretions
E. Laryngospasm

5. The following data have been collected from a patient breathing on a ventilator in the control mode.

Ventilator Settings		ABG Results	
V_T	800 ml	pH	7.50
Rate	15/min	$PaCO_2$	30 torr
FIO_2	0.45	PaO_2	98 torr

In order to increase this patient's $PaCO_2$ to 40 torr, the ventilator rate should be adjusted to what level?

A. 10 breaths/min
B. 11 breaths/min
C. 12 breaths/min
D. 13 breaths/min
E. 14 breaths/min

6. The following data have been collected from a patient breathing with a Bennett 7200 ventilator in the control mode.

Ventilator Settings		ABG Results	
V_T	700ml	pH	7.44
Rate	10/min	$PaCO_2$	42 torr
FIO_2	0.4	PaO_2	58 torr

Based on this information, the respiratory therapist should recommend which of the following ventilator changes?

A. Increase FIO_2 to 0.6
B. Increase V_T to 800 ml
C. Add 5 cm of water PEEP
D. Place on continuous positive airway pressure (CPAP) of 4 cm of water and 50% oxygen
E. Increase inspiratory flow

*See answers at the end of the chapter.

127

Ventilator Management

I. NEGATIVE- VERSUS POSITIVE-PRESSURE VENTILATORS

A. **Negative-pressure ventilators**
 1. **Iron lung** (body tank respirator)

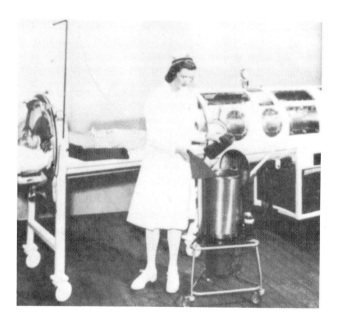

 a. Patient is placed in an airtight cylinder up to the neck (head is exposed to ambient conditions).
 b. The underside of the cylinder has a bellows that is powered by an electric motor or operates manually.

 c. As the bellows descends, it drops the pressure within the airtight chamber to below atmospheric pressure. This sets up a pressure gradient between the inside of the cylinder and the patient's mouth (at atmospheric pressure), and air flows into the airway.
 d. Gas flow stops as the bellows moves upward and pressures equalize. The patient exhales normally because of the elastic recoil of the lungs. (The motor moves the bellows up and down in response to a timing mechanism. Therefore, the iron lung is a **time-cycled ventilator**.)
 e. The iron lung was used extensively during the polio epidemic of the 1950s. It is not commonly used to ventilate patients at present.
 f. Negative pressures of up to **15 cm of water** were commonly used to ventilate the patient.
 g. **Disadvantages of the iron lung:**
  (1) Difficult patient care
  (2) Strictly a control ventilator—no means of assisting, but patient may breathe spontaneously between machine breaths
  (3) Difficult to clean
  (4) Large and cumbersome
  (5) No means of regulating flow
  (6) "Tank shock"—pooling of abdominal blood, resulting in decreased venous return

2. **Cuirass** (chest respirator)

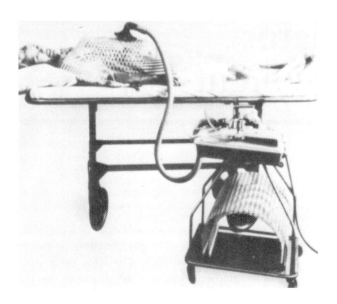

a. A plastic shell that covers the chest that was designed to minimize the disadvantages of the iron lung.

b. A flexible hose connects to the shell and is attached to an electric pump, which creates a negative extrathoracic pressure.

c. Since only the thorax receives negative pressure, and not the abdomen, "tank shock" is eliminated. Therefore, venous return is enhanced during inspiration.

d. It is used to wean patients off the iron lung or for home use in paralyzed patients.

e. **Disadvantages of the cuirass:**
   (1) Noisy
   (2) No means of regulating flow
   (3) Difficult to maintain a tight fit
   (4) Difficult patient care

f. **Advantages of the cuirass (over the iron lung):**
   (1) Patient care is easier
   (2) A flow-sensing device may be used to allow patient-triggered breaths.

B. **Positive-pressure ventilators**
   1. Types of positive-pressure ventilators:
      a. Preset volume ventilators (volume-limited or volume-cycled)
      b. Preset pressure ventilators (pressure-limited or pressure-cycled)
   2. **Volume-cycled ventilators**
      a. A preset V_T is delivered to the patient with each machine breath, and once it is delivered, inspiration ends.
      b. The volume-cycled ventilator is capable of developing an inspiratory pressure that can maintain the present V_T when changes in air-

way resistance and compliance occur (volume constant, pressure variable).
   c. They are used for mechanical ventilation of adult patients.
   3. **Pressure-cycled ventilators**
      a. A preset inspiratory pressure is delivered to the patient, and once it is reached inspiration ends.
   ** b. The delivered V_T is unknown but varies with changes in airway resistance and lung compliance (volume varies, pressure constant).
   ** c. When lung compliance decreases, delivered V_T decreases. In other words, as the patient's lungs become stiffer and harder to ventilate, the delivered V_T decreases.
      d. The pressure control is used like the volume control. When inspiratory pressure is increased, delivered V_T is increased and *vice versa*.
      e. They are used to ventilate infants and postoperative patients (wake up) and to administer intermittent positive-pressure breathing (IPPB) treatments. Inspiration ends on most infant ventilators when a preset time is reached. The set inspiratory pressure is reached during that time.

II. VENTILATOR CONTROLS

A. **Ventilator modes (volume ventilators)**
   1. **Control mode**
      a. The patient cannot initiate inspiration.
      b. Inspiration is initiated by a timing device. Example: **Control rate of 10**—the ventilator delivers a breath every **6 seconds** (60/10). Minute volume remains constant, as rate cannot be altered.
      c. The patient should be heavily sedated or paralyzed.
   2. **Assist mode**
      a. The patient initiates inspiration by creating a preset negative pressure, which causes the ventilator to deliver the set V_T.
   ** b. The sensitivity control determines how much negative pressure is required to initiate inspiration. It should be adjusted to **−0.5 to −2 cm of water**.
      c. The patient **must** initiate inspiration. There is no back-up rate should the patient become apneic. This mode is seldom used.
   3. **Assist/control mode**
      a. The patient initiates inspiration by creating a negative pressure, but if the patient fails to cycle the ventilator into inspiration, a back-

up rate is set and a machine V$_T$ breath will be delivered.

b. This is a commonly used mode of ventilation.

c. The patient can receive as many machine breaths as required above the set rate; therefore, the patient's minute volume is not consistent.

4. **Intermittent mandatory ventilation (IMV)**

a. The ventilator delivers a set number of machine breaths, but the patient is able to breathe spontaneously between machine breaths.

b. IMV is set up on the Bennett MA-1 ventilator by turning off the sensitivity control so that the patient cannot initiate machine breaths. A separate gas source (either a nebulizer or reservoir bag) is attached to the inspiratory side of the circuit, providing gas for the patient to breathe spontaneously.

c. **Reservoir bag IMV setup**

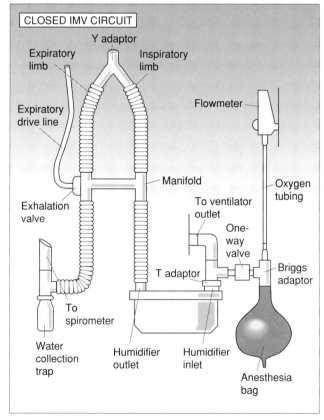

From Persing G. *Entry Level Respiratory Care Review.* Philadelphia: WB Saunders; 1992.

d. **Nebulizer IMV setup**

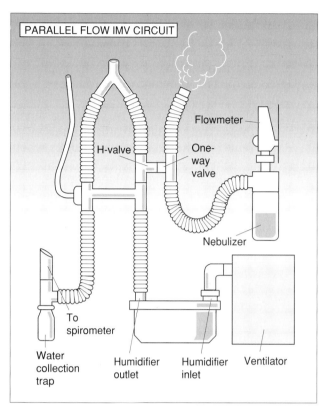

From Persing G. *Entry Level Respiratory Care Review.* Philadelphia: WB Saunders; 1992.

e. One-way valves (H valves) are incorporated into the setup so that gas flows only in the direction of the patient from the inspiratory limb of the ventilator circuit.

** f. To ensure adequate flow for spontaneous breaths, the reservoir bag should remain one-third to one-half full at all times. If a nebulizer setup is used, mist should be visible exiting the H valve reservoir at all times. If these conditions are not observed, **increase the IMV flow**.

** g. The one-way valve must be placed correctly to open **toward** the patient. If placed backward, the patient will not be able to open the valve and receive gas flow for spontaneous breathing. This is recognized by observing increased work of breathing and excessive negative pressure on the ventilator pressure manometer during inspiration.

** h. During spontaneous inspiration, the manometer needle should be observed deflecting no more than −2 cm of water. If it is greater than −2 cm of water, make sure the one-way valve is opened toward the patient. If it is, increase the flow.

i. IMV was designed to aid in the ventilator weaning process.

j. This IMV system allows "breath-stacking" to occur. This means that the ventilator (being time-cycled) will deliver a breath at a specific time, depending on the dialed-in rate. It may come while the patient is breathing spontaneously.

5. **Synchronized intermittent mandatory ventilation (SIMV)**

   a. SIMV allows spontaneous breathing along with positive-pressure ventilator breaths. It is built into the ventilator and senses when the patient is breathing spontaneously; therefore, no "breath-stacking" occurs.

   b. It is used both as a weaning technique and for ventilation prior to weaning.

   c. The sensitivity control is left on, as the patient must open a demand valve to obtain gas flow for spontaneous breathing.

6. **Pressure support ventilation (PSV)**

   a. This is a relatively new mode of ventilation found on the new generation of ventilators that aids in the weaning process from the ventilator.

   b. It is a patient-assisted, pressure-generated, flow-cycled breath that may be augmented with SIMV or used by itself.

   c. It was designed to make spontaneous breathing through the endotracheal (E-T) tube during weaning more comfortable by overcoming the high resistance and increased inspiratory work caused by the E-T tube.

   d. An inspiratory pressure is set (usually 2 to 10 cm of water for weaning purposes). As the patient initiates inspiration, the preset pressure is reached and holds constant until a certain inspiratory flow is reached. The pressure is then terminated.

   e. The inspiratory pressure level may be set to achieve a specific V_T.

   f. Pressure support ventilation may be used in patients who are ventilating well but are intubated to protect the airway, or in patients on CPAP who have oxygenation deficiencies.

7. **Continuous Positive Airway Pressure (CPAP)**

   a. May be achieved with the use of a CPAP mask, nasal prongs, or intubation and placement on a ventilator.

   b. A preset pressure is maintained in the airway as the patient breathes totally independently. No positive-pressure breaths are delivered.

   c. Patients whose PaO_2 cannot be maintained within normal limits on an **oxygen mask delivering 60% oxygen or more, and who have normal $PaCO_2$ levels, should be

placed on CPAP. Patients with **obstructive sleep apnea benefit from CPAP** to relieve obstruction in the upper airway.

   d. Uses **low-pressure alarm in case of leaks.

   e. CPAP separate from the ventilator, such as a CPAP mask, may be accomplished as shown in the diagram below:

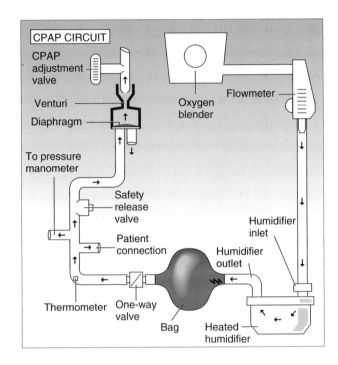

   (1) In this type of setup, the patient's exhaled gas flow enters the expiratory limb of the circuit, at which point it meets an opposing gas flow entering through a Venturi.

   (2) This opposing gas flow causes a resistance to exhalation that the patient must overcome.

   (3) The pressure the patient must generate to overcome this resistance results in a positive pressure that is read on a manometer placed in-line. This pressure is the CPAP level.

   (4) The CPAP level may be increased or decreased by adjusting the opposing gas flow passing through the jet in the expiratory limb.

NOTE: These types of CPAP setups should have low-pressure alarms incorporated to warn of potential leaks in the system.

   f. The indications and hazards of CPAP are the same as those listed for PEEP later in this chapter.

8. **Bilevel positive airway pressure (BiPAP)**

   a. This is a relatively new mode of intermittent mechanical ventilation that may be delivered to non-intubated patients through a nasal mask or to intubated patients.

b. BiPAP has been used to reverse chronic hypoventilation in patients with neuromuscular dysfunction and chest wall deformities such as kyphoscoliosis.

c. BiPAP is gaining popularity for its use in avoiding placing a patient with respiratory distress on a conventional volume-cycled ventilator.

d. BiPAP is a time-cycled, pressure-limited ventilator that allows the patient to trigger inspiration and expiration similar in nature to pressure support ventilation.

e. Inspiratory and expiratory airway pressures are controlled by adjustment of the inspiratory positive airway pressure (IPAP) control ranging from 2 to 25 cm H_2O and expiratory positive airway pressure (EPAP) control ranging from 2 to 20 cm H_2O.

f. The frequency control ranges from 6 to 30 cycles/min, and a %IPAP control adjusts the proportion of each cycle spent at IPAP and ranges from 10 to 90%.

g. Exhaled tidal volume is also measured through the device.

B. **Tidal volume (V_T)**

1. Tidal volume control on ventilator determines the delivered V_T to the patient in milliliters or liters (variable from 50 to 2200 ml)

** 2. Should be set at **10 to 15 ml/kg of ideal body weight; for children: 8 to 10 ml/kg; for infants: 6 to 8 ml/kg**

3. **Increasing the V_T increases alveolar ventilation while also increasing the minute volume. This decreases the $PaCO_2$.**

4. **Decreasing the V_T decreases alveolar ventilation while also decreasing the minute volume. This increases the $PaCO_2$.**

EXAMPLE: A patient breathing 10 times/min with a V_T of 600 ml has a minute volume of 6 L. **(Minute volume is calculated: respiratory rate × tidal volume.)**
If the patient begins breathing 20 times/min with a V_T of 300 ml, the minute ventilation remains the same but the **alveolar ventilation has decreased because of the decreased V_T.**

5. On volume ventilators:
   a. Increasing the V_T → increases the inspiratory time
   b. Decreasing the V_T → decreases the inspiratory time
6. The preset machine V_T is not the actual volume reaching the patient's lungs.
   a. Volume is "lost" in the ventilator circuit because of airway resistance from gas flow.

b. Tubing compliance may be calculated to determine how much volume is being lost in the circuit.

c. With the ventilator set on a specific V_T and the high-pressure limit turned up completely, the machine is cycled into inspiration with the patient wye occluded. Observe the manometer pressure reading.

d. Compliance $= \dfrac{\text{volume}}{\text{pressure}}$

EXAMPLE: Set tidal volume—200 ml (0.2L); peak pressure reached—40 cm of water

$$\text{Compliance} = \frac{200\ \text{ml}}{40\ \text{cm}\ H_2O} = 5\ \text{ml/cm}\ H_2O$$

**This means that once the patient is placed on the ventilator, 5 ml of the dialed-in volume will be lost in the tubing for every centimeter of water registering on the manometer.

EXAMPLE: Tubing compliance—5 ml/cm of water; V_T—800 ml; Peak inspiratory pressure—20 cm of water

Lost volume = tubing compliance × peak inspiratory pressure
5 ml/cm H_2O × 20 cm H_2O = **100 ml**
Dialed-in V_T = 800 ml − 100 ml (lost volume) = **700 ml**

e. Lost volume is affected by the water level in the humidifier. Lower water levels allow more compressed volume into the walls of the humidifer—hence, more lost volume or less delivered volume to the patient.

f. More volume will be lost in the patient's conducting airways (trachea, bronchi, and so on) because of resistance to gas flow. This part of the patient's airway is called the **anatomic deadspace**. It is the part of the airway in which no gas exchange occurs and is often called "wasted air."

NOTE: Anatomic deadspace is equal to a 1 ml/lb of the patient's ideal body weight but is reduced by 50% in the intubated patient. Thus, anatomic deadspace is equal to 1 ml/kg.

EXAMPLE: A **75-kg** (165 lb) patient has an anatomic deadspace of approximately **75 ml**. This means that 75 ml of the patient's V_T does not reach the alveoli to take part in gas exchange. This may also be subtracted from the ventilator V_T setting to obtain a corrected V_T.
NOTE: When using the formula for selecting ventilator V_T as **10 to 15 ml/kg of body weight**, this lost volume is taken into account and this is usually an adequate V_T.

7. Exhaled V_T is measured with a bellows spirometer (MA-1) or by a digital readout. It is most

accurately measured with a respirometer placed between the E-T tube and the ventilator wye or at the exhalation valve. **The V$_T$ delivered by the ventilator should be measured at the ventilator outlet.**

** 8. Volume may be lost from other causes:
    a. Loose humidifier jar or tubing connections—will register a low exhaled V$_T$ reading on spirometer
    b. Leak around E-T tube cuff—low exhaled V$_T$ reading

** 9. If the bellows spirometer on the Bennett MA-1 ventilator rises during inspiration (it should drop), the most likely cause is a hole in the exhalation diaphragm or a disconnected exhalation drive line.

**10. If the bellows spirometer (Bennett MA-1) fails to empty during inspiration, check dump valve or reconnect dump valve tubing.

C. **Respiratory rate**
  1. Normal initial setup is 8 to 12 breaths/min.
  2. **Adjusting the rate control alters the expiratory time and therefore alters the I:E ratio.**
    a. Increasing rate → decreases expiratory time
    b. Decreasing rate → increases expiratory time
  3. **Adjusting the rate alters the minute ventilation.**
    a. Increasing rate → increases minute ventilation
    b. Decreasing rate → decreases minute ventilation
  4. **Adjusting the rate affects the PaCO$_2$ level.**
    a. Increasing rate → decreases PaCO$_2$
    b. Decreasing rate → increases PaCO$_2$

NOTE: Adjusting the rate to alter the patient's PaCO$_2$ level is more beneficial for patients on controlled ventilation or on SIMV/IMV. On assist/control, the patient may obtain as many machine breaths as needed no matter what the set rate.

  5. Adjustable on most ventilators from 0.5 to 60 breaths/min

D. **Flowrate**
  1. Normal setting—40 to 60 L/min
  2. Adjusting the flowrate alters the inspiratory time, therefore altering the I:E ratio.
    a. Increasing flowrate → decreases inspiratory time
    b. Decreasing flowrate → increases inspiratory time
  3. Adjustable on most ventilators from 20 to 120 L/min

E. **I:E ratio**
  1. It is a comparison of the inspiratory time to the expiratory time.
  2. **The normal I:E ratio for the adult is 1:2.** This means that expiration should be twice as long as inspiration.

3. The normal I:E ratio for the infant is 1:1.
4. The I:E ratio is established by the use of **three** ventilator controls on the volume ventilator.
  a. **Volume control**
    (1) Increasing volume → increases inspiratory time
    (2) Decreasing volume → decreases inspiratory time
  b. **Flowrate control**
    (1) Increasing flowrate → decreases inspiratory time
    (2) Decreasing flowrate → increases inspiratory time
  c. **Respiratory rate control**
    (1) Increasing rate → decreases expiratory time
    (2) Decreasing rate → increases expiratory time

5. Calculation of I:E ratio uses the following formula:

$$\frac{\text{inspiratory flowrate (L/min)}}{\text{minute ventilation (L/min)}} - 1 \text{ (for inspiration)}$$

EXAMPLE:

    V$_T$ 800 ml (0.8 L)
    Rate   12/min
    Flow   40 L/min

$$\text{I:E ratio} = \frac{40 \text{ L/min}}{9.6 \text{ L/min}} = 4.2 - 1 = \textbf{1:3.2}$$
$$\textbf{(0.8 L} \times \textbf{12)}$$

6. Inspiratory time should generally not exceed expiratory time. This is termed **an inverse I:E ratio.** It may greatly compromise venous blood return to the heart.
  a. If the I:E ratio alarm is sounding on the ventilator, three controls may be adjusted to correct it:
    (1) Rate—decrease to lengthen expiratory time
    (2) Volume—decrease to shorten inspiratory time
  **(3) Flow—increase to shorten inspiratory time.

Most common adjustment to correct an inverse I:E ratio

F. **Oxygen percentage control**
  1. Adjustable from 21% to 100% to maintain normal PaO$_2$ levels
  **2. Oxygen percentage should be increased to a maximum of 60% to maintain normal PaO$_2$ levels. Once 60% is reached and PaO$_2$ is low, PEEP should be added or increased.
  **3. Oxygen should be reduced first to a level of 60% before decreasing PEEP levels in hyperoxygenated patients.

G. **Sensitivity control**
1. This determines the amount of patient effort required to cycle the ventilator into inspiration.
2. Should be set so that the patient will pull a **negative 0.5 to 2 cm of water pressure**.
3. If the ventilator self-cycles, the sensitivity control is adjusted too high. Decrease the sensitivity.
**4. If it takes more than −2 cm of water pressure to cycle the ventilator into inspiration, increase the sensitivity.
5. In the control mode of ventilation, the sensitivity control is turned off, not allowing the patient to trigger a machine breath.
6. The sensitivity is also turned off on the MA-1 ventilator when using an external gas source for the IMV mode.
**7. When PEEP is added or increased on the Bennett MA-1, the sensitivity must be increased accordingly and decreased if PEEP is decreased to maintain the patient effort at −2 cm of water to trigger a machine breath.

H. **Sigh controls**
1. Sigh rate should be set at 6 to 12 sighs/hour.
2. Sigh volume should be set at 1½ to 2 times the V_T.
3. Sighs aid in preventing atelectasis.
4. Usually not functional in the SIMV mode.

I. **Inflation hold**
1. Adjustable from 0 to 2 seconds.
2. Mechanism keeps the exhalation valve closed, causing the ventilator V_T to be held in the lungs for a preset time.
3. Used to improve oxygenation by reducing atelectasis and shunting and increasing the diffusion of gases.
4. Using the inspiratory hold or plateau causes an increased intrathoracic pressure.
5. Used to calculate static lung compliance by obtaining a plateau pressure.

J. **Expiratory retard**
1. Used to prevent premature airway collapse during expiration. (Used on Bennett MA-1 or various intermittent positive-pressure breathing setups.)
2. Increases the expiratory time and therefore alters the I : E ratio and increases intrathoracic pressure

K. **PEEP**
1. It is used to maintain positive pressure in the airway following a ventilator breath.
2. **Indications for PEEP**
   a. Atelectasis
   **b. Hypoxemia with patient receiving 60% oxygen or more
   c. Decreased functional residual capacity

d. To lower oxygen percentage to safe levels (<60%)
e. Decreased lung compliance
f. Pulmonary edema
3. **Hazards of PEEP**
   a. Barotrauma
   b. Decreased venous return
   c. Decreased cardiac output
   d. Decreased urinary output
4. Excessive PEEP levels may lead to decreases in $PaCO_2$ and lung compliance by overdistending already open alveoli and shunting blood to collapsed alveoli.
5. If PEEP causes a decreased cardiac output, it will be evidenced by a drop in blood pressure and $P\overline{v}O_2$ values.
6. **Optimal PEEP—the level of PEEP that improves lung compliance without decreasing the cardiac output
7. A mixed venous PO_2 ($P\overline{v}O_2$) may be obtained from the pulmonary artery via the Swan-Ganz catheter.
   a. **Normal $P\overline{v}O_2$ is 35 to 45 torr**
   b. **A $P\overline{v}O_2$ of less than 35 torr indicates a possible decrease in cardiac output. If the $P\overline{v}O_2$ drops after initiation of PEEP, it is a good indicator of reduced venous return and cardiac output caused by the PEEP.**
   c. The $P\overline{v}O_2$ value represents the adequacy of tissue oxygenation.
   d. **Use the PEEP level that provides the best lung compliance and $P\overline{v}O_2$ value.
8. PEEP pressure curves compared with other curves:

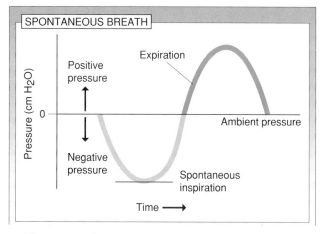

Figure continues on next page.

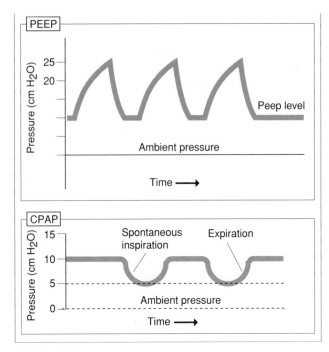

From Persing G. *Entry Level Respiratory Care Review.* Philadelphia: WB Saunders; 1992.

III. VENTILATOR ALARMS AND MONITORING

A. **Low-pressure alarm**
1. Should be set 5 to 10 cm of water below peak inspiratory pressure
****2. This alarm is activated as a result of leaks in the ventilator circuit or by patient disconnection.

B. **High-pressure alarm**
1. Should be set 5 to 15 cm of water above peak inspiratory pressure
2. When this pressure is reached on a volume ventilator, inspiration ends prematurely, decreasing delivered V_T.
**3. This alarm may be activated by:
   a. Decreasing lung compliance
   b. Increasing airway resistance caused by:
      (1) Airway secretions
      (2) Bronchospasm
      (3) Water in the ventilator tubing
      (4) Kink in the ventilator tubing
      (5) Patient coughing

C. **Low PEEP/CPAP alarm**
1. Should be set 2 to 4 cm of water below the baseline level
2. This alarm is activated as a result of leaks in the ventilator circuit or by patient disconnection.

D. **Apnea alarm**
1. Set according to the patient's respiratory rate
2. This alarm is activated after a preset time passes with no inspiratory flow through the tubing.

3. Important alarm for patients on the ventilator in the CPAP mode

E. **Mean airway pressure monitoring**
NOTE: Mean airway pressure (MAP) is also abbreviated P_{aw}.
1. MAP is the average pressure applied to the airway over a specific time.
2. MAP is directly affected by:
   a. Ventilator rate
   b. Peak inspiratory pressure
   c. Inspiratory time
   d. Inspiratory hold
   e. Expiratory retard
   f. PEEP level
   g. Pressure waveform
   h. I : E ratio
3. MAP is commonly measured by a digital reading on a MAP monitor, or it may be calculated using the following equation:

$$MAP = 0.5 \ [\text{Peak inspiratory pressure} - \text{PEEP} \times (\text{inspiratory time/total respiratory cycle})]$$

**4. Optimal MAP is the MAP level that improves oxygenation and ventilation without resulting in cardiovascular embarrassment and barotrauma.
5. Studies have shown that MAP levels greater than 12 cm of water result in a greater risk of barotrauma.
6. Provided that there has been no change in dynamic compliance or ventilator parameters, if the MAP decreases it indicates that less pressure is needed to ventilate the patient or that there is an increased static lung compliance. An increased MAP indicates that higher pressure is needed to ventilate the patient or there is decreased static lung compliance.

F. **End-tidal carbon dioxide monitoring (capnography)**
NOTE: End-tidal carbon dioxide is abbreviated $P_{ET}CO_2$.
1. Capnography is a technique by which exhaled carbon dioxide is measured. This measurement is obtained by the use of a mass spectrometer.
2. Normal end-tidal carbon dioxide is approximately the same as alveolar carbon dioxide, which is equal to arterial PCO_2. Capnography, therefore, is a noninvasive technique to obtain the patient's $PaCO_2$.
3. End-tidal carbon dioxide may be expressed as partial pressure or a percentage. A normal end-tidal carbon dioxide level is 35 to 45 torr or **4.5% to 5.5%.
4. There is a difference of approximately 2 to 5 torr between normal $PaCO_2$ and end-tidal carbon dioxide.

5. End-tidal carbon dioxide readings may decrease as a result of the following:
   a. Hyperventilation
   b. Apnea (reading falls to zero)
   c. Total airway obstruction (reading falls to zero)
   d. Conditions in which perfusion is decreased (hypotension, pulmonary embolism, decreased cardiac output)—low reading results from decreased perfusion to the pulmonary capillaries rendering an inaccurate end-tidal carbon dioxide reading. $PaCO_2$ may be increasing.
6. End-tidal carbon dioxide readings may increase as a result of the following:
   a. Hypoventilation
   b. Hyperthermia (increased carbon dioxide production)
7. Continuous end-tidal carbon dioxide monitoring with tracings is becoming an important technique in monitoring critically ill patients. The tracing records carbon dioxide readings during inspiration (should be zero, since there is little carbon dioxide in inspired air) and during expiration when carbon dioxide begins to increase.
8. An end-tidal carbon dioxide measurement by itself should not be used to predict $PaCO_2$ in patients with left ventricular failure (decreased cardiac output), pulmonary embolism, and chronic obstructive pulmonary disease because of inaccurate readings in these conditions.

IV. INDICATIONS FOR MECHANICAL VENTILATION

A. **Apnea**
B. **Acute ventilatory failure**
   1. $PaCO_2$ of greater than 50 torr indicates ventilatory failure and a need for mechanical assistance.
   2. To determine ventilatory failure in a patient with chronic obstructive pulmonary disease who chronically retains carbon dioxide, the pH will be below normal, signaling the need for ventilator assistance.
C. **Impending acute ventilatory failure**
   1. Sometimes normal arterial blood gas (ABG) results can be deceiving. A patient may have normal ABG values but is breathing 30 to 40 times/min to achieve this normal PCO_2 level.
   2. This patient is likely to tire soon, with an elevated $PaCO_2$ level resulting in ventilatory failure.
   ****3. A patient with a neuromuscular disease such as Guillain-Barré syndrome, must be monitored

closely for lung muscle involvement. **Measurement of the patient's negative inspiratory force (pressure) and vital capacity will best determine the lung status.**
D. **Oxygenation**
   1. Patient may be ventilating adequately but oxygenating poorly.
   2. Mechanical ventilation is indicated if oxygen deficiency is directly related to an abnormal ventilatory pattern or an increased work of breathing.
   **3. A patient receiving **60% of oxygen or more through a mask who is ventilating well (normal or decreased $PaCO_2$) but is not oxygenating adequately (low PaO_2) is probably exhibiting a large intrapulmonary shunt. This may be corrected by the use of CPAP. Mechanical ventilation may not be necessary initially.

V. COMMON CRITERIA FOR INITIATION OF MECHANICAL VENTILATION

A. Vital capacity of less than 15 ml/kg (normal is 65 to 75 ml/kg)
B. Alveolar-arterial (A-a) gradient of greater than 450 torr on 100% oxygen (normal is 25 to 65 torr)
   1. When the PaO_2 is low and the A-a gradient is normal for ambient conditions and the patient's age, the hypoxemia is most likely the result of hypoventilation.
   2. When the PaO_2 is low and the A-a gradient is high, the hypoxemia is most likely the result of a ventilation/perfusion (V/Q) mismatch, diffusion defect, or shunting. In this type of situation, the patient may be hyperventilating to compensate for the hypoxemia.
C. $V_D : V_T$ ratio of greater than 60% (normal is 25% to 35%)

$$\frac{V_D}{V_T} = \frac{PaCO_2 - PECO_2}{PaCO_2}$$

V_D = deadspace

($PECO_2$ = exhaled CO_2)

D. Negative inspiratory force of less than −20 cm of water (normal is −50 to −100 cm of water)
E. Peak expiratory pressure of less than 40 cm of water (normal is 100 cm of water)
NOTE: A negative inspiratory force of <−20 cm of water or a positive expiratory pressure of <40 cm of water indicates the patient cannot generate an adequate cough to maintain clearance of secretions.
F. Respiratory rate of greater than 35 breaths/min (normal is 10 to 20 breaths/min)

VI. GOALS OF MECHANICAL VENTILATION

A. Increased minute ventilation
B. Decreased work of breathing
C. Increased alveolar ventilation
D. Maintenance of ABG values within normal range
E. Improved distribution of inspired gases—it has been shown that positive-pressure breaths on 21% oxygen increase the PaO_2 slightly

VII. COMPLICATIONS OF MECHANICAL VENTILATION

A. **Barotrauma**
   1. Pneumothorax—may be evident because of **subcutaneous emphysema** (air in the subcutaneous tissues)
   2. Pneumomediastinum
   3. Pneumopericardium
B. **Pulmonary infection**
   1. Debilitated patients have lower resistance
   2. Contaminated equipment
   3. Improper airway care (tracheostomy care, suctioning, and so on)
   4. Retained secretions due to E-T tube and poor cough
   5. Ciliary dysfunction due to E-T tube
NOTE: The most cost-effective method of preventing cross-contamination of patients and equipment is by proper handwashing techniques.
C. **Atelectasis**
   1. Use a minimum V_T of 10 ml/kg of body weight to prevent atelectasis.
   2. Instituting a sigh breath periodically reduces the potential of atelectasis.
D. **Pulmonary oxygen toxicity**
   1. Also referred to as adult respiratory distress syndrome
   2. Results from using high oxygen concentrations for prolonged periods
   3. It is characterized by:
      a. Impaired surfactant production
      b. Capillary congestion
      c. Edema
      d. Fibrosis
      e. Thickening of alveolar membranes
      f. Decreased lung compliance resulting in high peak pressures required to ventilate the patient
NOTE: See Chapter 12 for more information.
E. **Tracheal damage**—usually at the cuff site
F. **Decreased venous blood return to the heart**
   1. Results from the positive airway pressures being transferred onto the large veins returning blood to the heart
   2. This results in decreased pulmonary blood flow, decreased cardiac output, and decreased blood pressure.
G. **Decreased urinary output**
   1. Results from decreased renal blood flow (due to decreased cardiac output)
   2. Also results from an increased production of antidiuretic hormone (ADH)
      a. ADH production is increased because of baroreceptors in the atria of the heart, which sense the decreased venous return.
      b. These receptors send a message to the hypothalamus, which stimulates the pituitary gland to secrete more ADH, thereby inhibiting urine excretion.
H. **Lack of nutrition**
   1. Malnutrition may lead to:
      a. Difficulty weaning from the ventilator because of weakened respiratory muscles
      b. Reduced response to hypoxia and hypercarbia
      c. Impaired wound healing
      d. Decreased surfactant production
      e. Infection
      f. Pulmonary edema due to decreased serum albumin levels
   2. Since oral feeding is not possible, nasogastric feedings should be implemented. Other feeding routes include intravenous or enteral feedings through a catheter in the stomach.
   3. High-protein, high-carbohydrate diets are recommended.

VIII. DEADSPACE

A. Deadspace is that portion of the V_T that does not take part in gas exchange.
B. Types of deadspace
   1. **Anatomic deadspace** (discussed earlier) consists of the conducting airways from the nose and mouth to the terminal bronchioles—air that does not reach the alveolar epithelium where gas exchange occurs.
      a. Anatomic deadspace = 1 ml/lb body weight
      b. **A tracheostomy decreases the anatomic deadspace by 50%** by bypassing the upper airway.
   2. **Alveolar deadspace**
      a. Air reaching the alveoli but not taking part in gas exchange
      b. Results from lack of perfusion to air-filled alveoli
      c. May result from hyperinflated alveoli in which blood is not able to use all the air.

3. **Physiologic deadspace**
   a. The sum of anatomic and alveolar deadspace
   b. The most accurate measurement of dead-space
4. **Mechanical deadspace**
   a. Ventilator circuits have a certain amount of deadspace, which ranges from 75 to 150 ml.
   b. Since anatomic deadspace decreases when a patient is intubated or has had a tracheostomy, the deadspace created by the circuit is balanced out.
   c. Additional mechanical deadspace may be added to the ventilator circuit <u>between the ventilator adaptor and the E-T tube adaptor</u> to increase **PaCO₂ levels.**
      (1) For every 100 ml of deadspace added, the $PaCO_2$ increases approximately 5 torr.
      (2) Mechanical deadspace should be added to the circuits of patients on control or assist/control only. **Never add deadspace if the patient is on SIMV/IMV or CPAP.**

IX. LUNG COMPLIANCE

A. Compliance is defined as the change in volume that corresponds to the change in pressure accompanying the volume change.

$$C = \frac{V}{P}$$

1. Lung compliance is the ease with which the lung expands.
2. The higher the compliance, the easier it is to ventilate the lung.
3. The lower the compliance, the stiffer the lung is and the harder it is to ventilate.
4. **Normal total lung compliance** (sum of lung tissue and thoracic cage) is **0.1 L/cm of water.**
B. **Calculation of lung compliance**
   1. **Dynamic compliance**
      a. $$\frac{V_T}{\text{Peak inspiratory pressure} - PEEP}$$

Given the following data, calculate the patient's dynamic lung compliance.

V_T	600 ml
Peak inspiratory pressure	35 cm of water
PEEP	5 cm of water

Dynamic compliance =

$$\frac{600 \text{ ml}}{30 \text{ cm H}_2\text{O}} = 20 \text{ ml/cm H}_2\text{O}$$
$$(35 - 5)$$

b. Dynamic compliance is measured as air is flowing through the circuit and airways; therefore, it is actually a measurement of airway resistance.
**c. Dynamic compliance will change with changes in airway resistance caused by:
   (1) Water in the ventilator tubing
   (2) Bronchospasm
   (3) Secretions
   (4) Mucosal edema
d. Dynamic compliance is not an accurate measurement of how compliant the lungs are.
2. **Static compliance**
   a. Static compliance is a more accurate measurement of lung compliance or how easily the lung is expanded, since it is measured with no air flowing through the circuit and airways (static conditions).
   b. Air flow may be stopped with the volume remaining in the lungs by adjusting a 1- to 2-second inspiratory hold or pinching off the expiratory drive line after inspiration has begun.
   c. Once the flow has stopped, a **plateau pressure** will occur after peak pressure has been reached.
   d. Static compliance is calculated as follows:

$$\frac{V_T}{\text{Plateau pressure} - PEEP}$$

EXAMPLE:

V_T	800 ml
Plateau pressure	25 cm of water
PEEP	5 cm of water
Peak pressure	45 cm of water

Calculate the static lung compliance:

$$\frac{800 \text{ ml}}{20 \text{ cm H}_2\text{O}} = \frac{\textbf{40 ml}}{\textbf{1 cm H}_2\textbf{O}}$$
$$\textbf{(25} - \textbf{5)}$$

C. **Important points concerning lung compliance**
   **1. Increasing plateau pressures indicate the lung compliance is decreasing or the lungs are harder to ventilate.
   **2. If the peak pressures are increasing, but the plateau pressure remains the same, lung compliance is not decreasing. Increased airway resistance is occurring (bronchospasm, secretions, and so on).

EXAMPLE:

Time	Peak Pressure	Plateau Pressure
6:00 AM	28 cm of water	10 cm of water
7:00 AM	34 cm of water	10 cm of water
8:00 AM	42 cm of water	10 cm of water

**In this example, the peak pressures are increasing while the plateau pressures remain stable. This indicates an increase in airway resistance and not a decreasing lung compliance.

EXAMPLE:

Time	Peak Pressure	Plateau Pressure
1:00 PM	34 cm of water	16 cm of water
2:00 PM	40 cm of water	22 cm of water
3:00 PM	44 cm of water	26 cm of water

In this example, the plateau pressures are increasing along with the peak pressures. **This indicates a decreasing lung compliance.

    3. Decreasing static lung compliance results from:
      a. Pneumonia
      b. Pulmonary edema
      c. Consolidation
      d. Atelectasis
      e. Air trapping
      f. Pleural effusion
      g. Pneumothorax
      h. Adult respiratory distress syndrome
    4. Normal static lung compliance in the ventilated patient is 60 to 70 ml/cm of water

X. VENTILATION OF THE HEAD TRAUMA PATIENT

A. Higher than normal flowrates should be used to make inspiratory time shorter, lessening the time of positive pressure in the airways. The longer the time of positive pressure in the airways, the more impedance of blood flow from the head, which increases intracranial pressure (ICP).

B. Maintain the **$PaCO_2$ between 25 and 30 torr,** as this reduces ICP by vasoconstriction of cerebral vessels. **ICP should be maintained at less than 15 torr (normal ICP is <10 torr).**

C. If the ICP begins to increase, the patient should be hyperventilated (preferably with a resuscitation bag) to reduce the cerebral blood flow, thus lowering ICP.

D. Caution must be exercised when suctioning, as this tends to increase ICP from hypoxemia.

XI. WEANING FROM MECHANICAL VENTILATION

A. **Criteria for weaning**
    1. V_T equal to three times the body weight in kilograms
    2. Vital capacity of >15 ml/kg or twice the V_T
    3. Negative inspiratory force >−20 cm of water
    4. $V_D : V_T$ ratio of <0.60

    5. A-a gradient <350 torr on 100% oxygen
    6. Respiratory rate of less than 25 breaths/min
    7. Patient should be alert and able to follow commands.
    8. Patient should not be taking any medication that may hinder spontaneous ventilation.
    9. Life-threatening situations such as shock or hypotension should not be present.
    10. Anemia, fever, or electrolyte imbalances should not be present.

B. **Weaning techniques**
    1. Use of SIMV/IMV to decrease the number of mechanical ventilator breaths while allowing for more spontaneous breathing.
      a. Patient should be on 40% oxygen or less prior to extubation.
      b. Patient should be on SIMV/IMV rate of 4 or less before removal from the ventilator.
      c. Postoperative patients may be weaned as they begin waking up. Provided that they have normal blood gas values and are beginning to arouse, the SIMV/IMV rate may begin to be decreased.

    2. **Time on–time off method**
      a. Patient is taken off the ventilator periodically and placed on flow-by for a specific length of time and then placed back on the ventilator.
      b. The time off the ventilator is gradually increased until the patient is spending more time off the ventilator than on it.
      c. Patient is often returned to the ventilator while asleep.
      d. Patient must be monitored closely (blood pressure, V_T, heart rate, respiratory rate, and oxygen saturation/ABG results)
      e. Oftentimes the oxygen percentage is increased 10% while on flow-by.

XII. HIGH-FREQUENCY VENTILATION

High-frequency ventilation (HFV) refers to breathing rates that are four times the normal rate (60/min in the adult). Smaller than normal tidal volumes are used, sometimes less than anatomic deadspace. HFV has been shown to improve gas exchange without the barotrauma and cardiovascular problems associated with conventional volume-limited and pressure-limited ventilation in both infants and adults.

A. **Three classifications of high-frequency ventilation**
    1. **High-frequency positive pressure ventilation (HFPPV)**
      a. Gas delivery to the patient occurs with the use of a time-cycled, pressure-limited, or

volume-limited device through ventilator tubing that has a very low compressible volume. This ensures that very little volume is lost in the tubing.

b. Gas is directed through an insufflation catheter that is placed through the E-T tube, and the rapid opening and closing of the exhalation valve determines gas flow into and out of the lungs.

c. The exhalation valve opens and closes in response to a pneumatic or electric source. Some pneumatic-type units incorporate fluidic gates to accomplish the opening and closing of the exhalation valve.

d. **Ventilatory rates with HFPPV are between 60 and 100 breaths/min with small tidal volumes of 3 to 5 ml/kg of body weight. I:E ratios of 1:3 or less are normally used.

**e. Delivery of small tidal volumes results in lower peak inspiratory pressure and lower MAP, at a much higher rate than conventional ventilation, and an improved distribution of gas.

f. PEEP may also be used with HFPPV to improve oxygenation with less cardiovascular embarrassment than with conventional positive-pressure ventilation and PEEP.

g. HFPPV has also been used during thoracic surgery such as lobectomy or pneumonectomy in which conventional ventilation may not be effective.

2. **High-frequency jet ventilation**

a. A high-pressure gas source injects short, rapid bursts of gas through a jet catheter, usually incorporated into a special E-T tube. Air is entrained through a separate channel during inspiration, increasing flow to the patient.

b. Frequency rates vary from about 100 to 600 cycles/min at an I:E ratio of 1:1 to 1:4. Peak inspiratory pressures are usually about 8 to 10 cm of water above baseline. Tidal volumes are usually a little bit larger than anatomic deadspace.

**c. A low-pressure alarm set 2 to 3 cm of water below peak inspiratory pressure should be incorporated to determine power loss or system leaks.

**d. A high-pressure alarm should be set 5 to 10 cm of water above peak inspiratory pressure. This alarm may be activated by a plugged E-T tube, air trapping (resulting from short exhalation time at high rates), pneumothorax, or airway secretions requiring suctioning.

e. The gas is most effectively humidified with the use of a heat exchanger that is designed to withstand high pressure. Water and the jet gas mix and then pass through the exchanger. This warms the gas and also humidifies it.

f. An infusion pump may also be used to humidify the inspired gas. The pump places water in front of the jet nozzle and as the gas passes through the jet it combines with the water just outside the jet, humidifying the gas.

g. Because low tidal volumes are delivered with HFV, resulting in an increased potential for atelectasis, PEEP should be employed to reduce the incidence of this.

3. **High-frequency oscillation**

a. High-frequency oscillation (HFO) uses an oscillating device that forces small impulses of gas into and out of the patient's airway.

b. Three types of oscillating devices are used:

(1) Piston—as the piston moves inward a small volume of gas is delivered to the patient. As the piston withdraws, the same amount of gas is drawn away from the patient (exhalation). A sine-type flowwave is usually produced.

(2) Diaphragm—audio loudspeakers have been used to accomplish HFO. As the diaphragm vibrates, the rapid movement, both forward and backward, moves a volume of gas into and out of the patient's lungs.

(3) Flow interrupter—as flow is being delivered to the patient's airways, it passes through a rotating bar with a hole in it. Gas flow periodically passes through the hole and is delivered in small bursts to the patient. Exhalation occurs by normal passive recoil of the lung.

c. Oscillations occur at a rate of 60 to 3600/min at tidal volumes less than anatomic deadspace.

d. HFO may be beneficial in treating patients with large degrees of intrapulmonary shunting. It is being used currently to ventilate infants with respiratory distress syndrome.

B. **Potential advantages of HFV over conventional ventilation**

1. Reduced risk of barotrauma

2. Reduced risk of cardiac embarrassment (decreased venous return and decreased cardiac output)

3. Less fluctuation in ICP

4. Improvement of mucociliary clearance

XIII. ESTIMATING DESIRED VENTILATOR PARAMETER CHANGES

A. Making changes in the FIO₂

$$\text{Desired } FIO_2 = \frac{PaO_2 \text{ (desired)} \times FIO_2 \text{ (current)}}{PaO_2 \text{ (current)}}$$

EXAMPLE: The following data are from a patient on a volume ventilator.

Ventilator Settings		ABG Results	
Mode	Control	pH	7.43
V$_T$	750 ml	PaCO₂	42 torr
Rate	12 breaths/min	PaO₂	53 torr
FIO₂	0.4		

In order to increase this patient's PaO₂ to 80 torr, to what level must the FIO₂ be changed?

$$\text{Desired } FIO_2 = \frac{80 \times 0.4}{53} = \frac{32}{53} = \textbf{0.60}$$

B. Making changes in the ventilator rate

$$\text{Desired rate} = \frac{\text{rate (current)} \times PaCO_2 \text{ (current)}}{PaCO_2 \text{ (desired)}}$$

EXAMPLE: The following data were collected from a patient in the control mode on a volume ventilator.

Ventilator Settings		ABG Results	
V$_T$	800 ml	pH	7.51
FIO₂	0.35	PaCO₂	26 Torr
Rate	16 breaths/min	PaO₂	94 torr

In order to raise the patient's PaCO₂ to 35 torr, the ventilator rate should be adjusted to what level?

$$\text{Desired rate} = \frac{16 \times 26}{35} = \frac{416}{35} = 11.8 \text{ or } \textbf{12/min}$$

C. Making changes in minute volume (V$_E$)
NOTE: **V$_E$ = rate × V$_T$**

$$\text{Desired } (V_E) = \frac{V_E \text{ (current)} \times PaCO_2 \text{ (current)}}{PaCO_2 \text{ (desired)}}$$

EXAMPLE: The following data were collected from a patient on a volume ventilator in the control mode.

Ventilator Settings		ABG Results	
V$_T$	700 ml (0.7 L)	pH	7.28
Rate	10 breaths/min	PaCO₂	54 torr
FIO₂	0.45	PaO₂	74 torr

Which of the following ventilator settings would decrease the patient's PaCO₂ to 45 torr?
A. V$_T$—650 ml, rate—10 breaths/min
B. V$_T$—700 ml, rate—12 breaths/min
C. V$_T$—700 ml, rate—14 breaths/min
D. V$_T$—750 ml, rate—10 breaths/min
E. V$_T$—800 ml, rate—10 breaths/min

In this question we use the preceding equation to derive the necessary minute volume to decrease the PaCO₂ to the desired level. Then we choose the answer with the appropriate minute volume that has been calculated.

$$\text{Desired } V_E = \frac{7 \times 54}{45} = \frac{378}{45} = \textbf{8.4 L}$$

The minute volume required to decrease the PaCO₂ to 45 torr is 8.4 L. In the example, **choice B** represents a minute volume of 8.4 L (700 × 12).

D. Making changes in alveolar ventilation (V$_A$)
NOTE: **V$_A$ = (V$_T$ − anatomic deadspace) × rate**

$$\text{Desired } V_A = \frac{V_A \text{ (current)} \times PaCO_2 \text{ (current)}}{PaCO_2 \text{ (desired)}}$$

EXAMPLE: The following data were recorded from a patient on a volume ventilator in the control mode.

Ventilator Settings		ABG Results	
V$_T$	800 ml (0.8 L)	pH	7.3
Rate	12 breaths/min	PaCO₂	50 torr
FIO₂	0.40	PaO₂	76 torr

Anatomic deadspace   150 ml

Which of the following ventilator settings would decrease the patient's PaCO₂ to 40 torr?
A. V$_T$—700, rate—15 breaths/min
B. V$_T$—800, rate—18 breaths/min
C. V$_T$—800, rate—15 breaths/min
D. V$_T$—850, rate—12 breaths/min
E. V$_T$—900, rate—12 breaths/min

In this question we use the preceding equation to derive the alveolar ventilation necessary to bring the PaCO₂ down to 40 torr. It is the same equation that we used in the previous problem except that we correct for anatomic deadspace, in this case 150 ml, which is subtracted from the V$_T$. This value is then multiplied by the rate to determine the alveolar ventilation.

(800 − 150 = 650 ml or 0.65 L)   0.65 × 12 = 7.8 L

$$\text{Desired } V_A = \frac{7.8 \times 50}{40} = \frac{390}{40} = \textbf{9.75 L}$$

Therefore, an alveolar volume of 9.75 L is required to decrease the $PaCO_2$ to 40 torr. You now choose the appropriate setting—in this case, **choice C.**

(800 − 150 = 650 ml or 0.65 L)
$$6.5L \times 15 = 9.75 L$$

XIV. PRACTICE VENTILATOR PROBLEMS

A. A 75-kg male patient is placed in the control mode on the Bear 2 ventilator. Appropriate data follow:

Ventilator Settings		ABG Results	
V_T	700 ml	pH	7.28
Rate	12 breaths/min	$PaCO_2$	54 torr
FIO_2	0.50	PaO_2	74 torr
PEEP	5 cm of water	HCO_3	23 mEq/L

1. Based on this information, the respiratory care practitioner should recommend which of the following ventilator changes?
   a. Increase PEEP to 10 cm of water
   b. Add 100 ml of mechanical deadspace
   c. Increase the FIO_2 to 0.60
   d. Increase the V_T to 800 ml
   e. Place the patient on CPAP of 4 cm of water

Answer: d. The patient is hypoventilating as a result of an inadequate V_T. The patient weighs 75 kg. Using 10 to 15 ml/kg of ideal body weight to determine adequate V_T, the ventilator should be set on a V_T between 750 and 1125 ml.

B. A patient on the Bennett 7200 is placed in the control mode of ventilation. Pertinent data follow:

Ventilator Settings		ABG Results	
V_T	800 ml	pH	7.41
Rate	12 breaths/min	$PaCO_2$	37 torr
FIO_2	0.60	PaO_2	137 torr
PEEP	8 cm of water	HCO_3	26 mEq/L

1. What is the most appropriate ventilator change to recommend at this time?
   a. Decrease the FIO_2 to 0.50
   b. Increase the V_T to 900 ml
   c. Decrease the rate to 10 breaths/min
   d. Add 50 ml of mechanical deadspace
   e. Decrease the PEEP to 6 cm of water

Answer: e. The patient is ventilating well but is hyperoxygenating on 60% oxygen. Since the oxygen precentage is at a relatively safe level, we may reduce the PaO_2 by decreasing the level of PEEP.

C. A 46-year-old, 80-kg (176-lb) male is being mechanically ventilated on a volume ventilator in the assist/control mode. A list of important data follows:

Ventilator Settings		ABG Results	
FIO_2	0.30	pH	7.46
Rate	12 breaths/min	$PaCO_2$	34 torr
V_T	900 ml	PaO_2	53 torr

1. What is the most appropriate recommendation at this time?
   a. Decrease the rate to 8 breaths/min
   b. Increase V_T to 950 ml
   c. Increase the FIO_2 to 0.50
   d. Place patient on PEEP of 8 cm of water
   e. No ventilator change is necessary

Answer: c. This patient is hyperventilating slightly as a result of hypoxemia. As the PaO_2 increases, hyperventilation should subside. Increasing the FIO_2 or adding PEEP will both elevate the PaO_2, but since the FIO_2 is 0.3, we can safely increase it to as high as 0.6 before adding PEEP.

D. A patient has been placed on a ventilator in the control mode. The following settings have been used.

Ventilator Settings		ABG Results	
V_T	800 ml	pH	7.5
Rate	10 breaths/min	$PaCO_2$	29 torr
FIO_2	0.35	PaO_2	97 torr
		HCO_3	25 mEq/L

1. What would be the most appropriate ventilator change to make at this time?
   a. Increase V_T to 900 ml
   b. Add 5 cm of water PEEP
   c. Increase the FIO_2 to 0.50
   d. Add mechanical deadspace
   e. Decrease the FIO_2 to 0.21

Answer: d. This patient is hyperventilating, and by adding deadspace we can elevate the $PaCO_2$.

E. A 60-kg (132-lb) female patient is on the MA-1 ventilator in the control mode. Pertinent data follow:

Ventilator Settings		ABG Results	
V_T	950 ml	pH	7.52
Rate	12 breaths/min	$PaCO_2$	28 torr
FIO_2	0.4	PaO_2	92 torr

1. What is the appropriate ventilator change at this time?
   a. Increase the FIO_2 to 0.50
   b. Increase V_T to 1000 ml
   c. Decrease rate to 4 breaths/min
   d. Decrease flowrate
   e. Decrease V_T to 700 ml

Answer: e. The V_T setting is greater than 15 ml/kg; therefore, the patient is being hyperventilated. Decreasing the V_T will increase the $PaCO_2$. Decreasing the rate will also increase the $PaCO_2$, but a rate of 4/min (choice c) in the control mode is much too low.

XV. VENTILATOR FLOW-WAVE CAPABILITIES

A. **Square wave (constant flow)**

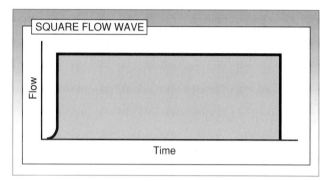

From Persing G. *Entry Level Respiratory Care Review.* Philadelphia: WB Saunders; 1992.

1. With this flow pattern, the flow remains constant throughout inspiration.
2. Changes in airway resistance and compliance will not change the flow pattern under normal circumstances.
3. This type of flow pattern is beneficial to patients with increased respiratory rates.

B. **Sine wave**

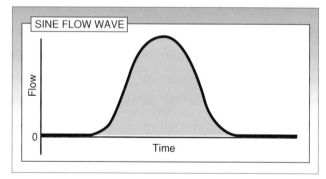

From Persing G. *Entry Level Respiratory Care Review.* Philadelphia: WB Saunders; 1992.

1. Flow gradually accelerates from the beginning of inspiration, then decelerates toward the end of inspiration.
2. This flow pattern benefits patients with increased airway resistance by decreasing airway turbulence produced with this type of flow.

C. **Decelerating flow wave**

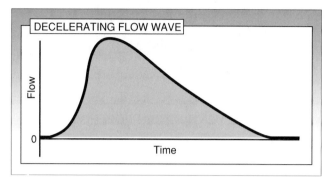

From Persing G. *Entry Level Respiratory Care Review.* Philadelphia: WB Saunders; 1992.

1. Initial flow is high and begins decelerating as inspiration continues.
2. Flow will never decrease more than 50% to 55% of initial flow.
3. Benefits patients with low compliance, as this pattern allows ventilation to occur at a decreased pressure.

D. **Accelerating flow wave**

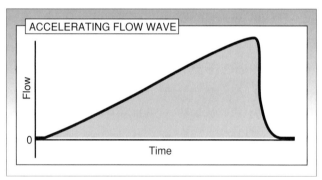

From Persing G. *Entry Level Respiratory Care Review.* Philadelphia: WB Saunders; 1992.

1. Flow is initially slow and accelerates to a peak flow by the end of inspiration.
2. This pattern creates less turbulence of flow at the beginning of inspiration; therefore, more volume may be delivered through narrowed or obstructed airways.

XVI. CHARACTERISTICS OF SPECIFIC MECHANICAL VENTILATORS

A. **Bennett MA-1**
1. An electrically powered, double-circuit, low-pressure–driven, volume ventilator
2. Exhaled volume measured with a bellows spirometer

3. PEEP attained with a separate PEEP valve connected to the side of the ventilator to obtain PEEP levels of up to 15 cm of water
4. IMV is accomplished with an external gas source (discussed earlier in this chapter) attached to the inspiratory limb of the circuit. The potential of "breath-stacking" occurs while in this mode.
5. A low-oxygen inlet pressure alarm will sound when the oxygen high-pressure hose is disconnected from the oxygen wall outlet. Should the high pressure hose be plugged into a compressed air wall outlet inadvertently, the alarm **will not sound**, since this is strictly a low-pressure alarm.
6. The Bennett MA-1 delivers a square flow wave only.
7. An expiratory resistance control may be used to prolong expiration, similar to pursed-lip breathing.
8. The sensitivity control must be adjusted with changes in PEEP levels.
9. The only alarm that alerts personnel of patient disconnection is the exhaled volume spirometer alarm.
10. The I : E ratio alarm will light and sound if inspiration is longer than expiration.

B. **Bennett MA-2**
1. The Bennett MA-2 is an electrically powered and controlled, double-circuit, low-pressure–driven, volume ventilator.
2. Followed the Bennett MA-1 with SIMV and CPAP modes added
3. Exhaled volume measured with a bellows spirometer
4. The Bennett MA-2 incorporates a built-in PEEP valve to provide PEEP levels of up to 45 cm of water.
5. Has the same I : E ratio alarm as the Bennett MA-1
6. Provides a low inspiratory pressure alarm, a high and low oxygen concentration alarm, and a high and low humidifier temperature alarm
7. Provides for only a square flow wave
8. Uses "continuous mandatory ventilation" (CMV) to designate control and assist control ventilation

C. **Bennett 7200, 7200a microprocessor ventilators**
1. The Bennett 7200 is an electrically powered and controlled, single-circuit, high-pressure–driven, volume ventilator.
2. The Bennett 7200 uses a microprocessor that controls the drive mechanism, volume, flow waveform, and oxygen percentage.
3. The Bennett 7200 uses push buttons to set

parameters, with a knob that only adjusts the PEEP/CPAP level.
4. Flow waves that may be used include square, descending ramp, and sine waves.
5. A 100% oxygen suction button may be pushed that increases the oxygen percentage to 100% for 2 minutes and then returns to the initial setting.
6. If the patient becomes apneic for 20 seconds, the machine switches to a V_T of 500 ml, a breath rate of 12 breaths/min, a peak inspiratory flowrate of 45 L/min, 100% oxygen, and a high-pressure limit of 20 cm of water above baseline. The alarm sounds until the alarm condition is reset.
7. Pressure support is available as an option to be used in the SIMV and CPAP modes.
8. Pressure ventilation is available in the continuous mandatory ventilation, SIMV, and CPAP modes. The mandatory breaths are pressure-limited rather than volume-limited.
9. The Bennett 7200 is compliance-compensated, meaning that the gas delivered to the patient has volume subtracted for the temperature change from room to body temperature and volume added to correct for volume lost in the ventilator tubing.
10. Each time the ventilator is turned on, a self-test occurs that checks the function of the microprocessor. An extended self-test may be performed, which also checks the function of the microprocessor and also computes tubing compliance and checks for system leaks.

D. **Siemens Servo 900 C**
1. The Servo 900 C is a pneumatically powered, electronically controlled, single-circuit, low-pressure–driven ventilator.
2. The modes available include volume control, pressure control, SIMV, CPAP, and pressure support.
3. By setting the minute volume control and the rate control, V_T is calculated. (There is no V_T control.)
   a. *EXAMPLE:* The physician writes an order for the patient to be placed on a V_T of 800 ml and a rate of 12 breaths/min.
      Minute volume = V_T × rate
      Minute volume = 0.8 L (800 ml) × 12 = **9.6 L**
      **This ventilator setting is accomplished by adjusting the minute volume control to 9.6 L and setting the rate on 12 breaths/min.
   b. The physician writes an order 8 hours later to decrease the rate to 10 breaths/min.
      **Remember, the rate control alone cannot

be decreased, as this would increase the V_T. By decreasing the rate to 10 breaths/min and leaving the minute volume on 9.6 L, the V_T is now 960 ml (9.6 L).

In order to maintain the same V_T and decrease the rate, multiply the V_T by the new rate and set the minute volume accordingly.

$$0.8 \text{ L (800 ml)} \times 10/\text{min} = 8 \text{ L}$$

**To accomplish the rate change, the rate is decreased to 10 breaths/min and the minute volume is decreased to 8 L.

c. In order to determine what V_T the patient is on given a minute volume and rate simply divide the minute volume by the rate.

EXAMPLE: The patient is on a rate of 15 breaths/min and a minute volume of 10.5 L. What is the patient's V_T?

$$\frac{10.5}{15} = \textbf{700 ml or 0.7 L}$$

4. There is no flowrate control, but there is an inspiratory time percentage control. This control is adjusted to 20%, 25%, 33%, 50%, 67%, or 80%.
5. Each inspiratory percentage time has a specific factor that is derived by dividing it into 100.

Inspiratory % Time	Factor
20	5
25	4
33	3
50	2
67	1.5
80	1.25

6. Inspiratory flowrate is calculated by the following formula:

**Flowrate =
minute volume × inspiratory time % factor**

**EXAMPLE: What is the inspiratory flowrate if the minute volume is 9 L and the inspiratory time percentage is 25%?

Flowrate = 9 × 4 = **36 L/min**

**NOTE: If the sine flow wave is being used, multiply the calculated flowrate by 1.5 (36 × 1.5 = 54 L/min).

7. Inspiratory hold may be accomplished by dialing in an inspiratory pause percentage of 5%, 10%, 20%, or 30%.

8. Sigh rates and volumes cannot be adjusted by the practitioner. When the mode switch is set to the *volume control plus sigh* position, a twice-normal V_T breath will be delivered every 100 breaths. Sighs are not available in any other mode.

E. **Sechrist IV-100B infant ventilator**
1. The Sechrist IV-100B is a pneumatically powered, electrically and *fluidically* controlled, time-cycled, time-limited, preset-pressure, continous-flow ventilator.
2. A microprocessor provides the inspiratory and expiratory times as the user adjusts the inspiratory time and expiratory time control knobs.
3. The inspiratory and expiratory times, the I:E ratio, and the respiratory rate are displayed digitally on the front of the unit.
4. The maximum rate available is 150 breaths/min.
5. Gas from the ventilator flowmeter flows continuously through the circuit, past the patient, and through the exhalation valve. As the fluidic gates close the exhalation valve, gas can no longer flow past it and is diverted to the patient's airway.
6. The exhalation valve remains closed (inspiration) until the preset inspiratory time ends. The inspiratory pressure reached is determined by the inspiratory pressure control setting (adjustable from 7 to 70 cm of water).
7. Because the ventilator is a continuous-flow ventilator, the infant is always breathing in the IMV mode if mandatory breaths are set. A CPAP mode is also available.
8. A PEEP/CPAP control (called the expiratory pressure control) may be adjusted to obtain PEEP/CPAP levels of up to 15 cm of water.
9. A flow-wave control, located above the exhalation valve, may be adjusted to obtain either a square wave or a sine wave.
10. An audible and visual **low-pressure alarm** is the main alarm system with this ventilator and detects leaks in the system or patient disconnection.
11. Although this unit is generally used as a pressure-controlled ventilator, if the pressure limit is not reached, a fairly consistent volume may be delivered with each mechanical breath. This **approximate** volume may be calculated by using the following formula:

**Approximate V_T =
$$\frac{\text{inspiratory time (sec)} \times \text{flow (L/min)}}{60}$$**

XVII. SUMMARY OF VENTILATOR ADJUSTMENTS ACCORDING TO ABG RESULTS

ABG Abnormality	Ventilator Adjustment
Decreased pH Increased $PaCO_2$ Decreased or normal PaO_2	Increase V_T (Maintain 10 to 15 ml/kg) Increase rate
Increased pH Decreased $PaCO_2$	Decrease V_T Decrease rate Add mechanical deadspace
Normal pH Increased $PaCO_2$ PaO_2 of 50 to 60 torr	No adjustment needed as this is a normal ABG result of a patient with chronic obstructive pulmonary disease May place on SIMV
Normal pH Normal $PaCO_2$ Decreased PaO_2 (on PEEP)	Increase FIO_2 if <0.6 Add or increase PEEP if FIO_2 is 0.6 or greater
Normal pH Normal $PaCO_2$ Increased PaO_2 (on PEEP)	Decrease FIO_2 if it is greater than 0.6 Decrease PEEP if FIO_2 is less than 0.6
Decreased pH Normal $PaCO_2$ Decreased bicarbonate	No ventilator changes are necessary Administer bicarbonate

REFERENCES

1. Eubanks D, Bone R. *Comprehensive Respiratory Care.* 2nd ed. St. Louis: CV Mosby; 1990.
2. Dupuis, YG. *Ventilators — Theory and Clinical Application.* St. Louis: CV Mosby; 1986.
3. McPherson SP. *Respiratory Therapy Equipment.* 4th ed. St. Louis: CV Mosby; 1990.
4. Pilbeam SP. *Mechanical Ventilation — Physiological and Clinical Applications.* St. Louis: CV Mosby; 1986.
5. Scanlan C, Spearman C. *Egan's Fundamentals of Respiratory Care.* 5th ed. St. Louis: CV Mosby; 1990.

PRETEST ANSWERS

1. D
2. D
3. B
4. C
5. B
6. A

Disorders of the Respiratory System

PRETEST QUESTIONS*

1. Pursed-lip breathing would be most beneficial in which of the following lung disorders?

A. Emphysema
B. Pulmonary edema
C. Pneumonia
D. Pleural effusion
E. Tuberculosis

2. Upon assessing a patient's laboratory results, you notice that a sputum culture reveals a high eosinophil count. This is characteristic of which of the following pulmonary conditions?

A. Tuberculosis
B. Asthma
C. Pneumonia
D. Pulmonary embolism
E. Cystic fibrosis

3. Which lung condition is characterized by consolidation on chest x-ray film?

A. Pulmonary edema
B. Emphysema
C. Pneumonia
D. Pleural effusion
E. Asthma

4. A 17-year-old asthmatic patient enters the emergency room in moderate respiratory distress. You would expect the blood gases to reveal

A. Acute respiratory acidosis with hypoxemia
B. Metabolic acidosis with hypoxemia
C. Acute respiratory alkalosis with hypoxemia
D. Chronic metabolic alkalosis
E. Normal acid-base status with hypoxemia

5. Which of the following causative agents for pneumonia is characteristically seen in patients with acquired immunodeficiency syndrome (AIDS)?

A. *Pneumocystis carinii*
B. *Klebsiella*
C. *Pseudomonas*
D. *Haemophilus influenzae*
E. *Legionella*

6. Streptokinase is used to treat which of the following lung disorders?

A. Pneumonia
B. Pleural effusion
C. Pneumothorax
D. Pulmonary embolism
E. Sleep apnea

---

*See answers at the end of the chapter.

Disorders of the Respiratory System

I. CHRONIC OBSTRUCTIVE PULMONARY DISEASE (COPD)
**A condition that results in chronic obstruction to air flow within the lungs
**Diseases classified as COPD:
Emphysema
Chronic bronchitis
Asthma
Cystic fibrosis
Bronchiectasis

A. Emphysema
1. **Definition**—permanent abnormal enlargement of the air spaces distal to the terminal bronchioles, which undergo destructive changes in the alveolar walls
   a. Panlobular (panacinar) type
      (1) An acinus is the gas exchange unit of the lung made up of the respiratory bronchiole, alveolar duct, alveolar sacs, and the alveoli.
      (2) The entire acinus is involved in this type of emphysema.
      (3) There is significant loss of lung parenchyma.
      (4) Alveoli are destroyed.
      (5) Bullae are present.
      (6) It is usually associated with emphysema resulting from alpha₁-antitrypsin deficiency.
   b. Centrilobular (centriacinar) type
      (1) Lesion is in the center of the lobules, which results in enlargement and destruction of the respiratory bronchioles
      (2) It usually involves the upper lung fields and is most commonly associated with chronic bronchitis.
   c. Bullous emphysema
      (1) Emphysematous changes are isolated, with the development of bullae.
      (2) A **bulla** is defined as an air space in its distended state that is more than 1 cm in diameter.
      (3) A **bleb** is defined as an air space adjacent to the pleura, usually less than 1 cm in diameter in its distended state.
2. **Etiology**
   a. Smoking
   b. Alpha₁-antitrypsin deficiency (hereditary)
3. **Pathophysiology**
   **a. Elastic recoil of the lung is diminished, resulting in premature airway closure.
   **b. Inspiratory flowrates are normal, whereas expiratory flowrates are reduced.
   c. Air trapping leads to chronic hyperinflation of the lungs and an **increased functional residual capacity (FRC).
   d. **Lung compliance is increased because of the loss of elastic lung tissue from the destructive process.
   e. Emphysema diminishes the area over which gas exchange occurs and is accompanied by regional differences in ventilation and perfusion. This accounts for increased physiologic deadspace and the abnormal arterial blood gas (ABG) results observed in emphysema patients.
4. **Clinical signs and symptoms**
   a. Dyspnea—initially on exertion; progressively worsens
   b. Digital clubbing—results from **chronic hypoxemia
   **c. Increased anterior-posterior chest diameter (barrel chest)
   **d. Use of accessory muscles during normal breathing
   **e. Elevated hemoglobin and hematocrit levels and red blood cell count
   **f. ABG results reveal chronic carbon dioxide retention and hypoxemia (advanced stages).
   g. Reduced breath sounds and resonance to percussion

h. Cyanosis
** i. **Right-sided heart failure (cor pulmonale)** in advanced stages
　(1) Cor pulmonale results from an increased workload on the right ventricle as it attempts to deliver blood through constricted pulmonary blood vessels.
　(2) These vessels are constricted (pulmonary hypertension) as a result of arterial hypoxemia and hypercarbia.
　(3) Chronic pulmonary hypertension results in right ventricular hypertrophy and eventually right-sided heart failure.
** (4) **Cor pulmonale will result in peripheral edema such as pedal edema (ankle edema), distended neck (jugular) veins, and an enlarged liver.**
** (5) **Oxygen therapy is essential in the prevention or treatment of cor pulmonale in patients with chronic respiratory failure.**
　(6) Diuretics and digitalis are indicated when right ventricular failure supervenes the underlying respiratory problems.

5. **X-ray characteristics**
** a. Flattened diaphragm
** b. Hyperinflation
　c. Reduced vascular markings
　d. Bullous lesions

6. **Pulmonary function studies**
** a. Increased residual volume and FRC
　b. Decreased diffusion capacity
　c. Decreased vital capacity
** d. Decreased FEV_1 (forced expiratory volume in 1 second) (decreased FEV_1/forced vital capacity [FVC])
　e. Prolonged nitrogen washout

7. **Treatment**
　a. Cessation of smoking
　b. Adequate hydration
　c. Postural drainage
　d. Bronchodilators
　e. Prevention of infections by immunizations
　f. Exercise (walking)
** g. Breathing exercise training
** (1) Diaphragmatic breathing exercises
** (2) **Pursed-lip breathing**—prevents premature airway closure by producing a back pressure into the airway on exhalation.
** h. Care must be taken when administering oxygen to emphysema patients who chronically retain carbon dioxide and who are chronically hypoxemic. PaO_2 levels should be maintained between 50 and 60 torr to avoid knocking out the patient's "hypoxic drive."

NOTE: If, after placing a patient with severe COPD on oxygen, the PaO_2 increases to greater than 60 to 70 torr and the $PaCO_2$ begins increasing, this should be recognized as knocking out the patient's "hypoxic drive" and the oxygen percentage should be decreased. **Remember, maintain the PaO_2 level at 50 to 60 torr.**
NOTE: If given a choice of which oxygen delivery device to use on a COPD patient—a nasal cannula or Venturi mask at approximately the same percentage—**choose the Venturi mask.**

B. **Chronic bronchitis**
1. **Definition**—chronic, excessive mucus production resulting from an increase in the number and size of mucous glands and goblet cells. It results in a cough and increased mucus production for at least 3 months of the year for more than 2 consecutive years.
2. **Etiology**
　a. Smoking
　b. Males are most commonly affected
3. **Pathophysiology**
　a. Increase in the size of mucous glands
　b. Increase in the number of goblet cells
　c. Inflammation of bronchial walls
　d. Mucous plugs in peripheral airways
　e. Loss of cilia
　f. Emphysematous changes in advanced stages
　g. Narrowing airways leading to air flow obstruction
4. **Clinical signs and symptoms**
　a. Cough with sputum production
　b. Dyspnea on exertion progressing to dyspnea with less effort
　c. Carbon dioxide retention and hypoxemia (advanced stages)
　d. Increased pulmonary vascular resistance (advanced stages)
　e. Increased hemoglobin, hematocrit and red blood cell levels (advanced stages)
　f. Right-sided heart failure (cor pulmonale) in advanced stages
5. **X-ray characteristics**
　a. Not significant in early disease
　b. Hyperinflation (advanced stages)
6. **Pulmonary function studies**
　a. Normal in early disease
　b. Increased residual volume
　c. Decreased FEV_1
　d. Decreased inspiratory flowrates in obstructive bronchitis
7. **Treatment**
　Same as emphysema—refer to previous section
C. **Asthma**
1. **Definition**—a disease characterized by an increased reactivity of the trachea and bronchi to various stimuli resulting in bronchoconstriction

(bronchospasm), increased mucus production, and mucosal swelling

2. **Etiology**
   a. **Extrinsic asthma (allergic asthma)**
      (1) Begins early in life
      (2) Caused by inhalation of airborne antigens (dust, pollen, and so on)
      (3) Exercise often precipitates bronchospasm
   b. **Intrinsic asthma (nonallergic asthma)**
      (1) A nonseasonal, nonallergic form of asthma occurring later in life
      (2) Caused by inhalation of pollutants (dust, fumes, smoke, and so on), by infections, and by emotional crisis
      (3) Usually is a chronic form of asthma that is persistent in nature as opposed to the episodic nature of extrinsic asthma

3. **Pathophysiology**
   a. Mast cells in the bronchial tree are stimulated, causing the release of:
      (1) Histamine
      (2) Leukotrienes
      (3) Slow-reacting substance of anaphylaxis
      (4) Eosinophilic chemotactic factor of anaphylaxis
      (5) Prostaglandins
   b. The release of these substances results in:
      (1) Bronchoconstriction
      (2) Mucosal edema
      (3) Increased mucus production
      (4) Accumulation of eosinophils in the blood
      (5) Vasodilation

4. **Clinical signs and symptoms**
   a. Mild wheezing and cough initially, which may progress to severe dyspnea if the attack is not arrested
   b. Cough is initially nonproductive, progressing to a productive cough by the end of the episode.
   **c. Secretions reveal high eosinophil levels.
   d. Intercostal and supraclavicular retractions
   e. Use of accessory muscles to breathe (severe attack)
   **f. Paradoxical pulse—systolic blood pressure is 10 torr higher on expiration than on inspiration.
   g. Tachycardia and tachypnea
   **h. ABG results initially reveal hypoxemia and low $PaCO_2$ ($PaCO_2$ will increase as attack worsens).
   i. Cyanosis

5. **X-ray characteristics**
   a. Hyperinflation (hyperlucency of lung fields)
   b. Atelectasis—less common
   c. Infiltrates

6. **Pulmonary function studies**
   **a. Decreased FEV_1
   **b. Decreased FVC
   **c. Decreased FEV_1/FVC
   **d. Increased residual volume

7. **Treatment (preventive)**
   a. Prevention (avoid known allergens or causative factors)
   b. Medications
      (1) Bronchodilators
      (2) Cromolyn sodium—prevents attacks by stabilizing the mast cell; not used during an attack**
      (3) Corticosteroids
      (4) Anticholinergic drugs (atropine)

8. **Treatment (during an attack)**
   a. Bronchodilators
   b. Intravenous (IV) fluids
   c. Oxygen therapy
   d. IV aminophylline

9. **Status asthmaticus**—severe asthmatic attack not responding to treatment with an adequate amount of routine medications within a few hours
   a. Patient should be hospitalized immediately.
   b. IV aminophylline
   c. Hydration
   d. IV corticosteroids
   e. Supplemental oxygen
   f. Close monitoring of ABG results and oxygen saturation
   g. Bronchodilators
   h. Chest physiotherapy (if tolerated) to remove mucous plugs and secretions
   i. If not controlled, intubate and institute mechanical ventilation

D. **Cystic fibrosis (mucoviscidosis)**
   Covered in detail in Chapter 13.

E. **Bronchiectasis**
   1. **Definition**—a dilation of the bronchi and bronchioles, chronic in nature, that results in inflammation and damage to the walls of these airways.
   2. **Etiology**
      a. Chronic respiratory infections
      b. Tuberculous lesion
      c. Patients with cystic fibrosis
      d. Bronchial obstruction
   3. **Pathophysiology**
      a. It is not clear whether the chronic dilation is a result of destructive changes in the bronchial walls due to inflammation and infection or possibly a congenital defect of the airways.
      b. Bronchial obstruction may render the mucociliary transport system ineffective, leading to an accumulation of thick secretions.

c. The bronchial wall is destroyed, with resultant atrophy of the mucosal layer.

4. **Clinical signs and symptoms**

**a. Productive cough with large amounts of thick, purulent secretions; may be foul smelling; often a layering of the sputum occurs

b. Tachypnea and tachycardia

c. Hemoptysis

d. Recurrent pulmonary infections

e. Digital clubbing

f. Cyanosis

g. Respiratory alkalosis with hypoxemia (early stage)

h. Chronic respiratory acidosis with hypoxemia (late stage)

i. Barrel chest

5. **X-ray characteristics**

a. Increased lung markings

b. Flattened diaphragm

c. Segmental atelectasis

6. **Pulmonary function studies**

a. Decreased FVC

b. Decreased FRC

c. Decreased FEV_1

d. Decreased forced expiratory flow $(FEF)_{25\%-75\%}$

*Because of the decreased values in both flows and volumes, this disease may be both obstructive and restrictive in nature.

7. **Treatment**

a. Chest physical therapy

b. Aerosol therapy

c. Bronchodilator therapy

d. Mucolytics—acetylcysteine (Mucomyst)

e. Antibiotics

f. Oxygen therapy

g. Expectorants

II. LOWER RESPIRATORY TRACT INFECTIONS

A. Pneumonia

1. **Definition**—acute inflammation of the gas exchange units of the lungs

2. **Etiology**

a. Variety of organisms (discussed later)

b. Decreased airway defense mechanisms due to:

(1) Ineffective cough

(2) Obtunded airway reflexes

(3) Impaired mucociliary transport system

(4) Obstructed airways

c. Various conditions result in predisposition to pneumonia:

(1) COPD

(2) Alcoholism

(3) Malnutrition

(4) Seizure disorders

(5) Chronic debilitating illnesses

(6) Major surgical procedures

(7) Old age

3. **Pathophysiology**

a. Pathogenic microorganisms that reach the gas exchange areas of the lung cause an intense tissue reaction, resulting in production of inflammatory exudates and cells.

b. The white blood cells phagocytize the invading organisms, leading to further inflammation.

c. As the lungs begin filling with the inflammatory exudates and cells, they become **consolidated**.

d. If tissue necrosis is not present, the lung will heal and return to normal functioning.

e. If necrosis occurs, healing is slow, with production of fibrous scar tissue, resulting in pulmonary fibrosis and loss of normal lung function.

4. **Clinical signs and symptoms**

a. Infection

b. Malaise

c. Fever

d. Chest pain

e. Dyspnea and tachycardia

f. Inspiratory crackles on auscultation

5. **X-ray characteristics**

**a. Consolidation

b. Air bronchogram

6. **Types of pneumonia**

a. Bacterial

(1) *Streptococcus pneumoniae* (pneumococcal pneumonia)—most common bacterial pneumonia**

(2) *Haemophilus influenzae*

(3) *Klebsiella pneumoniae*

(4) *Legionella pneumoniae*

(5) *Pseudomonas aeruginosa*

b. *Mycoplasma pneumoniae*—smaller than bacteria and more common in children

c. Viral

(1) Influenza

(2) Adenovirus

(3) Chickenpox

d. Protozoan

(1) **Pneumocystis carinii pneumonia

(a) Pneumonia commonly seen in patients with acquired immunodeficiency syndrome (AIDS).

(b) This severe complication is diagnosed in about 60% of AIDS cases.

(c) Definitive diagnosis is made from cultures of lung secretions and lung tissue.

(d) *P. carinii* is commonly treated with the antiprotozoan drug **pentamidine via aerosolization.

7. **Treatment** (pneumonias in general)
   a. Antibiotics
   b. Supplemental oxygen
   c. Chest physiotherapy
   d. Adequate hydration
   e. Adequate nutrition
   f. Tracheal suctioning (if removal of secretions is poor because of ineffective cough)

B. **Lung abscess**
1. **Definition**—an infection of the lung that is characterized by a localized accumulation of pus with destruction of the surrounding tissue.
2. **Etiology**
   a. Most common cause is anaerobic bacteria
   b. Aerobic bacteria, including staphylococci, streptococci, and some gram-negative bacteria may be less common causes.
   c. May follow aspiration
   d. Associated with lung cancer
3. **Pathophysiology**
   a. In the acute phase, it looks much like pneumonia.
   b. As progression occurs, necrosis is evident, which may spread to adjacent lung tissue.
4. **Clinical signs and symptoms**
   a. Fever
   b. Productive cough (initially nonproductive or minimal production followed by production of **purulent, foul-smelling secretions**)
   c. Chest pain
   d. Weight loss
   e. Hemoptysis
   f. Digital clubbing
   g. Tachycardia
   h. Tachypnea
5. **X-ray characteristics**
   a. Localized area of consolidation
   b. Most common sites include the superior segments of lower lobes and posterior segments of upper lobes (due to position during an aspiration event).
6. **Laboratory findings**
   a. Increased white blood cell count
   b. Anemia (decreased red blood cell count)
   c. Sputum culture reveals pus cells and necrotic material.
7. **Treatment**
   a. Antibiotics
   b. Postural drainage
   c. Adequate nutrition

NOTE: If an abscess ruptures into the pleura, pus will accumulate in the pleural space. This is called an **empyema** and it should be drained prior to chest physiotherapy.

C. **Tuberculosis (TB)**
1. **Definition**—a granulomatous bacterial infection, chronic in nature, affecting the lungs and other organs of the body.
2. **Etiology**—caused by the inhalation or ingestion of the bacteria *Mycobacterium tuberculosis*. These organisms are known as **acid-fast bacilli** and are usually spread through coughing and sneezing. Diagnosis is obtained from skin tests, chest x-ray studies, and sputum culture showing the presence of acid-fast bacilli.
3. **Pathophysiology**
   a. After the bacilli are inhaled, they enter the alveoli, resulting in an inflammatory reaction similar to that seen with pneumonia (discussed earlier in this chapter).
   b. Macrophages enter the infected area and engulf the bacilli without fully killing them.
   c. The lung tissue surrounding this area encapsulates the bacilli, providing a protective covering. This is called a granuloma or tubercle.
   d. The granuloma fills with necrotic material and is referred to as a caseous (cheese-like) granuloma.
   e. If the patient's immunologic system controls this process or if antituberculosis drugs are given, the lung tissue will fibrose and calcify as healing occurs. This may result in stiffness or decreased lung compliance in the affected area.
   f. In most cases, the patient's own immunologic mechanisms keep the bacilli in check, but they will remain dormant in the lungs for many years, resulting in a positive TB skin test. These encapsulated bacilli can escape in later years, causing infection.
   g. Chronic dilation of the bronchi (bronchiectasis) may result during the healing process of TB.
   h. In uncontrolled cases, the tubercles increase in size and combine to form larger tubercles that may rupture, permitting air and the infected material to enter the pleural space, bronchi, and bronchioles.

NOTE: It is important to note that most individuals infected with TB bacteria often have few if any symptoms. The primary TB heals completely, possibly leaving a small scar, which could calcify later in life.

4. **Clinical signs and symptoms**
   a. Cough

**b. Sputum production—positive for acid-fast bacilli
  c. Tachycardia
  d. Increased cardiac output
  e. Chest pain
  f. Hemoptysis
  g. Dull percussion note
  h. Rales and rhonchi
  i. Hyperventilation and hypoxemia (early stages)
  j. Chronic respiratory acidosis with hypoxemia (late stages)
  k. Cyanosis (severe cases)

5. **X-ray characteristics**
  a. Enlarged lymph nodes in hilar region (lymphadenopathy)
  b. Pleural effusion
  c. Cavitation
  d. Ghon's complex (lung lesion and lymph node involvement)
  e. Fibrosis
  f. Infiltrates

6. **Pulmonary function studies**
  a. Decreased vital capacity
  b. Decreased FRC
  c. Decreased residual volume
  d. Decreased total lung capacity

NOTE: These pulmonary function findings are characteristic of the restrictive lung processes that occur in tuberculosis.

7. **Treatment**
  a. Supplemental oxygen
  b. Antituberculosis drugs
    (1) Rifampin
    (2) Isoniazid (INH)
    (3) Ethambutol
    (4) Streptomycin

NOTE: These drugs are used in combination for 2 to 4 months.

  c. Placement in respiratory isolation
  d. Routine airway maintenance

III. OTHER LUNG DISORDERS

A. **Pulmonary edema (cardiogenic)**
  1. **Definition**—an excessive amount of fluids in the lung tissues and/or alveoli due to an increase in pulmonary capillary pressure resulting from abnormal left heart function.
  2. **Etiology**
    a. Left heart failure
    b. Aortic stenosis
    c. Mitral valve stenosis
    d. Systemic hypertension

NOTE: These four causes result in the backup of fluid from the heart into the pulmonary capillaries, which become engorged, leading to pulmonary edema.

    e. Alveolar capillary membrane leak due to injury, such as seen in adult respiratory distress syndrome (noncardiogenic pulmonary edema)

  3. **Pathophysiology**
    a. Fluid is maintained within the capillaries by two forces:
      (1) **Plasma oncotic pressure** (pressure trying to keep fluid in the capillaries)
      (2) **Capillary hydrostatic pressure** (pressure trying to push fluid out of the capillaries)
    b. Oncotic pressure is normally much higher than capillary hydrostatic pressure, keeping fluid in the capillaries.
    c. As fluid from the heart backs up into the pulmonary circulation, capillary hydrostatic pressure increases to greater than plasma oncotic pressure, and fluid leaks out into the interstitial spaces.
    d. Excess fluid overwhelms the lymphatics (which normally drain the interstitial spaces) and drains into the alveoli, resulting in **decreased lung compliance**.
    e. Airway resistance increases because of excess fluid.
    f. A widened A-a gradient due to intrapulmonary shunting and ventilation/perfusion (V/Q) mismatch results.

  4. **Clinical signs and symptoms**
  **a. Dyspnea
    (1) **Orthopnea—dyspnea while lying down (relieved by sitting upright in semi-Fowler's or Fowler's position)
    (2) **Paroxysmal nocturnal dyspnea—severe attack of dyspnea occurring during sleep that awakens the patient (relieved by sitting up in semi-Fowler's position)
  **b. Productive cough with thin, pink, frothy secretions
  **c. Rales auscultated in bases (all lung fields in severe edema)
    d. Tachypnea
    e. Cyanosis
  ** f. Diaphoresis—sweating
    g. Distended neck veins
    h. Tachycardia or other arrhythmias

  5. **X-ray characteristics**
    a. Increased vascular markings
    b. Interstitial edema
    c. Enlarged heart shadow

  6. **Treatment**

a. Oxygen administration (percentage based on PaO$_2$)

b. Cardiac glycosides

c. Ventilatory support with positive end-expiratory pressure (PEEP) (if severe)

d. Maintain adequate airway

e. Morphine

f. Intermittent positive pressure breathing with ethyl alcohol (40% to 50%)

g. Diuretics (furosemide [Lasix])

B. **Pulmonary embolism**

1. **Definition**—obstruction of the pulmonary artery or one of its branches by a blood clot. An **embolus** is a clot that travels through the bloodstream from another vessel and lodges in a smaller one, thus obstructing blood flow.

2. **Etiology**

a. The blood clot usually originates in deep veins of the legs or pelvic area, dislodges, and travels back to the heart through the venous system, lodging in the pulmonary artery.

b. The clot originally forms because of stagnation or venous stasis from prolonged bed rest, immobility because of pain of trauma or surgery, or paralysis.

c. Seen in patients with COPD and venous stasis resulting from the increased viscosity of the blood.

3. **Pathophysiology**

a. Blood flow is obstructed to areas of the involved lung, contributing to deadspace ventilation (ventilation without perfusion).

b. Lung compliance decreases

c. Widened A-a gradient results from intrapulmonary shunting and V/Q mismatch.

d. Lung volumes decrease.

4. **Clinical signs and symptoms**

a. Dyspnea

b. Chest pain

c. Tachypnea

d. Cough

e. Pleuritic pain

f. Hemoptysis

g. Tenderness and swelling in lower extremities due to thrombophlebitis

h. Tachycardia

i. Cyanosis

j. Decreased breath sounds over the affected area (wheezing and rales may be heard)

5. **X-ray characteristics**

a. May be normal

b. Decreased lung volume

c. Linear densities of atelectasis

d. Pleural effusion

e. Elevated hemidiaphragm

6. **Treatment**

a. Prevention

(1) Use of elastic stockings

(2) Leg elevation

(3) Ambulation

(4) Small doses of heparin (anticoagulant)

b. Anticoagulation therapy

(1) Heparin

(2) Sodium warfarin (Coumadin)

(3) Streptokinase or urokinase in massive embolus

c. Supplemental oxygen

d. Hypotensive treatment

(1) Vasopressors

(2) Fluids

C. **Adult respiratory distress syndrome**

1. **Definition**—a group of symptoms causing acute respiratory failure resulting from pulmonary injury from various causes

2. **Etiology**

a. Diffuse lung injury

(1) Sepsis

(2) Aspiration

(3) Near drowning

(4) Oxygen toxicity

(5) Shock

(6) Thoracic trauma

(7) Extensive burn

(8) Inhalation of toxic gases

(9) Fluid overload

(10) Fat embolism

(11) Narcotic overdose

b. Most patients have no previous pulmonary problems.

3. **Pathophysiology**

a. Lung injury occurs followed by an inflammatory process.

b. Alveolar capillary membrane begins to leak, causing noncardiogenic pulmonary edema.

c. Fluid builds up in the interstitial spaces, alveoli, and distal airways.

d. Surfactant production decreases and along with excessive fluid in the alveoli and airways, atelectasis results.

**e. Because of inflammatory cells, fibrin, and cellular debris resulting from the inflammatory process, the lungs become stiff and lung compliance decreases.

f. In severe cases, the lungs may become almost entirely atelectatic, leading to large intrapulmonary shunting.

4. **Clinical signs and symptoms**

**a. Hypoxemia—in severe cases it is refractory (not responsive) to oxygen therapy

b. Cyanosis

c. Severe dyspnea and cough

**d. Decreased lung compliance
  e. Suprasternal and intercostal retractions
  f. Widened A-a gradient on 100% oxygen (severe cases)
  g. Tachypnea
5. **X-ray characteristics**
  a. Interstitial edema
  b. Alveolar edema (fluffy infiltration)
6. **Treatment**
  a. Usually not managed well on high oxygen concentrations alone because of decreased lung compliance
  **b. Mechanical ventilation with PEEP
    **(1) Because the lungs are noncompliant, peak inspiratory pressures are quite elevated.
    **(2) Add PEEP if PaO_2 is below normal with an FIO_2 of 0.6 or greater.
  c. Monitor heart pressures (pulmonary artery pressure, pulmonary capillary wedge pressure (PCWP)) with Swan-Ganz catheter
  d. Diuretics
  e. Routine airway maintenance
D. **Pneumothorax**
  1. **Definition**—the presence of air in the pleural space
  2. **Etiology**
    a. Spontaneous pneumothorax
      (1) Develops without trauma having occurred
      (2) Seen most commonly in tall, thin young males and results from bleb rupture
      (3) Seen in COPD patients as a result of bullous disease and bleb rupture
    b. Traumatic pneumothorax
      (1) Broken ribs
      (2) Puncture wound
      (3) Chest or neck surgery
  3. **Pathophysiology**
    a. Negative pressure is normally present in the pleural space. Any communication between the atmospheric air and the pleural space will draw air into the space, causing the lung to collapse.
    b. A **tension pneumothorax** occurs if the opening in the lung to the pleural space acts as a one-way valve permitting air to enter the space but not allowing the air to exit.
      (1) Ventilation of the affected lung diminishes.
      **(2) The trapped air increases pressure on the affected side, pushing the trachea and mediastinum to the unaffected side.
      (3) The **immediate action to take is to relieve the pressure in the pleural space by inserting a needle into the second or third intercostal space.

  c. The volume of the unaffected lung will increase and more blood will perfuse it, which helps prevent severe hypoxemia.
4. **Clinical signs and symptoms**
  a. Chest pain
  b. Dyspnea
  c. Decreased breath sounds over affected lung
  d. Hyperresonant percussion note over affected lung
  e. Asymmetric chest excursion
  f. Tachypnea (severe cases)
  g. Cyanosis (severe cases)
5. **X-ray characteristics**
  **a. Hyperlucency
  **b. Deviation of heart, trachea, and mediastinum to the opposite (unaffected) side if tension pneumothorax is present
NOTE: Although a chest x-ray study makes a definitive diagnosis for a pneumothorax in patients of all ages, **transillumination** with a fiberoptic probe has been successful for the diagnosis of a pneumothorax in infants. The transilluminator has a light on its distal tip, and when placed over areas of free air in the pleural space, transillumination will be greater than in other areas.
6. **Treatment**
  a. Needle aspiration—immediate if tension pneumothorax**
  b. Placement of chest tube
  c. Supplemental oxygen as needed (monitor oxygen saturation or ABG results)
E. **Pleural effusion**
  1. **Definition**—excessive fluid in the pleural space
    a. Transudate—fluid caused by an imbalance between transcapillary pressure and plasma oncotic pressure
    b. Exudate—fluid caused by increased capillary permeability as in inflammation
  2. **Etiology**
    a. Transudative pleural effusion
      **(1) Congestive heart failure (most common)
      (2) Cirrhosis of the liver
      (3) Kidney disease
    b. Exudative pleural effusion
      (1) Infections
      (2) Trauma
      (3) Surgery
      (4) Tumors
      (5) Pulmonary embolism
  3. **Pathophysiology**
    a. Fluid accumulates in the pleural space as a result of an imbalance between the formation of the fluid and how much is absorbed.
    b. Increased fluid formation may cause pleural effusion.

c. Decreased absorption may cause pleural effusion.
4. **Clinical signs and symptoms**
   a. Chest pain
   b. Dyspnea
   c. Dullness to percussion
   d. Lack of breath sounds over the fluid
5. **X-ray characteristics**
   a. Blunting of costophrenic angle
   b. Homogeneous density in dependent part of the hemithorax

NOTE: For small effusions, a lateral decubitus x-ray film should be taken.

6. **Treatment**
   a. Drain fluid by thoracentesis.
   b. Chest tube drainage may be necessary in chronic cases.
   c. Supplemental oxygen as needed (monitor ABG results or oxygen saturation)

III. SLEEP APNEA

A. Sleep apnea is diagnosed in patients who have at least 30 episodes of apnea over a 6-hour period of sleep.
B. The apneic period may last from 20 seconds to more than 1.5 minutes.
C. **Types of sleep apnea**
   1. **Obstructive sleep apnea**
      a. Apnea due to upper airway anatomic obstruction
      b. During the apneic period, the patient exhibits **strong and often intense respiratory effort (no respiratory effort seen with central sleep apnea).
      c. Although sleep posture (sleeping on side rather than supine) has some benefits, **the use of continuous positive airway pressure (CPAP) while sleeping is the most effective method for treating obstructive sleep apnea.
      d. Obstructive sleep apnea may be associated with:
         (1) Obesity
         (2) Excessive pharyngeal tissue
         (3) Deviated nasal septum
         (4) Laryngeal web
         (5) Laryngeal stenosis
         (6) Enlarged adenoids or tonsils
      e. **Symptoms of obstructive sleep apnea**
         (1) Loud snoring
         (2) Hypersomnolence (excessive daytime sleeping)
         (3) Morning headache
         (4) Nausea
         (5) Personality changes
   2. **Central sleep apnea**
      a. Apnea occurs because of the failure of the central respiratory centers (medulla) to send signals to the respiratory muscles.
      b. **It is characterized by the lack of inspiratory effort with no diaphragmatic movement (unlike obstructive sleep apnea).
      c. This type of sleep apnea is associated with central nervous system disorders.
      d. Central sleep apnea may be associated with:
         (1) Hypoventilation syndrome
         (2) Encephalitis
         (3) Spinal surgery
         (4) Brainstem disorders
      e. **Symptoms of central sleep apnea**
         (1) Insomnia
         (2) Mild snoring
         (3) Depression
         (4) Fatigue during the day

NOTE: Some patients may have a combination of both obstructive and central sleep apnea, which is defined as mixed sleep apnea.

D. **Sleep studies to diagnose sleep apnea**
   1. Recently sleep studies have become a very effective method in the diagnosis of sleep apnea and other breathing disorders such as sudden infant death syndrome.
   2. Sleep studies are also valuable in determining the causes, severity, and pathophysiologic effects of the breathing disorder during sleep.
   3. **Polysomnography refers to events that are recorded graphically while the individual is sleeping.
   4. Continuous recordings on graph paper **(polysomnogram) during the sleep study include:
      a. Eye movement (electrooculogram)
      b. Brain wave activity (electroencephalogram)
      c. Electrocardiogram
      d. Lack of air flow (apnea)—determined with the use of a carbon dioxide analyzer, thermistor, tracheal sound recorder, or pneumotachygraph
      e. Chest and abdominal movement
      f. Oxygen saturation using an ear oximeter.

REFERENCES

1. Des Jardins T. *Clinical Manifestations of Respiratory Disease.* 2nd ed. Chicago: Year Book Medical Publishers; 1990.
2. Farzan S. *A Concise Handbook of Respiratory Diseases.* 3rd ed. Norwalk, CT: Appleton & Lange, 1992.
3. Mitchell R, Petty T. *Synopsis of Clinical Pulmonary Disease.* 3rd ed. St. Louis: CV Mosby; 1982.

PRETEST ANSWERS

1. A

2. B

3. C

4. C

5. A

6. D

Neonatal/Pediatric Respiratory Care

PRETEST QUESTIONS*

1. An APGAR score of 5 is determined 5 minutes following delivery of a term infant. Which of the following should be done at this time?

A. Stimulate and deliver low to moderate oxygen concentration.
B. Intubate and place on mechanical ventilation.
C. Intubate and place on continuous positive airway pressure (CPAP) and 80% oxygen.
D. Place on nasal CPAP and 100% oxygen.
E. Conduct routine observation and send infant to normal newborn nursery.

2. The foramen ovale and ductus arteriosus remain patent in infants with persistent fetal circulation as a direct result of which of the following?

A. Hypocarbia
B. Pulmonary hypertension
C. Hyperoxia
D. Arterial hypotension
E. Cor pulmonale

3. Which of the following *is not* an indication for nasal CPAP in an infant?

A. To increase static lung compliance
B. To decrease functional residual capacity (FRC)
C. To decrease pulmonary vascular resistance (PVR)
D. To decrease intrapulmonary shunting
E. To decrease the work of breathing

_____
*See answers at the end of the chapter.

4. Which of the following are complications of an umbilical artery catheter (UAC)?
   I. Pneumothorax
   II. Thromboembolism
   III. Infection

A. I only
B. II only
C. I and III only
D. II and III only
E. I, II, and III

5. Which of the following may occur as a result of cold stress to an infant?
   I. Hypoxemia
   II. Metabolic acidemia
   III. Hypoglycemia
   IV. Decreased oxygen consumption

A. I and III only
B. II and IV only
C. I, II, and III only
D. I, II, and IV only
E. II, III, and IV only

6. An elevation in the level of chloride in the perspiration is diagnostic for which of the following lung conditions?

A. Bronchiolitis
B. Cystic fibrosis
C. Hyaline membrane disease
D. Epiglottitis
E. Croup

CHAPTER 13
Neonatal/Pediatric Respiratory Care

I. NEONATAL RESPIRATORY CARE

A. **The "high-risk infant"**
1. The term high-risk infant describes an infant who is at greater risk for death, either before or after birth, or in whom there is a higher probability of a permanent disability.
2. Maternal factors involved with high-risk infants:
   a. Age (less than 16 years or more than 35 years)
   b. Diabetes
   c. Drug, alcohol, or tobacco abuse
   d. Infections
   e. Previous cesarean section
   f. High blood pressure
   g. Previous history of infant with respiratory problems or anomalies
   h. Lack of adequate prenatal care
3. Other factors associated with high-risk infants
   a. Premature rupture of membranes—increases the risk for fetal infection, especially pneumonia
   b. Premature delivery (<38 weeks)
   c. Postmature delivery (>42 weeks)
   d. Meconium in amniotic fluid
   e. Prolapsed cord
   f. Prolonged labor
   g. Abnormal fetal presentation (i.e., breech)
B. **Assessment of the neonate**
1. Assessing gestational age
   a. The **Dubowitz** scoring system is one of the most accurate means of estimating the baby's gestational age.
   b. The Dubowitz system scores the infant on 11 neuromuscular signs and 10 external characteristics.
   c. Each specific sign is worth a given number of points, and the infant is given all or part of those points depending on the assessment of that particular sign or characteristic.

   d. Points from each assessed area are totaled and plotted on a graph, which determines the infant's gestational age.
   e. Areas assessed include skin thickness, color and transparency, amount of vernix present, plantar creases, posture, and muscle tone.
   f. Normal gestational age is 38 to 42 weeks.
   g. The calculated gestational age can then be plotted on a graph along with the infant's birth weight to determine if the infant is appropriate for gestational age (AGA), small for gestational age (SGA), or large for gestational age (LGA).
2. **APGAR scoring system**
   a. This system evaluates the infant's general condition within 1 to 5 minutes following birth.
   b. The areas of assessment and point system are listed below:

Assessed sign	Score		
	0	**1**	**2**
Heart rate	None	<100	>100
Respiratory effort	None	Slow, irregular	Strong cry
Color	Pale, blue	Body pink, extremities blue	Totally pink
Reflex irritability	No response	Grimace	Sneeze or cough
Muscle tone	Limp	Some flexion	Active flexion

   c. The APGAR score is taken at 1 minute after delivery to determine if immediate intervention is required and again at 5 minutes after birth.

d. APGAR results (1 minute) and proper intervention:
   (1) **7 to 10** = normal; routine observation, suction upper airway with bulb syringe, dry the infant and place under a warmer
   (2) **4 to 6** = moderate asphyxia; stimulation and oxygen administration
   (3) **0 to 3** = severe asphyxia; immediate resuscitation with ventilatory assistance
e. The 5-minute APGAR score is useful in determining the infant's response to intervention, and a score of less than 6 is associated with major complications, with the infant being treated in an intensive care nursery.
f. The five assessed signs in the APGAR scoring system may be more easily remembered by using the following reference:
   "A"—appearance (color)
   "P"—pulse (heart rate)
   "G"—grimace (reflex irritability)
   "A"—activity (muscle tone)
   "R"—respiration (respiratory effort)

NOTE: Acrocyanosis, or cyanosis in the hands and feet, is normal following birth, but cyanosis observed in the mucous membranes or lips indicates oxygen therapy must be administered immediately.

3. **Silverman scoring system**
   a. This system helps determine the severity of respiratory distress.
   b. The infant is assessed in five areas:
      (1) Intercostal retractions
      (2) Xiphoid retractions
      (3) Chest lag/paradoxical breathing
      (4) Nasal flaring—often the first and/or only sign of respiratory distress
      (5) Grunting—an audible expiratory grunt, caused by the infant partially closing the glottis during exhalation in order to prevent alveolar collapse, is a common sign of respiratory distress.
   c. Each assessed area is worth from 0 to 2 points, with the lowest score indicating minimal distress (as opposed to the highest score being the best on the APGAR).

4. **Other clinical assessments**
   a. Respiratory rate—normally 40 to 60 breaths/min
   b. Blood pressure—normal systolic = 60 to 90 torr
      normal diastolic = 30 to 60 torr
   c. Arterial blood gas (ABG) levels (normal on room air)

pH   7.35–7.45 (no less than 7.25 immediately after birth)

PaCO$_2$	35–45 torr
PaO$_2$	50–70 torr
Bicarbonate	20–26 mEq/l
B.E.	−5–+5

C. **Oxygen delivery devices for neonates**
   1. Incubators (Isolette)

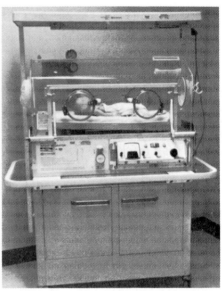

From Scanlon C, Spearman C, Sheldon R. *Egan's Fundamentals of Respiratory Care.* 5th ed. St. Louis: CV Mosby; 1990.

   a. Inlet nipples on the incubator allow attachment of oxygen tubing, which supplies the flow of oxygen to the inside of the incubator.
   b. Low levels (21% to 40%) and high levels (40% to 100%) are obtainable on most models by adjusting a lever that alters the amount of room air entrainment. Most units have a red lever that identifies low or high levels of oxygen use. If the lever is in a vertical position, the oxygen percentage is greater than 40%. If the lever is in a horizontal position, it indicates oxygen percentages of less than 40%.
   c. Oxygen may also be delivered into the incubator via aerosol tubing from a nebulizer set on a specific percentage. The tubing is placed through one of the port holes of the incubator.
   d. The disadvantage of using an incubator with an infant on supplemental oxygen is the inconsistent oxygen percentage resulting from leaks in the incubator when it is opened to administer care to the infant.

2. **Oxygen hood**

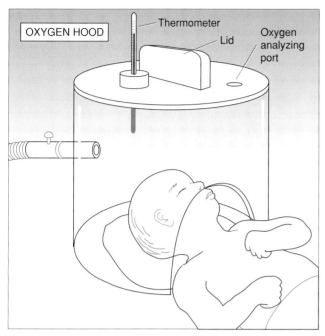

From Persing G. *Entry Level Respiratory Care Review.* Philadelphia: WB Saunders; 1992.

a. The oxygen hood is the recommended method for delivering oxygen to the infant in the range of 21% to 100%.

b. A heated nebulizer connected to an oxygen blender is the most common method of oxygen delivery. The aerosol tubing connects to the back of the hood. If a blender is used to regulate the oxygen percentage, the nebulizer must be set on 100% so that no air entrainment occurs, which would alter the blender percentage.

c. A heated humidifier (Cascade or passover) is often used rather than a nebulizer to prevent overhydration of the infant.

d. The percentage of oxygen should be analyzed continuously with an oxygen analyzer. A port in the top of the hood makes analyzing possible.

** (It should be noted that the oxygen should be analyzed as close to the infant's airway as possible, since the percentage of oxygen is somewhat higher at the bottom of the hood than at the top.)

e. A heated nebulizer or humidifier should be used because cold gas blowing on the infant's face may induce apnea, and colder temperatures in the hood may increase the infant's oxygen consumption.

f. Flows into the hood should be at least 5 L/min in order to prevent carbon dioxide buildup in the hood.

g. Temperatures inside the hood should be closely monitored through a port in the top of the hood to avoid overheating or underheating the infant.

h. It has been proved that noise levels inside the hood are a source of hearing loss in the infant. To keep noise levels to a minimum, nebulizers that entrain air should not be used because of the increased noise level they produce.

3. **Nasal catheter/cannula**

a. Nasal catheters and cannulas are available in infant sizes and are most commonly used for long-term oxygen therapy in the treatment of bronchopulmonary dysplasia (BPD) and other chronic diseases.

b. The flowmeters used to deliver oxygen through the catheter or cannula should be calibrated in small increments so that 0.25 or 0.5 L/min is available.

4. **Nasal CPAP**

a. CPAP is most commonly administered to infants through the use of nasal prongs.

b. CPAP may also be administered with a mask, endotracheal (E-T) tube, or nasopharyngeal tube.

c. **Indications for nasal CPAP**

(1) To improve oxygenation
   **NOTE: In order to prevent pulmonary tissue damage (e.g., BPD) from high FIO_2 levels, CPAP should be administered. The FIO_2 should be no higher than 0.6 to maintain normal PaO_2 levels if possible.

(2) To increase static lung compliance

(3) To increase FRC

(4) To decrease the work of breathing

(5) To decrease intrapulmonary shunting

(6) To decrease PVR

d. **Complications of nasal CPAP**

(1) Barotrauma (pneumothorax)

(2) Decreased venous return resulting in decreased cardiac output
   NOTE: These two complications are less likely to occur if the infant has respiratory distress syndrome (RDS) from the reduced static lung compliance. Infants with normal lungs would be more prone to these complications.

(3) Air trapping

(4) Pressure necrosis

(5) Loss of CPAP from crying or displacement

e. When CPAP is used, ABGs should be obtained occasionally to determine the $PaCO_2$.

If PaCO$_2$ levels begin to rise, mechanical ventilation will be necessary.

f. The idea of nasal CPAP on infants is based on the fact that infants are obligate nose breathers. If the baby cries, CPAP will be lost.

D. **Hazards of oxygen therapy in the neonate**
1. **Retrolental fibroplasia (RLF)**
   a. This condition is also called neonatal retinopathy.
   **b. RLF is caused by high levels of oxygen in the blood (PaO$_2$ of >100 torr).
   c. RLF occurs primarily in premature infants who have very fragile retinal blood vessels.
   d. Initially, the high arterial oxygen levels cause constriction of the retinal vessels. As the vessels remain constricted, new vessels form in an attempt to oxygenate the retina.
   e. This growth of new vessels leads to hemorrhaging within the retina, retinal detachment, and blindness.
   f. The degree of blindness varies in each situation, and infants exposed to supplemental oxygen should have an eye examination before discharge.
   g. Arterial blood samples should be obtained frequently while the infant is on oxygen therapy to determine the oxygen level in the blood. **If the infant has a ductal shunt** (discussed later in this chapter), **the blood must be drawn from the right radial, brachial, or temporal artery to measure the PaO$_2$ of the blood going to the head.** If no shunt exists, blood may be drawn from the umbilical artery catheter or any peripheral artery.
2. **Bronchopulmonary dysplasia (BPD)**
   a. BPD is caused by long-term supplemental oxygen and mechanical ventilation.
   b. Damage occurs in the alveolar epithelium, causing destruction of pulmonary tissues.
   NOTE: BPD is discussed in detail later in this chapter.
E. **Sites for obtaining arterial blood**
1. **Umbilical artery**
   a. **UAC** is normally placed in critically ill infants who will require frequent ABG analysis.
   b. The catheter is inserted into one of the two umbilical arteries. After insertion, the position of the catheter should be determined by x-ray studies.
   c. The tip of the catheter should rest in the **descending aorta** at either one of the following vertebral levels on x-ray film:

(1) T-6 to T-10 (thoracic aorta)
(2) L-3 to L-4 (lumbar aorta)
   d. The catheter may be secured in place by umbilical tape or sutures attached to the umbilical stump and the catheter than taped to the abdominal wall.
   e. **Advantages of the UAC**
   (1) Frequent blood gas determinations are easily obtained.
   (2) Prevents frequent peripheral artery punctures
   (3) Allows continuous monitoring of blood pressure
   (4) Allows the infusion of drugs and fluids
   f. **Complications of the UAC**
   (1) Infection
   (2) Thromboembolism (flush line with heparin after a blood sample is drawn)
   (3) Air embolism
   (4) Hemorrhage
   g. UACs should be left in place for no longer than **7 to 10 days** to help avoid these complications.
   h. Generally, no more than 0.5 ml of blood is necessary for the analysis of ABGs.
   i. If there is a perfusion problem to the lower extremities, blanching or cyanosis of the legs or feet will be evident. The catheter should be withdrawn or replaced.
2. **Peripheral artery puncture**
   a. Arterial blood may be drawn from one of several arteries in the neonate, including the radial, brachial, temporal, and posterior tibial arteries.
   b. The radial artery is the most common site because of its easy accessibility, good collateral circulation, and lack of nerves or veins closely adjacent.
   c. A 25- or 26-gauge needle is generally used to puncture the artery at a 35° to 45° angle to the artery. The bevel of the needle should be facing up if radial puncture is performed.
   d. Location of the radial artery is determined by a radial pulse or by placing a **transilluminator** under the back of the wrist. This lighted device will aid in the location of the artery.
   e. Since the radial artery in a neonate is very small, it is not uncommon to insert the needle completely through the artery. If after advancing the needle no blood is obtained, withdraw the needle slightly until blood enters it.
   f. When an adequate amount of blood has been obtained, the needle is withdrawn and pressure applied to the puncture site for approximately 5 minutes.

g. Any air bubbles in the sample should be removed prior to analysis. If this is not done, the blood gas analysis will come back with erroneous values indicating a high PaO_2 and low $PaCO_2$

3. **Arterialized capillary blood sampling**
   a. Arterialized capillary blood is normally obtained from the heel of the neonate using a lancet to puncture the capillary.
   b. The infant's foot should be warmed for several minutes (usually by wrapping a warm, moist diaper around it) to cause peripheral vasodilation, which improves capillary perfusion and arterializes the capillary blood.
   c. The heel should then be cleaned with alcohol, followed by the capillary puncture using a lancet. The blood is withdrawn into a heparinized glass capillary tube.
   d. Care should be taken not to squeeze the heel, as this may cause damage to the foot as well as contamination of the sample with venous blood and interstitial fluid.
   e. The capillary tube should be as close to the puncture site as possible to avoid contaminating the sample with room air.
   f. Once the sample is obtained, pressure should be applied to the heel until the bleeding stops and then an adhesive bandage applied to the puncture site.
   g. Capillary blood samples offer fairly reliable correlations for arterial pH and PCO_2, but are unreliable for PO_2 values. Although the capillary PO_2 (PC_{O_2}) may be low, the PaO_2 may actually be high, which increases the risk of RLF or BPD. It is also possible to have a high PC_{O_2} when the PaO_2 is actually low, risking hypoxic damage. **Arterial PO_2 levels must be monitored periodically to prevent this potential hazard! Normal PC_{O_2} is 40 to 50 torr.

F. **Transcutaneous blood gas monitoring**
   1. By applying blood gas electrodes over the skin, the neonate's PaO_2 and $PaCO_2$ may be monitored continuously without having to perform arterial sticks as frequently.
   2. The probe is attached to the skin and warmed to 42 to 44°C, which results in vasodilation and increased perfusion to the dermal layer of the skin. Oxygen and carbon dioxide diffuse through the skin in concentrations similar to those in the arterial blood.
   3. **Disadvantages of transcutaneous monitoring**
      a. The heated probe may burn the skin; the location of the probe should be changed every **3 to 4 hours to prevent this. In the more immature infant with very fragile skin, the probe position should be changed every **2 hours**.
      **b. The infant must have adequate perfusion to the area of the skin where the probe is attached in order for accurate readings to be obtained.
      **c. Inaccurate readings will occur if the probe is inadequately heated, the monitor is not calibrated properly, or the probe becomes loose and air comes between the probe and the skin.
   4. The monitor requires calibrating during the initial setup and after probe position changes. Following calibration, the monitor will take 20 to 30 minutes to equilibrate before accurate readings will be displayed.

G. **Oximetry**
   1. Monitoring arterial oxygen saturation (SaO_2) is becoming a very popular method to determine the oxygenation status of infants.
   2. Oximetry uses photometrics (use of a light beam shining through the skin or nailbed) to determine SaO_2; therefore, burning of the skin associated with transcutaneous monitoring is not a factor.

NOTE: For more detailed information on oximetry, see Chapter 10.

H. **Thermoregulation of the infant**
   1. It is very important that infants are kept in a **thermal neutral environment**, which is an environment that keeps the infant's body temperature normal, resulting in a normal level of oxygen consumption.
   2. The neonate is unable to shiver if exposed to a cold environmental temperature. The infant becomes cold stressed. In order to generate heat, the infant begins to break down brown fat that is stored mainly in the neck and thorax. This is called nonshivering thermogenesis.
   **3. As brown fat is metabolized, oxygen consumption increases, which may result in hypoxemia. This leads to lactic acidosis (metabolic acidosis). This cold stress will also result in apnea and hypoglycemia.
   4. Incubators are common devices used to maintain a thermal neutral environment.
   5. **Radiant warmers** are also used as a way of controlling temperature. These devices deliver warm air from above the infant in an open-type bed. The infant is therefore more easily accessible.
   **6. A skin probe is applied to the infant's right upper abdomen. The probe measures the infant's temperature, which should be maintained around 36.5°C. Should the infant's body tem-

perature increase or decrease, a **servo control** will adjust the amount of heat needed to maintain the temperature that is set on the control (usually 36.5°C).

II. NEONATAL CARDIOPULMONARY DISORDERS

A. **Respiratory distress syndrome (RDS)**
1. **Definition**—a syndrome associated with premature infants caused by inadequate amounts of pulmonary surfactant, leading to massive atelectasis and hypoxemia (also known as hyaline membrane disease).
2. **Etiology**
   a. Immature lungs with surfactant deficiency
   b. **Lecithin:sphingomyelin ratio of less than 2:1. These lipid levels may be obtained from amniotic fluid to determine the maturity of the surfactant. A ratio of greater than 2:1 indicates mature surfactant.
   c. Infants born earlier than 35 weeks' gestation are at risk for the development of RDS.
3. **Pathophysiology**
   a. Surfactant lines the inner surface of alveoli, decreasing the surface tension and thereby reducing their tendency to collapse.
   b. Immature surfactant or decreased surfactant production, as seen with RDS, leads to alveolar collapse, decreased lung compliance, hypoxemia, and metabolic acidosis.
   c. Alveolar surface tension increases because of lack of surfactant, resulting in fluid being pulled into the alveoli. Because of damage to the capillary endothelial cells by acidosis and hypoxemia, the fluid entering the alveoli contains protein and the blood clotting component fibrin. This makes the alveoli very stiff (noncompliant) and causes the hyaline membrane formation.
4. **Clinical manifestations**
   a. Nasal flaring
   b. Grunting
   c. Retractions
   d. Tachypnea
   e. Cyanosis
   f. ABG results reveal hypercapnia and hypoxemia with a mixed respiratory/metabolic acidosis
5. **Chest x-ray findings**
   a. "Ground glass" appearance
   b. Diffuse atelectasis
   c. Air bronchograms
6. **Treatment**
   a. Oxygen therapy to maintain PaO_2 at greater than 50 torr

   b. Nasal CPAP or E-T CPAP if infant's PaO_2 remains less than 50 torr on 60% oxygen
   c. Positive-pressure ventilation with positive end-expiratory pressure if $PaCO_2$ exceeds 60 torr with a pH of less than 7.25
   d. Surfactant replacement
   e. Thermoregulation
   f. Adequate fluids to prevent dehydration
   g. Packed red blood cells to prevent anemia and blood loss from frequent ABG sampling

B. **Bronchopulmonary dysplasia (BPD)**
1. **Definition**—a form of chronic lung disease seen in infants with severe RDS following prolonged positive-pressure ventilation and supplemental oxygen therapy. Dysplasia refers to abnormal development, in this case to the bronchi and lungs.
2. **Etiology**
   a. Although the cause of BPD is widely debated, it is thought to be caused by prolonged (>7 days) exposure to high concentrations of oxygen with positive-pressure ventilation.
   b. High inspiratory pressures associated with mechanical ventilation leading to barotrauma are thought to be a major cause of BPD.
   c. It occurs more frequently in infants weighing less than 1500 g.
3. **Pathophysiology**
   There are four stages involved in BPD
   a. **Stage 1:** occurs 2 to 4 days following birth and includes:
      (1) Hyaline membrane formation
      (2) Atelectasis
      (3) Necrosis of bronchiolar mucosa
      (4) Bronchiolar metaplasia
   b. **Stage 2:** occurs 4 to 10 days following birth and includes:
      (1) Necrosis and repair of alveolar and bronchial epithelium
      (2) Emphysematous changes
   c. **Stage 3:** occurs 10 to 20 days following birth and includes:
      (1) Interstitial fibrosis
      (2) Atelectasis
      (3) Continuation of bronchiolar metaplasia
      (4) Increased mucus production
      (5) Bullae formation
   d. **Stage 4:** occurs 30 days following birth and includes:
      (1) Formation of emphysematous alveoli
      (2) Atelectasis
      (3) Continuation of interstitial fibrosis

NOTE: Large amounts of mucus are produced leading to air trapping with resultant atelectasis.
4. **Clinical manifestations**

a. Increased airway resistance

b. Decreased dynamic lung compliance

c. Normal or increased static lung compliance

d. Ventilation/perfusion mismatch

e. Hypoxemia on room air

f. Hypercapnia

g. Tachypnea

h. Barrel chest

i. Retractions

5. **Chest x-ray findings**

a. Ground glass appearance

b. Opacification

c. Atelectasis

d. Hyperlucency

e. Presence of bullae

6. **Treatment**

a. Oxygen therapy to maintain PaO_2 between 50 and 70 torr (helps prevent pulmonary hypertension resulting from hypoxemia)

b. Pressure-limited, time-cycled ventilator may be required to maintain normal ABG levels

c. Adequate humidification to prevent mucus plugging in the airways or E-T tube

d. Chest physiotherapy and suctioning

e. Adequate nutrition

f. Maintenance of fluid balance and/or diuretics because of the infant's increased risk of cor pulmonale, pulmonary edema, and congestive heart failure

g. Bronchodilator therapy

C. **Meconium aspiration**

1. **Definition**—aspiration of meconium most commonly associated with full-term or post-term infants. Meconium is discharged in the first fetal bowel movement and is composed of mucus, vernix, epithelial cells, and amniotic fluid.

2. **Etiology**

a. If while *in utero* the infant becomes hypoxic, meconium will be passed into the amniotic fluid.

b. Infants breathe very shallowly *in utero*, moving amniotic fluid into and out of the oropharynx. If the infant is stressed or asphyxiated, however, the breaths are much deeper, and meconium may be aspirated through the vocal cords and into the lungs.

c. The postterm infant is at greater risk for meconium aspiration because less amniotic fluid is present and therefore there is less dilution of the meconium.

d. Even if the meconium is present only in the mouth or the glottic area, aspiration may occur with the infant's first few breaths.

3. **Pathophysiology**

a. The substances that make up meconium cause it to be very thick and, therefore, if aspirated it will plug airways, leading to atelectasis and an increased airway resistance.

b. Most generally, air flow passes through the obstruction during inspiration but gets trapped during expiration as the airway diameter decreases, resulting in hyperinflation.

c. This air trapping often leads to a pneumothorax.

d. Infants with this condition often present with patent ductus arteriosus (discussed later) due to intrauterine hypoxia. Hypoxia causes pulmonary vasoconstriction, which prevents the ductus arteriosus and foramen ovale from closing, resulting in a right-to-left shunt.

4. **Clinical manifestations**

a. Long fingernails and peeling skin (signs of postmaturity)

b. Hypoxemia

c. Hypercarbia

d. Tachypnea

e. Retractions, nasal flaring, grunting

f. Barrel chest (from air trapping)

g. Cyanosis

h. Rales and rhonchi on chest auscultation

5. **Chest x-ray findings**

a. Patchy infiltrates

b. Atelectasis

c. Consolidation

d. Pneumothorax (commonly observed)

e. Hyperinflation

6. **Treatment**

a. If meconium is observed during delivery, the infant's oronasopharynx should be suctioned once the head is delivered and before the first cry to prevent aspiration of the meconium.

b. Immediately after delivery, the infant should be intubated and suctioned to remove meconium from the lower airway.

c. Positive-pressure ventilation should not be started until all meconium is cleared because this would push it farther into the airways.

d. Oxygen therapy or mechanical ventilation depending on severity of the condition

e. Chest physiotherapy

f. Frequent suctioning

D. **Persistent fetal circulation (PFC)**

1. **Definition**—a condition whereby fetal blood circulation through the heart persists following birth. PFC is also referred to as **persistent pulmonary hypertension of the neonate.**

Normal fetal circulation: blood flow through the heart of the infant *in utero* differs from the pathway the blood takes following birth. Only about 10% of blood returning to the right side of the infant's heart flows on into the pulmonary circulation. The other 90% or so of the blood volume in the right side of the heart shunts over to the left side via two pathways. One is through the foramen ovale, a pathway that allows blood to flow from the right atrium into the left atrium. The second area in which shunting occurs is through the ductus arteriosus, which is a communication between the pulmonary artery and the descending aorta.

These two communications between the right and left sides of the heart are kept open *in utero* because of the high pressure found in the pulmonary vasculature. After the infant is delivered and begins breathing oxygen from the air, pulmonary vasodilation occurs, reducing the pulmonary hypertension and allowing the foramen ovale and ductus arteriosus to gradually close.

If closure of these two pathways does not occur, blood will bypass the lungs and be shunted directly into the left side of the heart and out to the body without oxygenation occurring.

2. **Etiology**
   a. Most common in full-term or postterm infants, as their pulmonary vessels are more reactive to hypoxia, leading to pulmonary vasoconstriction
   b. Conditions associated with PFC:
      (1) Perinatal asphyxia
      (2) Meconium aspiration
      (3) Pneumonia
      (4) Sepsis
      (5) Congenital heart defects
      (6) Diaphragmatic hernia
      (7) Hypoplastic lungs
      (8) Hypoglycemia

NOTE: Any condition that results in increased PVR can cause PFC.

3. **Pathophysiology**
   a. The foramen ovale and ductus arteriosus remain patent as a result of pulmonary hypertension.
   b. This results in right-to-left shunting, causing hypoxemia not responsive to oxygen therapy.

4. **Clinical manifestations**
   a. Tachypnea
   b. Hypoxemia
   c. Cyanosis (not in all cases)
   d. >15 torr difference in the PaO_2 between preductal blood (radial or temporal artery) and postductal blood (umbilical artery) on 100% oxygen
   NOTE: Even though this difference is diagnostic of a right-to-left shunt, PFC should not be ruled out if this is not observed. PFC may still be present.

e. Significant increase in PaO_2 (>100 torr) when $PaCO_2$ is maintained at 20 to 25 torr
NOTE: Maintaining low $PaCO_2$ levels results in pulmonary vasodilation, which should allow less blood flow through the ductus arteriosus and foramen ovale. If shunting is occurring, PaO_2 levels would increase during this test.

5. **Chest x-ray findings**
   a. May be normal
   b. Decreased pulmonary vasculature

6. **Treatment**
   a. Mechanical hyperventilation to maintain $PaCO_2$ levels at 20 to 25 torr with an alkaline pH
   b. Maintenance of PaO_2 levels >100 torr
   NOTE: Maintaining $PaCO_2$ and PaO_2 levels as mentioned previously should be done only for the first few days of therapy.
   c. Drug therapy
      (1) Tolazoline (Priscoline)—vasodilator
      (2) Sodium nitroprusside (Nipride)—vasodilator
      (3) Sodium bicarbonate—to produce alkalemia
      (4) Dopamine—increases systemic vascular resistance, thus reducing right-to-left pressure gradient, which decreases shunting
   d. Weaning from mechanical ventilation should be done slowly, as small decreases in ventilator rates, peak inspiratory pressure, and FIO_2 may result in a return to shunting, which will require even higher ventilator parameters (rate, peak inspiratory pressure, FIO_2) than before the changes.

III. AIRWAY DISORDERS OF THE PEDIATRIC PATIENT

A. **Epiglottitis**
1. **Definition**—a bacterial infection of the epiglottis most commonly affecting children 3 to 7 years of age, resulting in inflammation and edema of supraglottic area
2. **Etiology**
   a. Bacterial infection
   b. Bacterial pathogens responsible for epiglottitis:
      (1) *Haemophilus influenzae*—most common cause
      (2) Streptococci
      (3) *Staphylococcus aureus*
      (4) Pneumococci

3. **Pathophysiology**
   a. Bacterial infection leads to inflammation of the epiglottis, glottis, and hypopharynx.
   b. Inflammation leads to swelling of the supra-glottic area, resulting in a sudden onset of severe respiratory distress often precipitating a life-threatening situation.
4. **Clinical manifestations**
   a. High fever
   b. Drooling
   c. Sore throat
   d. Dyspnea
   e. Tachycardia
   f. Inspiratory stridor
   g. Intercostal and sternal retractions
   h. Use of accessory muscles during inspiration
   i. Hoarseness
   j. As swelling progresses, child sits up and leans forward to maintain an open airway.
   k. Epiglottis is swollen and red upon direct visualization.
   l. Initial ABG results reveal hypoxemia and respiratory alkalosis progressing to respiratory acidosis if hypoxemia is not reversed.
5. **X-ray findings**
   a. Lateral neck x-ray study reveals swollen epiglottis known as thumb's sign, as it resembles the distal end of a thumb.
6. **Treatment**
   a. Tracheal intubation
      (1) Tracheotomy performed if nasal or oral intubation is impossible
      (2) Usually the patient is able to undergo extubation within 36 to 48 hours
   b. Oxygen therapy in uncomplicated cases
   c. Antibiotics (for *H. influenzae*)
   d. Mechanical ventilation is rarely necessary
B. **Laryngotracheobronchitis (croup)**
   1. **Definition**—upper airway obstruction resulting from inflammation of the larynx and subglottic area most commonly seen in children 8 months to 4 years of age
   2. **Etiology**
      a. Primarily parainfluenza virus
      b. May result from adenovirus or respiratory syncytial virus
   3. **Pathophysiology**
      a. Swelling and edema of the laryngeal and subglottic area result from inflammation, leading to a narrowing airway lumen.
      b. With the subglottic area being the narrowest portion of the infant's or child's airway, a small degree of edema causes a significant reduction in the cross-sectional area.
      c. The inflammation results in increased mucus production from the mucous glands.
   4. **Clinical manifestations**

a. Tachypnea
b. Tachycardia
c. Cyanosis
d. Inspiratory stridor
e. Intercostal and sternal retractions
f. Use of accessory muscles
g. Barking cough
h. Fever
i. Initial ABG results reveal hypoxemia and respiratory alkalosis progressing to respiratory acidosis if hypoxemia is not reversed.
5. **X-ray findings**
   a. Lateral neck x-ray indicates haziness in the subglottic region.
6. **Treatment**
   a. Oxygen therapy
   b. Cool aerosol to reduce swelling
   c. Aerosolized racemic epinephrine to reduce swelling
   d. Adequate hydration
C. **Foreign body aspiration**
   1. **Definition**—inhalation of a foreign body into the tracheobronchial tree
   2. **Etiology**
      a. Young children often place objects in their mouths and in some instances aspirate the object into the respiratory tract.
      b. The most common aspirated objects are seeds, peanuts, and coins.
   3. **Pathophysiology**
      a. The aspirated object usually lodges in the right mainstem bronchus because of its angle of bifurcation from the trachea.
      b. Certain objects (especially peanuts) may result in a chemical bronchitis resulting in mucosal swelling and edema.
      c. Commonly, infection distal to the obstruction occurs, resulting in abscess, pneumonia, or bronchiectasis.
   4. **Clinical manifestations**
      a. Choking and/or coughing, depending on severity
      b. Dyspnea
      c. Cyanosis
      d. Wheezing (normally unresponsive to bronchodilator therapy)
      e. Hemoptysis (uncommon)
   5. **X-ray findings**
      a. Chest x-ray study may indicate hyperinflation of the affected lung.
      b. Mediastinal shift away from the side of aspiration during expiration as affected lung becomes hyperinflated
      NOTE: Inspiratory and expiratory chest x-ray films should be taken to determine if mediastinal shift is present.
   6. **Treatment**

a. Abdominal thrusts (severe cases of obstruction)
b. Bronchoscopy to remove foreign object
c. Bronchodilator therapy followed by postural drainage and percussion is often successful in removing the object prior to the use of bronchoscopy.

D. **Bronchiolitis**

1. **Definition**—an inflammation of the bronchioles most commonly seen in children during the first 2 years of life

2. **Etiology**
   ** a. Most commonly results from **respiratory syncytial virus** (RSV)
   b. Adenovirus and influenza virus (less commonly)

3. **Pathophysiology**
   a. The virus causes inflammation of the bronchioles, mucosal edema, and spasm of the bronchiolar smooth muscle.
   b. In severe cases, mucus and fibrin may accumulate in the lumen of the affected bronchioles.
   c. Inspiratory and expiratory flows become obstructed, increasing FRC.
   d. Atelectasis may result from the inflammation in severe cases.

4. **Clinical manifestations**
   a. Recent upper respiratory tract infection
   b. Fever
   c. Cough
   d. Tachypnea
   e. Dyspnea
   f. Rales and wheezing on chest auscultation
   g. Apnea (in infants)
   h. Sternal and intercostal retractions
   i. Hypoxemia

5. **Chest x-ray findings**
   a. Marked hyperradiolucency
   b. Infiltrates

6. **Treatment**
   a. Mild cases will not require hospitalization.
   In more severe cases:
   (1) Oxygen therapy (via hood or tent depending on age of the child)
   (2) CPAP—to treat more severe hypoxemia
   ** (3) **Ribavirin (antiviral drug) administered via a small-particle aerosol generator (SPAG) for 12 to 18 hours daily through an oxygen hood for 3 to 7 days**
   (4) Mechanical ventilation if ribavirin treatment is unsuccessful
   (5) Adequate hydration

E. **Cystic fibrosis (mucoviscidosis)**

1. **Definition**—a hereditary disease affecting the exocrine glands of the body that results in the production of thick mucus from these glands. The glands most commonly affected are located in the pancreas, the sweat glands, and the lungs. It is classified as a chronic obstructive lung disease.

2. **Etiology**
   a. A genetically transmitted disease
   b. The mother and father must both be carriers of this recessive gene. Each birth renders a one in four chance of producing a child with the disease.

3. **Pathophysiology**
   a. Large amounts of thick mucus are produced as a result of the abnormally large numbers of bronchial glands and goblet cells located in the tracheobronchial tree.
   b. Thick mucus stagnates in the airways, leading to airway obstruction and facilitation of bacterial growth.
   c. Mucus plugging results in atelectasis, hyperinflation, and pneumonia.
   d. Abnormalities in the pancreatic ducts and glands result in inadequate absorption and digestion of food, causing malnutrition if not properly treated.

4. **Clinical manifestations**
   a. Tachypnea
   b. Tachycardia
   c. Cough with thick mucus production
   d. Increased anterior-posterior chest diameter
   e. Digital clubbing
   ** f. Elevated chloride levels in the perspiration (diagnostic of this disease)
   g. Use of accessory muscles during normal breathing
   h. Early in disease process, ABG results indicate hypoxemia with respiratory alkalosis.
   i. Late stages of disease reveal ABG results that indicate chronic ventilatory failure with hypoxemia.
   j. Cyanosis
   k. Cor pulmonale in late stage
   l. Pulmonary function studies reveal decreases in expiratory flow values and increased FRC values.

5. **X-ray findings**
   a. Hyperinflation
   b. Flattened diaphragm
   c. Increased lung markings
   d. Cardiomegaly

6. **Treatment**
   ** a. Aerosolized bronchodilator with mucolytic agent (acetylcysteine [Mucomyst]) followed by postural drainage and percussion

b. Oxygen therapy
c. Expectorants
d. Continuous aerosol mask
e. Antibiotics

REFERENCES

1. Aloan C. *Respiratory Care of the Newborn.* Philadelphia: JB Lippincott; 1987.
2. Burgess W. and Chernick V. *Respiratory Therapy in Newborn Infants and Children.* 2nd ed. New York: Thieme; 1986.
3. Carlo W., Chatburn R. *Neonatal Respiratory Care.* 2nd ed. Chicago: Year Book Medical Publishers; 1988.
4. Lough M. *Newborn Respiratory Care.* Chicago: Year Book Medical Publishers; 1983.

PRETEST ANSWERS

1. A
2. B
3. B
4. D
5. C
6. B

Respiratory Medications

PRETEST QUESTIONS*

1. For which of the following lung disorders would acetylcysteine be indicated?

   I. Emphysema
  II. Bronchiectasis
 III. Cystic fibrosis
 IV. Pulmonary edema

A. I and II only
B. II and III only
C. III and IV only
D. I, II, and III only
E. II, III, and IV only

2. A patient with glottic edema after extubation is in mild respiratory distress. Which of the following medications would be of benefit in this situation?

A. Cromolyn sodium
B. Succinylcholine
C. Racemic epinephrine
D. Pentamidine
E. Ribavirin

3. You are having difficulty intubating a combative patient in the emergency room. The respiratory therapist should recommend the delivery of which drug in order to facilitate intubation?

A. Succinylcholine
B. Cromolyn sodium
C. Atropine
D. Epinephrine
E. Lidocaine

4. Which of the following aerosolized medications is used in the treatment of respiratory syncytial virus?

A. Succinylcholine
B. Amoxicillin
C. Pentamidine
D. Amphotericin B
E. Ribavirin

5. Which of the following airway disorders may be successfully treated with dexamethasone?

   I. Asthma
  II. Glottic edema
 III. Pulmonary edema

A. I only
B. II only
C. I and II only
D. I and III only
E. II and III only

---

*See answers at the end of the chapater.

Respiratory Medications

I. CLASSIFICATION OF RESPIRATORY MEDICATIONS

A. **Diluents**
 1. **Normal saline (0.9% sodium chloride)**
  a. Used to dilute bronchodilators
  b. Used to dilute secretions for improved expectoration—often instilled through endotracheal (E-T) tubes and tracheostomy tubes 3 to 5 ml at a time
 2. **Hypotonic saline (0.4% sodium chloride)**
  a. Used in ultrasonic nebulizers because smaller particles are produced, resulting from a lower concentration
  b. More stable than sterile water
 3. **Hypertonic saline (1.8% sodium chloride)**
  a. Larger aerosol particles are produced because of the higher concentration of the solution
  b. Used to stimulate coughing and induce sputum, as it is irritating to the airway
 4. **Sterile distilled water**
  a. Used to dilute other medications
  b. Used to hydrate secretions, thereby decreasing the viscosity for easier expectoration
  c. Used to humidify dry gases
B. **Mucolytics**—drugs that break the sputum down chemically for more effective expectoration
 1. **Acetylcysteine (Mucomyst)**
  a. Available in 10% or 20% solutions
  b. Breaks the **disulfide bonds** in the sputum, which decreases its viscosity
 ** c. Often used with bronchodilators, since a common side effect is **bronchospasm**
 ** d. Should be used in patients with **thick secretions that are difficult to mobilize**
  e. Often used in patients with cystic fibrosis or bronchiectasis
  f. May be nebulized (1 to 3 ml t.i.d. to q.i.d.) or instilled directly into the trachea

** g. Should bronchospasm occur, stop the treatment immediately and administer a bronchodilator.
 h. Irritating to mucosal tissues—patient should rinse mouth after treatment
 2. **Sodium bicarbonate (2%)**
  a. Increases the pH of the sputum, thereby decreasing its viscosity
  b. May be used to improve the mucolytic actions of acetylcysteine
  c. Dosage: 2 to 5 ml via aerosol or 2 to 10 ml instilled directly into the trachea every 4 to 8 hours
C. **Sympathomimetic bronchodilators**
NOTE: These medications stimulate one or more of the following receptors:

Receptor	Location	Response
Alpha	Mucosal blood vessels; bronchial smooth muscle	Vasoconstriction, bronchoconstriction
Beta$_1$	Heart muscle	Increased heart rate and cardiac output; arrhythmias
Beta$_2$	Bronchial smooth muscle; peripheral mucosal blood vessels; central nervous system (CNS) and peripheral limb muscles	Bronchodilation, vasodilation, nervousness (CNS), tingling in fingers

NOTE: The ideal bronchodilator is one that is a pure beta$_2$ receptor stimulator.
 1. **Epinephrine (Adrenalin, Sus-Phrine)**
  a. Stimulates all three receptors, but beta$_1$ the strongest
  b. Duration of action is 0.5 to 2 hours
  c. Used to stimulate the heart—not commonly used as a bronchodilator
  d. Adverse effects:
   (1) Increased heart rate
   (2) Hypertension

(3) Anxiety

(4) Mild bronchoconstriction

e. Dosage: aerosol—0.1 to 0.5 ml (1:100) in 3 to 5 ml of diluent

2. **Racemic epinephrine (Micronefrin, Vaponefrin)**

a. Stimulates all three receptors, but beta$_1$ is the strongest

b. Duration of action is 0.5 to 2 hours

**c. Used to decrease mucosal edema and inflammation after extubation or in children with croup

d. Has milder effects than epinephrine (one-half strength)

e. Dosage: aerosol—0.2 to 0.5 ml in 3 to 5 ml of diluent every 3 to 4 hours

3. **Isoetharine (Bronkosol, Dilabron)**

a. Stimulates beta$_1$ and beta$_2$ receptors

b. Duration of action is 1 to 4 hours

c. Used to decrease airway resistance

d. Adverse effects:

(1) Increased heart rate

(2) Increased blood pressure

(3) Anxiety

(4) Paresthesia

(5) Dizziness

e. Dosage: 0.25 to 0.5 ml in 3 to 5 ml of diluent t.i.d. to q.i.d.

4. **Isoproterenol (Isuprel)**

a. A strong beta$_1$ and beta$_2$ stimulator

b. Duration of action is 1 to 2 hours

c. Used to decrease airway resistance

d. Adverse effects:

**(1) Increased heart rate

(2) Increased blood pressure

(3) Anxiety

(4) Tingling in fingers

(5) Nervousness

e. Dosage: 0.25 to 0.5 ml in 3 to 5 ml of diluent t.i.d. to q.i.d.

5. **Metaproterenol (Alupent, Metaprel)**

a. Very minor beta$_1$ and mild beta$_2$ stimulator

b. Duration of action is 4 to 6 hours

c. Used to decrease airway resistance

d. Adverse effects:

(1) Mild cardiac effects

(2) Mild CNS effects

e. Dosage: 0.1 to 0.3 ml in 3 to 5 ml of diluent, every 4 hours

6. **Terbutaline sulfate (Brethine, Bricanyl)**

a. Very minor beta$_1$ and moderate beta$_2$ stimulator

b. Duration of action is 3 to 7 hours

c. Used to decrease airway resistance

d. Adverse effects

(1) Mild cardiac effects

(2) Mild CNS effects

e. Dosage: 0.25 to 0.5 mg in 3 to 5 ml of diluent, every 4 to 8 hours

7. **Albuterol (Proventil, Ventolin)**

a. **Mild beta$_1$ and strong beta$_2$ stimulator**

b. Duration of action is 4 to 6 hours

c. Used to decrease airway resistance

d. Adverse effects

(1) Mild cardiac effects

(2) Mild CNS effects

e. Dosage: 0.1 to 0.2 mg in 3 to 5 ml of diluent, every 6 to 8 hours

D. **Parasympatholytic bronchodilators**

1. **Atropine sulfate**

a. It is an anticholinergic drug. It blocks the cholinergic constricting influences on the airway and potentiates the adrenergic influences (beta$_2$ stimulation), resulting in bronchodilation.

b. It also inhibits secretion production and increases secretion viscosity.

NOTE: There is more potential for mucus plugging in patients with thick secretions who are administered atropine **systemically**. Given as an aerosol, it has little effect on lung secretions but may dry out the oral mucosa.

c. Used to decrease airway resistance, congestion, and cardiac arrhythmias

d. Adverse effects

(1) Increased secretion viscosity

(2) Dry mouth

(3) CNS stimulation

e. Dosage: 1 mg in 3 to 5 ml of diluent, every 4 to 6 hours.

E. **Phosphodiesterase inhibitors**

These drugs are called xanthines and they inhibit the cellular production of phosphodiesterase, an enzyme that readily breaks down cyclic adenosine monophosphate (cAMP). It is cAMP, another cellular enzyme, that when produced results in bronchodilation. It is by the increased production of cAMP that sympathomimetic bronchodilators work.

1. **Theophylline (aminophylline)**

a. Stimulates respiratory rate and depth of breathing and produces pulmonary vasodilation and bronchodilation

**b. Used to decrease airway resistance, especially in asthmatics

c. Duration of action is 4 to 6 hours.

d. Adverse effects:

(1) Cardiac effects

(2) CNS effects

(3) Nausea and vomiting

(4) Diuresis

e. Dosage: Intravenous (IV) loading dose—6

mg/kg; maintenance dose—0.5 mg/kg/hour—average dose is 250 mg every 6 hours

NOTE: Therapuetic serum level is 10 to 20 mg/L.

F. **Miscellaneous respiratory drugs**
   1. **Cromolyn sodium (Intal)**
      a. It stabilizes the mast cell, making it less sensitive to specific antigens, and inhibits the release of histamine.
      b. Duration of action is 2 to 6 hours
      c. Used as a **preventive therapy for asthma **(it is not effective during an asthma attack)**
      d. Adverse effects:
         (1) Bronchospasm (when delivered in powdered form)
         (2) Cough (powdered form)
         (3) Local irritation (powdered form)

NOTE: Cromolyn sodium is now available in aerosolized form and is tolerated much better than the powdered form. The powdered form was delivered through a device called a **spinhaler**. The capsule was punctured and placed in the device and the patient inhaled deeply, which delivered the powder into the airway. **Bronchospasm is a common complication when cromolyn sodium is delivered in this form.**

      e. Dosage: one capsule (20 mg) q.i.d. (powdered form); nebulized form—20 mg q.i.d.
   2. **Ethanol (ethyl alcohol)**
      a. An antifoaming agent used to decrease the surface tension of frothy, bubbly secretions observed with **pulmonary edema
      b. **Used in the treatment of pulmonary edema to disperse the edema bubbles, making the airway more patent
      c. Adverse effects:
         (1) Mucosal irritation
         (2) Dry mouth
      d. Dosage: 3 to 15 ml of a 40% to 50% solution

NOTE: 100 proof vodka is 50% ethyl alcohol and may be used.

G. **Neuromuscular blocking agents**
   1. **Succinylcholine (Anectine)**
      a. It is a depolarizing agent that competes with acetylcholine for cholinergic receptors of the motor end plate of a muscle. If these receptors remain occupied by the depolarizing agent, further stimulation cannot occur, and paralysis persists.
      b. Onset of action is 1 minute with a duration of action of only **5 minutes**.
      **c. Used as a short-term paralyzing agent to facilitate E-T intubation
      d. Adverse effects:
         (1) Decreased heart rate
         (2) Decreased blood pressure
            NOTE: Atropine may be administered to

counteract the paralyzing effects of this drug.
      e. Dosage: 20 mg IV (2 to 3 mg/min)
   2. ***d*-Tubocurarine (curare)**
      a. A nondepolarizing agent that blocks the transmission of acetylcholine at the postjunctional membrane
      b. Onset of action is 3 to 5 minutes with a duration of action of 40 to 90 minutes
      c. Used to paralyze patients who are "fighting" mechanical ventilation
      d. Adverse effects:
         (1) Bronchospasm (due to histamine release)
         (2) Decreased blood pressure
   3. **Pancuronium bromide (Pavulon)**
      a. A nondepolarizing agent that is five times stronger than curare and much more commonly used
      b. Onset of action is 2 to 3 minutes with a duration of action of up to 1 hour
      c. Used to paralyze patients who are "fighting" mechanical ventilation
      d. Adverse effects:
         (1) Increased heart rate (mild)
         (2) Increased blood pressure (mild)

NOTE: Pancuronium does not cause the release of histamine as curare does; therefore, bronchospasm is not a complication.

      e. Dosage: 4 to 5 mg IV in intervals of 1 to 3 hours

NOTE: The paralyzing effects of the nondepolarizing agents (curare and pancuronium) may be reversed with the administration of edrophonium chloride (Tensilon) or neostigmine (Prostigmine).

H. **Antibiotics (aerosolized)**

NOTE: Since a variety of organisms are found in patients with different pneumonias, as well as in patients with bronchiectasis, cystic fibrosis, and sinusitis, these medications can be very beneficial in combating these invading organisms.
   1. **Gentamicin**
      a. Commonly used in patients with cystic fibrosis
      b. Effective against *Pseudomonas aeruginosa*
      c. May be combined with carbenicillin
      d. May be instilled directly down the E-T tube
   2. **Amoxicillin**
      a. Used in patients with bronchiectasis
      b. Reduces the purulence of the sputum
   3. **Amphotericin B**
      a. Used for the treatment of fungal infections
      b. Improvement seen in the treatment of pulmonary aspergillosis and *Candida albicans*
   4. **Pentamidine**

a. An antiprotozoan agent

**b. Used in the treatment of *Pneumocystis carinii* (type of pneumonia commonly seen in patients with acquired immunodeficiency syndrome; see Chapter 12)

c. Bronchodilator therapy prior to the administration of pentamidine will help control the bronchospasm caused by this agent.

d. The nebulizer setup used to deliver pentamidine should incorporate a one-way valve that directs the exhaled air through a bacteria filter to prevent contaminating the personnel and surrounding air with this agent.

5. **Ribavirin (Virazole)**

a. An antiviral agent

**b. Used specifically to treat respiratory syncytial virus in neonatal and pediatric patients (see Chapter 13)

c. Delivered through a small-particle aerosol generator (see Chapter 2)

d. The medication is delivered continuously for 12 to 18 hours a day for 3 days to 1 week, generally through an oxygen hood, oxygen tent, or face tent.

e. Hazards of ribavirin

(1) Worsening of respiratory status

(2) Bacterial pneumonia (contamination)

(3) Occlusion of E-T tube or ventilator tubing by the hygroscopic particles— particle filters may decrease the potential of this hazard

I. **Corticosteroids (aerosolized)**

NOTE: These antiinflammatory agents are used in respiratory care to prevent or reduce airway inflammation in asthma and the upper airway swelling that accompanies glottic edema. Administering these agents via aerosol (usually metered dose inhaler [MDI]) reduces the systemic side effects such as cushingoid symptoms (edema, moon face) and adrenal suppression

1. **Dexamethasone sodium phosphate (Decadron)**

a. One of the first steroids administered successfully as an aerosol

b. May be administered in MDIs or in aerosol solution

c. Systemic side effects are common even when delivered via aerosol.

2. **Beclomethasone dipropionate (Vanceril, Beclovent)**

a. Commonly used in asthma and other chronic lung diseases

b. Fewer system side effects than dexamethasone

c. Delivered by MDI

3. **Flunisolide (Aerobid)**

a. Effective treatment for asthmatics

b. Delivered by MDI

NOTE: Patients on MDI steroid therapy must be well educated on the proper use of MDI and the possible side effects of the drugs if overused.

II. DRUG CALCULATIONS

A. **Percentage strengths**

1. Percentage strength is the number of parts of the solute (ingredient)/100 parts of solution.

2. To convert from ratio strength to percentage strength:

a. **What is the percentage strength of a 1:2000 solution?**

*Change 1:2000 to a fraction: 1/2000

*Change this to a percentage by dividing 2000 into 1 and multiply by 100

(*1 ÷ 2000) × 100 = **0.05%**

b. **What is the percentage strength of a 1:500 solution?**

*Change 1:500 to a fraction: 1/500

*Change this to a percentage by dividing 500 into 1 and multiplying by 100

(*1 ÷ 500) × 100 = **0.2%**

3. To convert from percentage strength to ratio strength:

a. What is the ratio strength of a 10% solution?

*Change 10% to 10/100 or 10:100

*10:100 is the same as 1:10 (10 goes into 100 10 times)

*Therefore a 10% solution has a **1:10 ratio strength**

B. **Dosage calculations**

NOTE: 1 ml of a 1% solution (1:100) = 10 mg of solute

1. **How many milligrams of a 1:100 solution of isoproterenol are in 0.5 ml of the drug?**

*A 1:100 solution is a 1% solution (1 divided by 100 times 100)

***1 ml of a 1% solution equals 10 mg (this is a standard rule)**

However, this question asks how many milligrams there are in **0.5 ml.**

*1 ml of a 1% solution = 10 mg

*0.5 ml of a 1% solution = 5 mg (half as much)

2. **How many milligrams is 0.2 ml of a 5% solution of metaproterenol?**

Always go back to the **standard rule: 1 ml of 1% = 10 mg**

*1 ml of a **1%** solution = 10 mg

*1 ml of a **5%** solution = 50 mg (five times as much)

*0.2 ml of 50 mg = **10 mg** (0.2 × 50 mg)

C. **Calculating children's dosages**

1. **Young's rule**—use child's age for 2- to 12-year-old children

$$\frac{\text{age of child}}{\text{age of child} + 12} \times \text{adult dose} = \text{child's dose}$$

2. **Clark's rule**—uses the weight of the child

$$\frac{\text{weight of child (lbs)}}{150 \text{ lb}} \times \text{adult dose} = \text{child's dose}$$

NOTE: 150 lb represents the average adult weight.

REFERENCES

1. Eubanks D, Bone R. *Comprehensive Respiratory Care.* 2nd ed. St. Louis: CV Mosby; 1990.
2. Oakes D. *Clinical Practitioner's Pocket Guide to Respiratory Care.* Rockville, MD: Health Educator Publications, 1984.
3. Scanlon C, Spearman C. *Egan's Fundamentals of Respiratory Care.* 5th ed. St. Louis: CV Mosby; 1990.
4. Rau J. *Respiratory Care Pharmacology.* 3rd ed. Chicago: Year Book Medical Publishers; 1989.

PRETEST ANSWERS

1. B

2. C

3. A

4. E

5. C

Respiratory Home Care

PRETEST QUESTIONS*

1. Which of the following oxygen systems would be indicated for a very active home care patient?

A. Oxygen concentrator
B. Liquid oxygen
C. H cylinder
D. E cylinder
E. Compressor

2. Which of the following is the least important area for the respiratory therapist to discuss with the home care patient?

A. Pathologic characteristics of the disease process
B. Cleaning of equipment
C. Side effects of prescribed therapy
D. Importance of proper therapy techniques
E. How to dispense aerosolized medications

3. Which of the following intermittent positive-pressure breathing (IPPB) machines is most convenient for use in the home because pressurized gas is not required?

A. Bird Mark 7
B. Bird Mark 8
C. Bennett PR-1
D. Bennett PR-2
E. Bennett AP-5

4. Diaphragmatic breathing exercises should result in which of the following?
   I. Increased tidal volume
   II. Less dependence on the use of the diaphragm during quiet breathing
   III. Increased functional residual capacity
   IV. Decreased respiratory rate

A. I and II only
B. I and IV only
C. II, III, and IV only
D. I, II, and IV only
E. I, II, III, and IV

---

*See answers at the end of the chapter.

CHAPTER **15**

Respiratory Home Care

I. HOME REHABILITATION

A. **Goals of rehabilitation**
1. Help the patient to become independent
2. Help the patient to improve his/her ability to cope with the disease
3. Help the patient to gain an understanding of the disease and the limitations that result from the disease
4. Help the patient to set realistic goals for life and then help him/her attain those goals

B. **Conditions requiring pulmonary rehabilitation**
1. Chronic lung diseases
   a. Emphysema
   b. Asthma
   c. Chronic bronchitis
   d. Cystic fibrosis
   e. Bronchiectasis
2. Neuromuscular diseases
   a. Myasthenia gravis
   b. Guillain-Barré syndrome
   c. Poliomyelitis
   d. Muscular dystrophy
3. Central respiratory center disorders
   a. Central nervous system injury
   b. Hypoventilation syndrome (pickwickian syndrome, sleep apnea)
   c. Ondine's curse

II. CARE OF THE REHABILITATION PATIENT

A. **Patient care plan**
1. Humidity therapy
2. Aerosol therapy
3. Oxygen therapy—**use of reservoir cannulas and pulse oxygen delivery systems aid in conserving oxygen use**
4. Bronchodilator therapy
5. Arterial blood gas sampling and analysis or oxygen saturation monitoring
6. Oropharyngeal and tracheal suctioning
7. Determination of breath sounds by chest auscultation
8. Postural drainage and percussion
9. Breathing exercises
10. Sputum induction
11. IPPB therapy—**Bennett AP-5 unit commonly used**

B. **Periodic evaluations**
1. Pulmonary function testing
2. Sputum collection and analysis
3. Arterial blood gas collection and analysis
4. Exercise tolerance testing
5. Chest x-ray studies

C. **Breathing exercises**
1. **Pursed-lip breathing**
   a. Should be taught to patients who experience premature airway closure
   b. Patient should be instructed to inhale through the nose and exhale through pursed lips.
   c. It aids in patient gaining control of dyspnea.
   d. It provides improved ventilation prior to a cough effort.
   e. It teaches the patient how to better control the rate and depth of breathing.
   f. It prevents premature airway collapse by generating a back pressure into the airways.
   g. It has psychologic benefits.
2. **Diaphragmatic breathing**
   a. It teaches the patient with chronic obstructive pulmonary disease to use the diaphragm rather than accessory muscles during breathing.
   b. The patient or respiratory care practitioner places a hand over the abdomen as the patient, while lying on the back, concentrates on moving the hand upward on inspiration.

185

(A book or weight may be used rather than a hand.)

   c. By increasing the use of the diaphragm, decreased respiratory rate, increased tidal volume, decreased functional residual capacity, and increased ventilation result.

3. **Segmental breathing**
   a. Similar to diaphragmatic breathing exercise except that a hand is placed over a specific lung area in which there is atelectasis, secretions, or decreased air flow
   b. The patient should concentrate on moving the hand outward on inspiration.

D. **Cough instruction**
**1. A forced vital capacity of less than 15 ml/kg of ideal body weight indicates an inadequate volume to provide for an effective cough.

2. **Proper cough instruction**
   a. Patient should inhale slowly and deeply through the nose and hold breath for 3 to 5 seconds (in sitting position).
   b. Patient should clasp arms across abdomen and give three sharp coughs without taking a breath while pressing arms into the abdomen.
   c. Use a pillow to "splint" incision sites (thorax, abdomen).

E. **Home oxygen administration**
1. **Oxygen cylinders**
   a. Probably the least expensive oxygen setup in the home at the present time depending on usage
   b. Disadvantages of oxygen cylinders in the home:
     (1) Heavy and difficult to move
     (2) High-pressure hazard
     (3) Difficult for older or debilitated patients to change cylinder or attach a regulator
     (4) Small cylinders are difficult to walk with.

2. **Liquid oxygen system**
   a. Can store more oxygen in liquid form than in gaseous form (860 times more)
   b. Liquid is safer than gas stored in high-pressure cylinders.
   c. Portable liquid walkers are much more convenient and easier for the patient to handle.

3. **Oxygen concentrators**

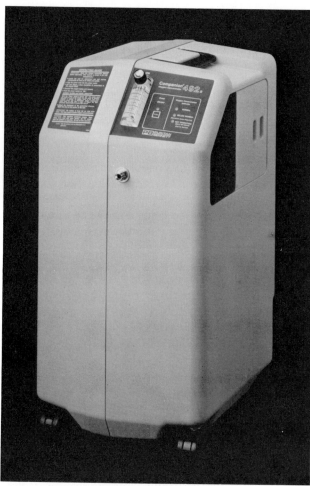

Courtesy of the Puritan-Bennett Corporation, Overland Park, KS.

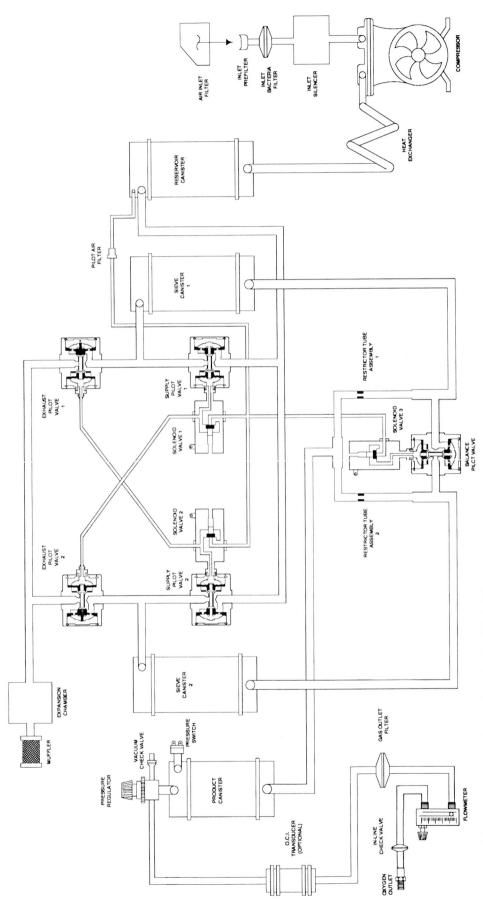

Courtesy of the Puritan-Bennett Corporation, Overland Park, KS.

a. They use the oxygen in the surrounding room air by drawing it into the concentrator and filtering out most of the gases except oxygen.

b. Two types of concentrators:
  (1) Membrane type—produces only about 40% oxygen out of the unit
  (2) Molecular sieve type—much more commonly used and produces 90% to 95% oxygen out of the unit

c. The concentrator should be placed in the home where air can freely be drawn into it.

d. The concentrator should not be placed near heater vents.

e. On the routine visit, the respiratory care practitioner should analyze the delivered oxygen from the concentrator and check all alarms, the flowrate, filters, and batteries.

f. A back-up oxygen system should be available, since concentrators are powered by electricity.

g. The higher the flow used on a concentrator, the less the delivered oxygen percentage.

NOTE: The patient and family should be instructed in all aspects of the proper care and safety of equipment used in the home.

F. **Cleaning equipment in the home**

1. All equipment designated "single use only" should be considered disposable and discarded after one use.

2. Nondisposable equipment, such as nebulizers and humidifiers, may be cleaned as follows:
  a. Clean first with mild soap
  b. Rinse
  c. Disinfect with a solution recommended by the manufacturer
  d. Rinse again
  e. Dry the equipment
  f. Repeat the process every 1 to 3 days

NOTE: Nebulizing 10 ml of 0.25% acetic acid (vinegar) through nebulizers and room humidifiers has been found to be an appropriate cleaning technique as well.

3. Cannulas should be cleaned with mild soap that does not leave a soap film and then rinsed prior to using a disinfectant. They should be replaced every 2 to 4 weeks.

4. Humidifers and nebulizers should be filled with sterile water and should incorporate safety relief devices.

5. If heated moisture is delivered, a thermometer should be placed in-line, close to the patient, to monitor the inspired gas temperature.

6. Medication nebulizers should be rinsed with water and dried following each treatment. They should be cleaned every day in a mild soap solution, rinsed, disinfected, rinsed again, and dried.

7. IPPB circuits (nondisposable) may be cleaned in mild soap, rinsed and disinfected, rinsed again, and dried every 1 to 2 days.

8. IPPB machines may be wiped down with a liquid disinfectant every few days.

G. **Respiratory care practitioner responsibilities in the home care of the pulmonary patient**

1. Helps set up and maintain equipment

2. Instructs the patient and family on use, care, and safety of all equipment used in the home setting

3. Instructs the patient and family in all therapy to be performed in the home, including the indications, contraindications, side effects, and hazards of the specific therapy

4. Assists in the delivery of therapy to the patient

5. Performs simple spirometry tests

6. Assesses the patient's present cardiopulmonary status and general well-being

7. Reports to the physician to discuss the present therapy and possible changes needed in current therapy

REFERENCES

1. Eubanks D, Bone R. *Comprehensive Respiratory Care.* 2nd ed. St. Louis: CV Mosby; 1990.
2. McPherson SP. *Respiratory Home Care Equipment.* St. Louis: CV Mosby; 1988.
3. Shapiro A. *Clinical Application of Respiratory Care.* 4th ed. St. Louis: Mosby-Year Book Medical Publishers; 1990.
4. Scanlan C, Spearman C. *Egan's Fundamentals of Respiratory Care.* 5th ed. St. Louis: CV Mosby; 1990.

PRETEST ANSWERS

1. B

2. A

3. E

4. B

CHAPTER **16**

Pulmonary Function Testing

1. Reversibility of obstructed airways and improved flowrates following a "before-and-after" bronchodilator study are considered significant at a minimum of what percentage increase?

A. 5%
B. 10%
C. 15%
D. 25%
E. 30%

2. In which of the following lung conditions would the functional residual capacity (FRC) be increased?
   I. Emphysema
  II. Cystic fibrosis
 III. Pneumonia

A. I only
B. I and II only
C. I and III only
D. II and III only
E. I, II, and III

3. A normal negative inspiratory force (NIF) for a healthy individual should be at least which of the following?

A. −10 cm of water
B. −20 cm of water
C. −30 cm of water
D. −40 cm of water
E. −50 cm of water

4. In order to evaluate the distribution of ventilation to perfusion with a ventilation/perfusion scan, the patient is instructed to inhale which of the following substances?

A. Helium
B. Carbon monoxide
C. Xenon
D. Argon
E. Carbon dioxide

5. The results of a patient's spirometry test before and after bronchodilator therapy follow:

	Before	*After*
FEV_1	32% of predicted	53% of predicted
FVC	38% of predicted	66% of predicted
FEV_1/FVC	50%	68%

FEV_1 = forced expiratory volume in 1 second; FVC = forced vital capacity

Which of the following is the correct interpretation of these results?

A. Mild restrictive disease with significant bronchodilator response
B. Severe obstructive disease with significant bronchodilator response
C. Severe restrictive disease with no significant bronchodilator response
D. Severe obstructive disease with no significant bronchodilator response
E. Obstructive and restrictive disease with significant bronchodilator response

---

*See answers at the end of the chapter.

Pulmonary Function Testing

I. LUNG VOLUMES AND CAPACITIES

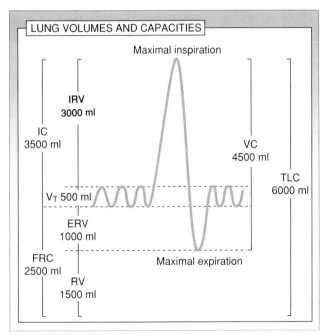

LUNG VOLUMES AND CAPACITIES

Maximal inspiration

IRV
3000 ml

IC
3500 ml

VC
4500 ml

TLC
6000 ml

V$_T$ 500 ml

ERV
1000 ml

Maximal expiration

FRC
2500 ml

RV
1500 ml

From Persing G. *Entry Level Respiratory Care Review.* Philadelphia: WB Saunders; 1992.

A. **Lung volumes**
  1. **Tidal volume (VT)**
     a. The volume of air (usually in milliliters) that is inhaled or exhaled during a normal breath
     b. The exhaled VT is usually measured with a respirometer at the bedside or by spirometry.
        **NOTE: When VT is measured at the bedside, it is most accurately achieved by the patient being instructed to breathe normally through a mouthpiece connected to a Wright's respirometer for 1 full minute. The volume reading is then divided by the patient's respiratory rate over that 1 minute to obtain the VT. Noseclips may be used to ensure mouth breathing only.
     **c. It is decreased or normal with restrictive disease and increased or normal with obstructive disease.
     d. Normal value—500 ml (3 ml/lb of body weight)
  2. **Residual volume (RV)**
     a. The volume of air left in the lungs following a maximal expiration
     b. It is derived after FRC is calculated using either the nitrogen washout test or the helium (He) dilution test. (See section on FRC in this chapter.)
     c. Once FRC is calculated, subtract the expiratory reserve volume (ERV) from the FRC; this equals the residual volume (**RV = FRC − ERV**).
     **d. It is increased in obstructive disease and decreased in restrictive disease.
     e. Normal value—1200 ml
  3. **Inspiratory reserve volume (IRV)**
     a. The maximum volume of air that can be inspired following a normal inspiration
     b. Normally not measured during simple spirometry but if it is measured, it should be from a slow vital capacity (SVC)
     c. It could be normal in both obstructive and restrictive disease; therefore, it is not clinically significant.
     d. Normal value—3000 ml
  4. **Expiratory reserve volume (ERV)**
     a. The volume of air exhaled following a normal expiration
     b. Measured directly by spirometry from an SVC (vital capacity [VC] − inspiratory capacity [IC])
     c. It may be normal or decreased in obstructive or restrictive disease.
     d. Normal value—1000 ml and is 20% to 25% of the VC

B. **Lung capacities**
  1. **Functional residual capacity (FRC)**
     a. The amount of air left in the lungs following a normal expiration (ERV + RV)
     b. Measured by the helium dilution test, nitrogen washout test, or body plethysmography
        (1) **Measurement of FRC by helium dilution test**
           (a) Also called the closed-circuit method
           (b) A spirometer is normally filled with about 600 ml of gas with about 10% helium added to the volume. The volume of the gas and the concentration of helium is measured and recorded prior to the test.
           (c) The patient is instructed to breathe normally and at the end of a normal exhalation is connected to the system.
           (d) The patient rebreathes the gas in the spirometer while carbon dioxide is removed by a carbon dioxide absorbant.
           (e) Helium is then diluted until equilibrium is reached. This normally takes about 7 minutes, but in patients with severe lung disease, it may take as long as 30 minutes for equilibrium to occur. This occurs as the helium analyzer falls to a stable level.
           (f) The final concentration of helium is then recorded.
           (g) From this information the following calculations can be made:

$$\text{system volume} = \frac{\text{He added (ml)}}{\text{\% He (first reading)}}$$

$$**\textbf{FRC} = \frac{(\% \text{ He}_1 - \% \text{ He}_2)}{\text{He}_2} \times$$
$$\text{system volume} \times$$
$$\text{BTPS correction factor}$$

He_1 = beginning helium concentration before patient is connected to the system

He_2 = final helium concentration when equilibrium has occurred

BTPS correction factor = a constant that is used to convert volume to body temperature and pressure saturated

        (2) **Measurement of FRC using the nitrogen washout test:**
           (a) Also called the open-circuit method
           (b) During this test, the patient breathes in 100% oxygen to wash out the nitrogen in the lungs. The nitrogen concentration in the lungs is approximately 79%.
           (c) The patient is instructed to breathe normally and **at the end of a normal exhalation the patient is connected to the 100% oxygen breathing system.**
           (d) During the procedure, the exhaled volume is monitored and recorded and the nitrogen percentages are also measured.
           (e) Complete nitrogen washout occurs in about 7 minutes.
           (f) FRC may now be calculated using this formula:

$$\textbf{FRC} = \frac{\text{expired volume} \times \text{N}_2}{\text{N}_1}$$

N_1 = nitrogen percentage in lungs at start of test

N_2 = nitrogen percentage in spirometer at end of test

        (3) **Measurement of FRC using body plethysmography**
           (a) The plethysmograph ("body box") is an airtight chamber in which the patient sits during the procedure.
           (b) While being tested, the patient is instructed to seal the lips tightly around around the mouthpiece and to breathe normally.
               NOTE: The patient may also be tested while being instructed to breathe in shallow panting-type breaths.
           (c) As the patient breathes, a pressure transducer measures pressure at the airway as well as inside the chamber.
           (d) An electrical shutter is used to periodically close the airway, causing the patient to breathe against a closed airway, at which time volume and pressure values are measured.
        ** (e) The technique of plethysmography is based on **Boyle's law**, which states that the volume of gas is inversely proportional to the pressure to which is it subjected.
           (f) FRC can then be calculated using this formula:

$$FRC = atmospheric\ pressure \times \frac{volume\ change}{pressure\ change}$$

(g) Body plethysmography also measures thoracic gas volume, total lung capacity, and RV.

NOTE: Since body plethysmography actually measures the total amount of gas in the thorax, FRC measurements may be higher than those measured by the helium dilution or nitrogen washout method.

** c. FRC is increased in obstructive disease and decreased in restrictive disease.
   d. Normal value—2400 ml
2. **Inspiratory capacity (IC)**
   a. The maximum amount of air that can be inspired following a normal expiration (VT + IRV)
   b. Measured by simple spirometry from a SVC
   c. Usually is decreased or normal in obstructive or restrictive disease
   d. Normal value—3000 to 4000 ml and is 75% to 85% of the VC
3. **Slow vital capacity (SVC) or vital capacity (VC)**
   ** a. The maximum amount of air that can be exhaled following a maximum inspiration (VT + IRV + ERV)
   b. Measured by simple spirometry or at the bedside using a respirometer
   NOTE: At the bedside, a mouthpiece connected to a Wright's respirometer is used. The patient is instructed to inhale as deeply as possible and then slowly completely exhale through the mouthpiece.
   ** c. Decreased in restrictive disease and normal or decreased in obstructive disease
   d. Normal value—4800 ml

NOTE: A decreased VC may be the result of pneumonia, atelectasis, pulmonary edema, or lung cancer.

4. **Forced vital capacity (FVC)**
   a. The maximum amount of air that can be exhaled as **fast and forcefully as possible** following a maximum inspiration.
   b. Measured by simple spirometry
   c. Used to measure FEVs and forced expiratory flows (FEFs)
   ** d. Decreased in both obstructive and restrictive disease.
5. **Total lung capacity (TLC)**
   a. The amount of air remaining in the lungs at the end of a maximal inspiration.
   b. Calculated by a combination of other measured volumes (FRC+IC or VC+RV)
   ** c. It is decreased in restrictive disease and increased in obstructive disease.
   d. Normal value—6000 ml

NOTE: TLC will decrease as a result of atelectasis pulmonary edema, and consolidation and will increase in emphysema.

6. **RV:TLC Ratio**
   a. The percentage of the TLC that remains in the lungs after a maximal expiration
   b. Measured by dividing the RV by the TLC and multiplying by 100 to obtain a percentage
   ** c. The RV:TLC ratio is decreased in restrictive disease and increased in obstructive disease.
   d. Normal value—20% to 35%

II. LUNG STUDIES

A. **Ventilation studies**
   1. **VT** (discussed earlier)
   2. **Respiratory rate**
      a. The number of breaths in 1 minute
      b. Measured by counting chest excursion for 1 minute
      c. Increased because of hypoxia and hypercarbia and decreased with central respiratory center depression or depressing hypoxic drive in a patient with chronic obstructive pulmonary disease
      d. Normal value—10 to 20 breaths/min
   3. **Minute volume (respiratory minute volume [VE])**
      a. The total volume of air (in liters) inhaled or exhaled in 1 minute; **calculated by multiplying the respiratory rate times the VT**
      b. Measured by simple spirometry or at bedside with a respirometer
      NOTE: When measuring VE at the bedside, a Wright's respirometer with mouthpiece is used. The patient is instructed to breathe normally through the mouthpiece as the practitioner times the breathing for 1 minute. The reading on the respirometer after 1 minute will be the VE.
      c. Increased from hypoxia, hypercarbia, acidosis, or decreased lung compliance; decreased from hyperoxia, hypocarbia, alkalosis, and increased lung compliance
      d. Normal value—5 to 10 L/min
B. **Flow studies**
   1. **Forced expiratory volume (FEV) (FEV$_{0.5}$, FEV$_1$, FEV$_3$)**
      ** a. The volume of air that is exhaled over a specific time interval during the FVC maneuver
      b. Measured over 0.5, 1, or 3 seconds; the FEV$_1$ is the most common measurement.
      ** c. The severity of airway obstruction may be determined because it is measured at speci-

fied time intervals. **FEV is usually decreased in both obstructive and restrictive disease.**

NOTE: FEV may be decreased in restrictive disease because the FVC is less than normal and the measurement of FEV is from the FVC. **A better indicator of an obstructive or restrictive disorder is determined from the FEV:FVC ratio.**

2. **FEV:FVC ratio**
   a. It is a percentage of the FEV to the FVC.
   b. Normal values:
      50% to 60% of the FVC is exhaled in 0.5 seconds
      75% to 85% of the FVC is exhaled in 1 second
      94% of the FVC is exhaled in 2 seconds
      97% of the FVC is exhaled in 3 seconds
   **c. Obstructive disease is indicated by less than normal values in the FEV:FVC ratio. Patients with restrictive disease have normal or greater than normal values.
   d. Since the FEV_1 is most commonly measured, look for an **FEV_1:FVC ratio of less than 75% to indicate an obstructive disease.

3. **Forced expiratory flow (FEF)$_{200-1200}$**
   a. The average flowrate of the exhaled air after the first 200 ml during an FVC maneuver
   b. Measured on the spirograph tracing between the 200-ml mark and the 1200-ml mark to determine the average flowrate from the FVC
   **c. Decreased in obstructive disease
   d. Normal value—6 to 7 L/sec (400 L/min)

4. **$FEF_{25\%-75\%}$**
   a. The average flowrate during the middle portion of the FEV
   b. The 25% and 75% points are marked on the spirographic curve from the FVC.
   **c. Values are decreased in obstructive disease.

5. **Peak flow**

   a. The maximum flowrate achieved during an FVC
   b. Measured from an FVC or by a peak flowmeter
   **NOTE: When measuring with a peak flowmeter at the bedside, the patient should be instructed to take as deep a breath as possible and exhale as hard and fast as possible through the mouthpiece. This test is often performed before a bronchodilator is administered and again afterward to determine its effectiveness.
   **c. Decreased in obstructive diseases
   d. Normal value—greater than 10 L/sec (600 L/min)

6. **Maximum voluntary ventilation (MVV)**
   a. The maximum volume of air moved into and out of the lungs voluntarily in 10, 12, or 15 seconds
   b. Tests for overall lung function and ventilatory reserve capacity and air trapping
   c. Decreased in obstructive disease and decreased or normal in restrictive disease (normal—170 L/min)

7. **Flow volume loop (curve)**
   a. A flow volume loop is displayed on a graph and represents the flow generated during an FEV maneuver followed by a forced inspiratory volume maneuver, both plotted against volume change.
   b. Using a flow volume loop, the following values may be measured:
      (1) Peak inspiratory flow
      (2) Peak expiratory flow
      (3) FVC
      (4) FEV (0.5, 1, and 3 seconds)
      (5) $FEF_{25\%-75\%}$
   c. Comparison of flow volume loops representing normal (top diagram), obstructive (middle diagram), and restrictive (bottom diagram) disorders:

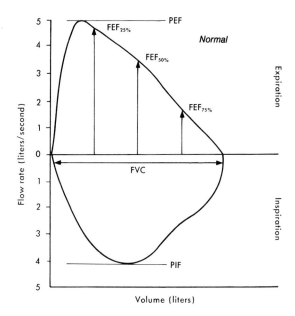

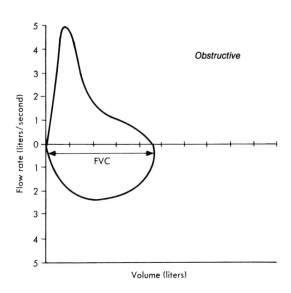

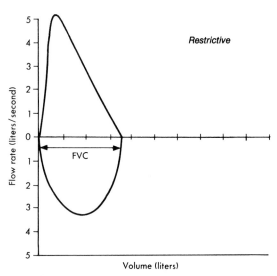

From Scanlon C, Spearman C, Sheldon R. *Egan's Fundamentals of Respiratory Care.* 5th ed. St. Louis: CV Mosby; 1990.

(1) The restriction pattern shows a decreased VC with normal expiratory flowrates.

(2) The obstructive pattern shows a decreased peak expiratory flowrate with a normal exhaled volume.

8. **Diffusion capacity of the lung (DL)**

a. The diffusion capacity is a measurement that represents the gas exchange capabilities of the lungs.

b. This procedure evaluates how well gas diffuses across the alveolar-capillary membrane into the pulmonary capillaries.

c. The most common method for measuring DL is the single-breath method.

d. The patient is connected to the system in which the inspired gas contains a mixture of 10% helium and 0.3% carbon monoxide (CO). Carbon monoxide is used because of its increased affinity for hemoglobin, which keeps the partial pressure of carbon monoxide in the capillaries low, and also because it diffuses rapidly across the alveolar-capillary membrane.

e. The patient is instructed to exhale completely to the RV level, place the mouthpiece in his/her mouth, inhale as deeply as possible, hold the breath for 10 seconds, and exhale.

f. The DL_{CO}, or the measurement of the amount of carbon monoxide diffusing from the alveoli to the pulmonary blood flow, is calculated using this formula:

$$DL_{CO} = \frac{\text{milliliters CO diffused/min}}{\text{A-a gradient of CO (torr)}}$$

g. Normal diffusion capacity is approximately 25 to 30 ml/min/torr

h. Diffusion capacity is typically decreased because of either a decreased surface area available for diffusion or thickening of the membrane itself.

** i. DL_{CO} is **decreased** as a result of the following:

(1) Oxygen toxicity

(2) Emphysema

(3) Sarcoidosis

(4) Edema

(5) Asbestosis

9. **Ventilation/perfusion scanning**

a. This type of x-ray study evaluates the distribution of ventilation to pulmonary perfusion in the lungs.

b. To determine gas distribution, the patient inhales the radioactive isotope **xenon** and holds the breath for 10 to 20 seconds. X-ray films, called photoscintigrams, are taken to observe how this substance is distributed in the lung.

  c. To determine pulmonary perfusion, the patient is injected with a radioactive iodine preparation, and photoscintigrams are taken as the blood perfuses the lungs.

III. OBSTRUCTIVE VERSUS RESTRICTIVE DISEASES

A. **Obstructive diseases**
  1. Emphysema
  2. Asthma
  3. Bronchitis
  4. Cystic fibrosis
  5. Bronchiectasis
  NOTE: These diseases result in **decreased flow studies** (FEV$_1$, FEF$_{25\%-75\%}$, FEF$_{200-1200}$).
B. **Restrictive diseases or disorders**
  1. Fibrotic disease
  2. Chest wall disease
  3. Pneumonia
  4. Neuromuscular disease
  5. Pleural disease
  6. Conditions in postsurgical patients
  NOTE: **These diseases result in decreased volumes (FRC, FVC, IC, IRV).**
C. **Severity of disease (by pulmonary function testing [PFT] interpretation)**
  Normal PFT: 80% to 100% of predicted value
  Mild disorder: 60% to 79% of predicted value
  Moderate disorder: 40% to 59% of predicted value
  Severe disorder: <40% of predicted value
D. **Predicted values are determined from:**
  1. Age
  2. Sex
  3. Height
  4. Ideal body weight
  5. Race

IV. MISCELLANEOUS PULMONARY FUNCTION STUDIES

A. **Before-and-after bronchodilator studies**
  1. Used to determine the reversibility of lung dysfunction and the effectiveness of the bronchodilator
  2. Patients, especially asthmatics, are instructed to perform a peak flow test prior to administration of a bronchodilator. The value is recorded. The patient is then administered a bronchodilator followed by another peak flow study.
  3. Reversibility of obstructed airways and improved flowrates are considered significant for **increases in flow studies of at least 15%.
B. **Methacholine challenge test**
  1. Determines the degree of airway reactivity to methacholine, a drug that stimulates bronchoconstriction
  2. May be performed in a before-and-after bronchodilator study or prior to exercise-induced asthma studies.
  3. The objective of the test is to determine the minimum level of methacholine that elicits a **20% decrease in FEV$_1$.
  4. A physician should be present during testing, and bronchodilators and resuscitation equipment should be readily available.
C. **Measurement of negative inspiratory force (NIF)**
  1. This measurement is also referred to as maximum inspiratory force.
  2. This value represents the maximum amount of negative pressure a patient can generate during inspiration.
  3. This is measured with the use of an aneroid manometer which connects to an endotracheal (E-T) tube via an adaptor. The patient is instructed to inhale as deeply as possible. The manometer will record the negative pressure.
  **NOTE: To prevent the reading from being inaccurate because of inadequate patient effort, a special adaptor may be used to connect the manometer to the E-T tube whereby a port may be occluded, cutting off air to the patient. The airway should be occluded for 20 seconds. As the patient becomes short of breath and tries to get air, a more accurate measurement of the NIF will be recorded.
  4. An adaptor attached to the manometer using a one-way valve that allows for exhalation but not for inspiration is also an effective method for obtaining NIF.
  NOTE: These two methods for determining NIF may cause agitation and anxiety in alert patients. The practitioner should always explain the procedure to the patient prior to beginning it.
  5. An NIF may also be obtained in patients not intubated by connecting the manometer to a mouthpiece and placing noseclips on the patient.
  **6. Normal NIF is approximately −50 to −100 cm of water.
  7. A patient who cannot generate at least **−20 cm of water pressure has inadequate respiratory

muscle strength. The patient will not be capable of generating the necessary NIF pressures required to cough and maintain a patent airway or to maintain adequate spontaneous ventilation; therefore, mechanical ventilation is most likely indicated.

D. **Measurement of maximal expiratory pressure (MEP)**

1. Also referred to as peak expiratory pressure
2. An aneroid manometer is attached to the patient's E-T tube and the patient is instructed to inhale as deeply as possible and exhale forcefully and completely.
3. The maximum pressure is observed and recorded.
4. MEP may be obtained in patients not intubated by attaching the manometer to a mouthpiece and placing noseclips on the patient.
**5. Normal MEP is 90 to 100 cm of water
6. Patients unable to generate an MEP of at least **40 cm of water pressure will not be able to maintain adequate spontaneous ventilation or secretion clearance, making mechanical ventilation necessary.

E. **Exercise stress testing**

1. Exercise stress testing is used to evaluate a patient's cardiopulmonary reserve capacity.
2. The cardiopulmonary stress test is usually conducted with the patient either pedaling a cycle **ergometer** or walking on a treadmill.
3. Prior to testing, a patient history and physical examination should be performed. The examination should include:
   a. Pulmonary function tests
   b. Carbon monoxide diffusion capacity (DL_{CO})
   c. Arterial blood determinations
   d. Blood pressure
   e. Before-and-after bronchodilator study (if airflow obstruction exists)
   f. Resting electrocardiogram (EKG)
4. Some patients are not ideal candidates for cardiopulmonary stress testing. Following is a list of conditions in which stress testing is contraindicated:
   a. Congestive heart failure
   b. Recent acute myocardial infarction
   c. Unstable angina
   d. Acute infection
   e. Uncontrolled cardiac arrhythmias
   f. Dissecting aneurysm
   g. Third-degree heart block
   h. Myocarditis
5. A physician should always be present during the stress test as should the following emergency equipment:
   a. Defibrillator

b. Oxygen source
c. Manual resuscitator with mask
d. Oral airway
e. Laryngoscope and E-T tubes
f. Intravenous line set up with 5% dextrose
g. Cardiac medications

6. There are two general types of stress tests that will be covered in this chapter:
   a. **The cardiac stress test**
      (1) The patient performs incremental work using either a cycle ergometer or a treadmill.
      (2) The patient's heart rate, blood pressure, and EKG are monitored prior to the test.
      (3) These same parameters are measured at the end of each stage of the test and for at least 15 minutes following the test or until any cardiopulmonary problems decline.
      (4) Most healthy individuals are able to complete all four stages of the exercise without difficulty. Patients with coronary artery disease may not be able to complete all stages because of dyspnea and angina.
      (5) This stress test is very useful in diagnosing and treating coronary artery disease but is limited in diagnosing other cardiopulmonary diseases.
   b. **The cardiopulmonary stress test**
      (1) This test requires a cycle ergometer or a treadmill, a system for analyzing exhaled gases, a device for recording ventilation parameters, and an oximeter for measuring oxygen saturation or an arterial line for obtaining blood gas measurements.
      (2) This test also requires the patient to exercise at certain work load increments.
      (3) Values measured during this test include:
         (a) Blood pressure
         (b) Heart rate
         (c) EKG
         (d) Respiratory rate
         (e) Oxygen saturation or blood gases
         (f) Oxygen consumption
         (g) Carbon dioxide production
         (h) Respiratory quotient
         (i) Oxygen pulse (volume of oxygen removed from the blood with each heartbeat—calculated by dividing oxygen consumption by the heart rate)
         (j) $V_D : V_T$ ratio (V_D = volume of dead space)

(k) MVV
(l) Anaerobic threshold (the point at which the oxygen requirements of the exercising muscles cannot be met and anaerobic metabolism begins providing an oxygen supply)
(4) The test is discontinued when the patient reaches a predetermined heart rate or if the following signs or symptoms occur:
(a) Physical exhaustion
(b) Excessive chest pain
(c) Excessive dyspnea
(d) Excessive fatigue in the legs
(e) Premature ventricular contractions
(f) Ventricular tachycardia
(g) Heart block
(h) Hypotension
(i) Patient requests the test to be stopped

V. INTERPRETATION CHART SUMMARY

	Obstructive	*Restrictive*
FVC	Decreased	Decreased
IC	Decreased or normal	Decreased
ERV	Decreased or normal	Decreased
VT	Increased	Decreased or normal
FRC	Increased	Decreased
RV	Increased	Decreased
RV : TLC	Increased	Decreased
FEV$_1$	Decreased	Normal (FEV$_1$/FVC)
FEF$_{200-1200}$	Decreased	Normal
FEF$_{25\%-75\%}$	Decreased	Normal
FEV : FVC	Decreased	Normal
MVV	Decreased	Decreased

VI. FLOW-SENSING DEVICES

A. **Wright's respirometer**

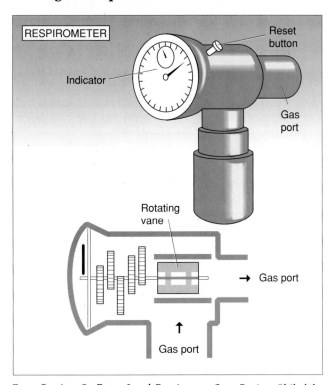

From Persing G. *Entry Level Respiratory Care Review.* Philadelphia: WB Saunders; 1992.

1. This respirometer is a hand-held device that is frequently used at the patient's bedside to measure VC, VT, and minute volume.
2. As the patient's exhaled gas flows through the respirometer, it rotates vanes within the device. Through a gearworks mechanism, the movement of the vane is indicated on a dial calibrated in liters.
3. This device may also be placed in-line to ventilator circuits to measure the patient's exhaled volume. When used for this purpose, it should be placed on the expiratory side of the circuit as close to the patient as possible.

B. **Pneumotachometers**
1. This type of flow-sensing device integrates flow signals to obtain volume measurements.
2. There are three types of pneumotachs that use different physical principles to measure flow:
   a. Pressure-drop pneumotach — air flows through the tube and meets a resistance that decreases pressure; the pressure drop is measured by a transducer that converts it into an electronic signal.
   b. Temperature-drop pneumotach — uses King's law, which states that the velocity of

gas flow over a heated element is proportional to the convective heat loss from the element. It can measure both flow and volume.

c. Ultrasonic-flow pneumotach—this tube has struts inside to cause a turbulence to gas flow. The turbulent flow waves hit the ultrasonic sound waves and change them. The changes in the ultrasonic sound waves are proportional to the flow of gas and are shown as liters per minute or liters per second.

REFERENCES

1. Eubanks D, Bone R. *Comprehensive Respiratory Care.* 2nd ed. St. Louis: CV Mosby; 1990.
2. Levitzky M. *Introduction to Respiratory Care.* Philadelphia: WB Saunders; 1990.
3. Ruppell G. *Manual of Pulmonary Function Testing.* 4th ed. St. Louis: CV Mosby; 1986.
4. Scanlan C, Spearman C. *Egan's Fundamentals of Respiratory Care.* 5th ed. St. Louis: CV Mosby; 1990.

PRETEST ANSWERS

1. C

2. B

3. E

4. C

5. B

Workbook

CHAPTER 17

Oxygen and Medical Gas Therapy

I. STORAGE AND CONTROL OF MEDICAL GASES

A. Storage and control of medical gases and cylinder characteristics

   1. Cylinders are constructed from what high-grade steel?

   2. List the maximum number of liters of oxygen capable of being stored in the following sized cylinders.
      H cylinder _____
      E cylinder _____

   3. How many liters of gaseous oxygen are equivalent to 1 cubic foot of liquid oxygen?

   4. Identify which safety system is used on the following sized cylinders.
      Small cylinders _____
      Large cylinders _____

   5. Identify the pinhole placement of a pin-indexed safety system for an oxygen cylinder.

   6. List the two types of safety relief devices found on oxygen cylinder valves and under what condition high pressure will be released.

      a.

      b.

   7. List the color of the cylinder for the following medical gases.
      Carbon dioxide _____
      Helium _____
      Oxygen _____
      Air _____
      Nitrous oxide _____
      Helium/oxygen _____
      Carbon dioxide/oxygen _____

8. How often are cylinders hydrostatically tested?

9. List three conditions that hydrostatic testing identifies.

   a.

   b.

   c.

10. At what temperature must liquid oxygen be stored in order to maintain it as a liquid?

11. What is the most common method used to produce liquid oxygen?

12. How can one determine the number of stages a regulator has?

13. Write the equation for determining how many minutes are left in an oxygen cylinder before it becomes empty.

14. Write the cylinder factors for the following cylinders.
    E cylinder ———————   H cylinder ———————

15. Calculate how long an E cylinder with 1900 psig will run at 5 L/min (see answer at bottom of page).

16. If an H cylinder containing 1400 psig runs at 8 L/min, how long will the contents last until the cylinder contains 300 psig? (See answer at bottom of page.)

17. Where is the needle valve located on an uncompensated flowmeter and what effect does back pressure have on the reading?

Answer to Question 15: 106 minutes or 1 hour and 46 minutes

Answer to Question 16: 7.2 hours or 7 hours and 12 minutes

18. Where is the needle valve located on a compensated flowmeter and what effect does back pressure have on the reading?

19. The diameter index safety system is used on equipment that operates on less than _____ psig.

20. What effect does back pressure have on the reading of a Bourdon gauge flowmeter?

21. List three types of air compressors and give examples of where they are used most commonly.

    a.

    b.

    c.

II. OXYGEN THERAPY

A. List three indications for oxygen therapy.

    1.

    2.

    3.

B. List seven signs and symptoms of hypoxemia.

    1.

    2.

3.

4.

5.

6.

7.

C. List five complications of oxygen therapy.

1.

2.

3.

4.

5.

D. In order to prevent retrolental fibroplasia in a premature infant, the PaO_2 should be kept below _____ torr.

E. In order to lessen the potential of knocking out the hypoxic drive in a patient with chronic obstructive pulmonary disease who is receiving oxygen, the PaO_2 should be maintained between _____ and _____ torr.

F. List the normal PaO_2 values for the following ages:

Age	*Normal PaO_2*
<60 years	
70 years	
80 years	
90 years	

G. List the four types of hypoxia and give examples of each type.

1.

2.

3.

4.

H. Given the following information, calculate the total oxygen content (See answer at bottom of page).

ABG Results

pH	7.37
PCO_2	37 torr
PO_2	82 torr
SaO_2	96%
Hb	13 vol%

I. What is meant by the term low-flow oxygen system?

J. List five types of low-flow oxygen delivery devices and the appropriate flows and percentages available with each.

1.

2.

Answer to Question H: $1.34 \times 0.96 \times 13 = 16.72$

$0.003 \times 82 = 0.246$

$16.72 + 0.246 = 16.966$ vol%

3.

4.

5.

K. What is the main indication for the use of a transtracheal oxygen catheter?

L. List the three criteria a patient must meet before a low-flow device is considered adequate for oxygen delivery.

1.

2.

3.

M. Define the term high-flow oxygen device.

N. List six types of high-flow oxygen delivery devices.

1.

2.

3.

4.

5.

6.

O. List the air:oxygen entrainment ratios for the following oxygen percentages.
24% _____
28% _____
30% _____
35% _____
40% _____
50% _____
60% _____

P. Write the equation for calculating air:oxygen entrainment ratios.

Q. What is the total flow being delivered to a patient receiving 40% oxygen through an aerosol mask running at 8 L/min? (See answer at bottom of page.)

R. A Venturi mask is set on 30% and an oxygen flow of 6 L/min. What is the total flow delivered by this device? (See answer at bottom of page.)

S. A patient has a total inspiratory flowrate of 48 L/min. What is the minimum flow necessary through a 40% aerosol mask to meet this patient's inspiratory flow demands? (See answer at bottom of page.)

T. How may you visibly observe that adequate flow is being delivered with an aerosol mask?

U. A face tent is most commonly used on what type of patient?

V. If the reservoir tube on a T-tube flow-by setup falls off, what effect will it have on the FIO_2?

Answer to Question Q: 32 L/min

Answer to Question R: 54 L/min

Answer to Question S: 12 L/min

W. A nebulizer set on the 60% dilution mode and connected to an oxygen flowmeter running at 12 L/min has an air bleed-in of 5 L/min downstream. Calculate the F_{IO_2} being delivered by this setup (see answer at bottom of page).

III. MIXED GAS THERAPY

A. What physical property makes helium beneficial for gas delivery to patients with airway obstructions?

B. List the two most commonly administered helium/oxygen (Heliox) mixtures.

C. An 80:20 mixture of helium/oxygen is running through an oxygen flowmeter at 6 L/min. What is the actual flow being delivered to the patient? (See answer at bottom of page.)

D. A 70:30 mixture of helium/oxygen is running through an oxygen flowmeter at 12 L/min. What is the actual flow being delivered to the patient? (See answer at bottom of page.)

E. The physician writes an order for an 80:20 helium/oxygen mixture to be delivered through a nonrebreathing mask at 10 L/min. If an oxygen flowmeter is used to deliver the gas, what must it be set at to deliver this ordered flow? (See answer at bottom of page.)

F. Describe the physiologic actions carbon dioxide has on respiration.

G. Describe the physiologic actions carbon dioxide has on the central nervous system.

H. What effect does an increased carbon dioxide level have on heart rate and cerebral blood flow?

Answer to Question W: 53%

Answer to Question C: $6 \times 1.8 = 10.8$ L/min

Answer to Question D: $12 \times 1.6 = 19.2$ L/min

Answer to Question E: $10/1.8 = 5.5$ L/min

I. List the most commonly administered carbon dioxide/oxygen mixture.

J. List five indications for carbon dioxide therapy.

   1.

   2.

   3.

   4.

   5.

K. List 10 side effects of carbon dioxide therapy.

   1.

   2.

   3.

   4.

   5.

   6.

   7.

8.

9.

10.

IV. HYPERBARIC OXYGEN THERAPY

A. Describe the difference between the multiplace hyperbaric chamber and the monoplace hyperbaric chamber.

B. The hyperbaric chamber is usually pressurized to _____ atmospheres.

C. Breathing 100% oxygen at 3 atmospheres will increase the patient's PaO_2 to approximately _____ torr.

D. List five physiologic effects of hyperbaric oxygen.

1.

2.

3.

4.

5.

E. List five indications for hyperbaric oxygen therapy.

1.

2.

3.

4.

5.

V. OXYGEN ANALYZERS

A. Which oxygen analyzer uses a wheatstone bridge in its operation?

B. Which oxygen analyzer uses the Pauling principle in its operation?

C. What conditions can affect the reading on the galvanic and polarographic analyzers?

VI. OXYGEN SATURATION MONITORING

A. What principle do pulse oximeters operate on?

B. List six causes of inaccurate pulse oximeter readings.

1.

2.

3.

4.

5.

6.

VII. CO-OXIMETRY

A. List three values that may be obtained with a co-oximeter.

1.

2.

3.

B. Carboxyhemoglobin levels of greater than _____% result in nausea and vomiting.

C. Carboxyhemoglobin levels of _____% to _____% are fatal.

CHAPTER 18

Humidity and Aerosol Therapy

I. HUMIDITY THERAPY

A. Define humidity.

B. List two clinical uses of humidity.

    1.

    2.

C. Fully saturated inspired air at body temperature contains how many milligrams of water per liter of air? How much vapor pressure (torr)?

    1. _____ mg of water/L of air

    2. _____ torr

D. Define the term absolute humidity.

E. Define relative humidity and give the equation used to calculate it.

F. What device is used to measure relative humidity?

G. The amount of moisture in a volume of air at 25°C contains 18 mg of water/L of air. Calculate the relative humidity. (Note: At 25°C the air can hold 23.04 mg of water/L of air; see answer at bottom of page.)

Answer to Question G: $18/23.04 = 0.78 \times 100 = 78\%$

H. The inspired gas of a patient contains 16 mg of water/L of gas. Calculate the humidity deficit in milligrams per liter and as a percentage (see answer at bottom of page).

I. A gas at 31°C has a relative humidity of 27%. Calculate the absolute humidity. (At 31°C the air can hold 32 mg of water; see answer at bottom of page.)

J. Calculate the percentage of body humidity of a patient inspiring air that contains 38 mg of water/L of gas (see answer at bottom of page).

K. List three factors that affect the efficiency of humidifiers.

    1.

    2.

    3.

L. Explain the operation of a pass-over humidifier.

M. Explain the operation of a bubble humidifier.

N. The bubble humidifier is capable of delivering a body humidity of _____% to _____%.

O. What body humidity (%) may be achieved with a heat moisture exchanger?

P. Explain how a heat moisture exchanger works.

Answer to Question H: $44 - 16 = 28$ mg/L; $28/44 = 0.64$ or 64%

Answer to Question I: $32 \times 0.27 = 8.64$ mg/L

Answer to Question J: $38/44 = 0.86$ or 86%

II. AEROSOL THERAPY

A. Describe the difference between an aerosol particle and a humidified particle.

B. What is the ideal aerosol particle size for delivery to the airway?

C. List six clinical uses of aerosol therapy.

1.

2.

3.

4.

5.

6.

D. List five factors that affect the penetration and deposition of aerosol particles.

1.

2.

3.

4.

5.

E. Describe the difference between a Pitot tube and a Venturi tube.

F. Explain the operation of a hydrosphere.

G. Explain the operation of a metered dose inhaler.

H. Describe the important points to emphasize to the patient regarding the proper use of the metered dose inhaler.

I. What is the purpose of using the small particle aerosol generator (SPAG) nebulizer?

J. Most aerosol particles produced by the SPAG nebulizer fall within what micron size range?

K. What principle does the ultrasonic nebulizer operate on?

L. What type of fluid should be placed into the couplant chamber of the ultrasonic nebulizer?

M. Which control on the ultrasonic nebulizer determines the particle size? Which controls the volume of aerosol output?

N. Aerosol output from the ultrasonic nebulizer may be as high as _____ ml/min.

O. List six hazards of ultrasonic nebulizer therapy.

1.

2.

3.

4.

5.

6.

III. IMPORTANT POINTS CONCERNING NEBULIZERS

A. Why should heated nebulizers be changed every 12 to 24 hours?

B. The pop-off valves on nebulizers are set at what level to release excess pressure?

C. If the capillary tube of the nebulizer becomes clogged, what effect will this have on its operation?

CHAPTER 19

Cardiopulmonary Patient Assessment

I. PATIENT HISTORY

A. What information should be obtained when getting a patient history?

II. ASSESSMENT OF SYMPTOMS

A. List five conditions that may result in a nonproductive cough.

1.

2.

3.

4.

5.

B. List four common symptoms that pulmonary patients frequently present with?

1.

2.

3.

4.

C. Describe what the following colors of sputum may indicate regarding a patient's illness.

1. White and translucent—

2. Yellow (purulent) —

3. Green—

4. Green and foul smelling—

5. Brown—

6. Red—

D. List nine causes of dyspnea.

1.

2.

3.

4.

5.

6.

7.

8.

9.

E. Define the term orthopnea.

F. Define the condition known as paroxysmal nocturnal dyspnea.

G. What is hemoptysis and with which disorders may you observe it?

H. List five sources from which chest pain may originate.

1.

2.

3.

4.

5.

III. OTHER PHYSICAL ASSESSMENTS

A. Give a brief description of the following breathing patterns and a condition in which the pattern may be observed.

1. Eupnea—

2. Bradypnea—

3. Apnea—

4. Tachypnea—

5. Hypopnea—

6. Hyperpnea—

7. Kussmaul's respiration—

8. Biot's respiration—

9. Cheyne-Stokes respiration—

B. What may asymmetric chest movement indicate?

1.

2.

3.

4.

C. What is a "barrel chest" indicative of?

D. What is paradoxical respiration and with what condition may it be observed?

E. List the factors that should be noted when observing the patient's breathing pattern.

   1.

   2.

   3.

   4.

   5.

   6.

   7.

   8.

   9.

F. What is digital clubbing and when is it observed?

G. Define pedal edema and explain what causes it.

H. Define the term cyanosis and explain what it results from.

I. Describe how to assess a patient's capillary refill and in what patients it is abnormally decreased.

J. Define the following chest deformities:

   1. Kyphosis—

   2. Scoliosis—

   3. Kyphoscoliosis—

   4. Lordosis—

   5. Pectus carinatum—

   6. Pectus excavatum—

K. Is kyphoscoliosis an obstructive or restrictive disease?

L. Why do patients with chronic lung disease use the accessory muscles during normal ventilation?

M. Under what three conditions may tactile fremitus be decreased?

   1.

2.

3.

N. A shift of the trachea to the affected side may indicate _____ _____.

O. A shift of the trachea to the unaffected side may indicate _____ _____.

P. A dullness to percussion over a specific lung segment may indicate what?

Q. Match the breath sound to the appropriate area in which it is heard.

1. Vesicular _____

2. Bronchial _____

3. Bronchovesicular _____

4. Tracheal _____

   a. Between the scapula and over the sternum

   b. Over the trachea

   c. Upper part of sternum, trachea, and mainstem bronchi

   d. Entire chest wall except the supraclavicular area

R. Give five examples of conditions in which rales may be heard on auscultation.

1.

2.

3.

4.

5.

S. What causes the wheezing sound heard on auscultation in asthmatics?

T. Describe where the mitral and tricuspid valves are located.

U. The first heart sound (S_1) represents the closing of the _____ valves.

V. Describe where the pulmonic and aortic valves are located.

W. The second heart sound (S_2) represents the closing of the _____ valves.

X. The atrioventricular valves consist of which two valves?

1.

2.

Y. The semilunar valves consist of which two valves?

1.

2.

Z. List four conditions that result in heart murmurs.

1.

2.

3.

4.

AA. A chest x-ray film showing consolidation may be indicative of what condition?

BB. At what level on a chest x-ray film should the tip of the endotracheal tube be placed?

CC. If an endotracheal tube is inserted too far, where would the tube most likely rest? How would you know the tube was inserted too far?

DD. List the four levels of consciousness and characteristics of each.

1.

2.

3.

4.

IV. ASSESSMENT OF LABORATORY VALUES

A. List the normal serum values for the following electrolytes:

1. Sodium (Na^+) —

2. Potassium (K^+) —

3. Chloride (Cl⁻)—

4. Calcium (Ca⁺)—

B. List eight causes of hyponatremia.

1.

2.

3.

4.

5.

6.

7.

8.

C. List five clinical symptoms of hyponatremia.

1.

2.

3.

4.

5.

D. List five causes of hypernatremia.

1.

2.

3.

4.

5.

E. List four clinical symptoms of hypernatremia.

1.

2.

3.

4.

F. List five causes of hypokalemia.

1.

2.

3.

4.

5.

G. List four clinical symptoms of hypokalemia.

1.

2.

3.

4.

H. List four causes of hyperkalemia.

1.

2.

3.

4.

I. List three clinical symptoms of hyperkalemia.

1.

2.

3.

J. List two causes of hypochloremia.

   1.

   2.

K. List two clinical symptoms of hypochloremia.

   1.

   2.

L. List four causes of hyperchloremia.

   1.

   2.

   3.

   4.

M. List five clinical symptoms of hyperchloremia.

   1.

   2.

3.

4.

5.

N. List five causes of hypocalcemia.

1.

2.

3.

4.

5.

O. List three clinical symptoms of hypocalcemia.

1.

2.

3.

P. List five causes of hypercalcemia.

1.

2.

3.

4.

5.

Q. List six clinical symptoms of hypercalcemia.

1.

2.

3.

4.

5.

6.

R. What is the normal blood urea nitrogen level and what does an elevated level indicate?

S. What is the normal glucose serum level and when are elevated levels observed?

T. What is the normal red blood cell level and what does a decreased level indicate?

U. List the normal values for hemoglobin and hematocrit. What is the importance of these values?
hemoglobin _____   hematocrit _____

V. What is the normal white blood cell count and what does an elevated level indicate?

CHAPTER 20

Management of the Airway

I. UPPER AIRWAY OBSTRUCTION

A. List six major causes of upper airway obstruction.

1.

2.

3.

4.

5.

6.

B. List six signs of partial upper airway obstruction.

1.

2.

3.

4.

5.

6.

C. List seven signs of complete upper airway obstruction.

1.

2.

3.

4.

5.

6.

7.

D. What are the steps to take in helping a conscious victim with a partial upper airway obstruction?

E. What is the best method of relieving an upper airway obstruction caused by the tongue falling into the back of the throat?

F. What maneuver is used to relieve an upper airway obstruction caused by food or other foreign body?

II. ARTIFICIAL AIRWAYS

A. Describe the proper insertion technique of an oropharyngeal airway.

B. List four hazards of the oropharyngeal airway.

    1.

    2.

    3.

    4.

C. Why should the oropharyngeal airway never be placed in a conscious victim?

D. Describe the proper insertion technique of the nasopharyngeal airway.

E. What are the two hazards of a nasopharyngeal airway?

    1.

    2.

F. When is the use of an esophageal obturator airway indicated?

G. Describe the steps taken for proper insertion of the esophageal obturator airway.

H. Describe the steps taken for proper removal of the esophageal obturator airway.

I. List five contraindications for the esophageal obturator airway.

1.

2.

3.

4.

5.

J. List four hazards of the esophageal obturator airway.

1.

2.

3.

4.

K. List four indications for endotracheal (E-T) tubes.

1.

2.

3.

4.

L. List the four normal airway reflexes and what response they elicit when stimulated.

1.

2.

3.

4.

M. List eight hazards of E-T tubes.

1.

2.

3.

4.

5.

6.

7.

8.

N. Describe the shape of the McIntosh and Miller laryngoscope blades.

O. Describe the steps for E-T intubation.

P. How far past the vocal cords should the E-T tube be advanced?

Q. What is the average distance from the teeth to the carina on the adult?

R. List eight complications of oral E-T tubes.

   1.

   2.

   3.

   4.

   5.

   6.

   7.

   8.

S. What are McGill forceps used for?

T. List the advantages and complications of nasotracheal tubes.

Advantages:

   1.

2.

3.

4.

5.

Complications:

1.

2.

3.

4.

5.

U. List five indications for tracheostomy tubes.

1.

2.

3.

4.

5.

V. List the immediate and late complications of tracheostomy tubes.

Immediate:

1.

2.

3.

4.

5.

Late:

1.

2.

3.

4.

W. Describe what a fenestrated tracheostomy tube is and its purpose.

X. Describe the tracheostomy button and its purpose.

Y. Describe how speaking tracheostomy tubes work.

III. MAINTENANCE OF ARTIFICIAL AIRWAYS

A. What type of cuff should be used on all E-T tubes and tracheostomy tubes?

B. Describe how to inflate a cuff using the minimal leak technique and the minimal occluding volume technique.

C. What is the importance of using the minimal leak or occluding volume technique for cuff inflation?

D. What pressure should the E-T tube cuff be kept below to prevent obstruction of arterial flow, venous flow, and lymphatic flow?

  1. Arterial flow—

  2. Venous flow—

  3. Lymphatic flow—

E. List the steps for E-T suctioning.

F. List the suctioning levels for adults, children, and infants.

  1. Adults—

  2. Children—

  3. Infants—

G. Describe how to determine what sized suction catheter is appropriate for a given E-T tube size.

H. A patient is intubated with a 6.5-mm E-T tube. What is the appropriate sized suction catheter to suction this tube?

I. What is a Coudé suction catheter used for?

J. List three indications for tracheal suctioning.

1.

2.

3.

K. List five hazards of tracheal suctioning and appropriate techniques to decrease the potential of these hazards.

1.

2.

3.

4.

5.

L. What is a Yankauer suction?

IV. EXTUBATION

A. Describe the steps in performing E-T tube extubation.

B. List two hazards of extubation and appropriate treatment of those hazards.

   1.

   2.

C. What type of oxygen delivery device is most appropriate following extubation and why?

V. LARYNGEAL AND TRACHEAL COMPLICATIONS OF E-T TUBES

A. What is the major clinical sign of glottic edema?

B. List four causes of glottic edema.

   1.

   2.

   3.

   4.

C. List three ways of treating glottic edema.

   1.

2.

3.

D. Describe subglottic edema.

E. Describe tracheal stenosis and where it is most commonly found in the airway.

F. How may tracheal stenosis at the cuff site be prevented?

CHAPTER 21

Special Respiratory Care Procedures

I. BRONCHOSCOPY

A. Describe the two types of bronchoscopes.

B. List seven indications for bronchoscopy.

 1.

 2.

 3.

 4.

 5.

 6.

 7.

C. How can bronchoscopy help in the control of pulmonary hemorrhage?

D. Describe how a bronchoscope is used in the performance of tracheal intubation.

E. List eight complications of bronchoscopy.

    1.

    2.

    3.

    4.

    5.

    6.

    7.

    8.

F. List five respiratory care practitioner duties relating to bronchoscopy.

    1.

    2.

    3.

    4.

5.

II. THORACENTESIS

A. Describe the technique used in performing a thoracentesis.

B. Upon fluid removal, it is analyzed for what six characteristics?

1.

2.

3.

4.

5.

6.

C. List three complications of thoracentesis.

1.

2.

3.

III. TRANSTRACHEAL ASPIRATION

A. Describe the technique for transtracheal aspiration.

B. List four complications of transtracheal aspiration.

1.

2.

3.

4.

IV. CHEST TUBE INSERTION AND MONITORING

A. List five substances that may accumulate in the pleural space.

1.

2.

3.

4.

5.

B. Describe the three types of chest tube drainage systems.

1. One-bottle system:

2. Two-bottle system:

3. Three-bottle system:

C. If no fluctuation is occurring in the water seal bottle, what must be suspected?

D. If a chest tube becomes obstructed, what may occur?

E. If an air leak is suspected, what action should be taken?

CHAPTER 22

Cardiopulmonary Resuscitation Techniques

I. CARDIOPULMONARY RESUSCITATION

A. What technique is preferred to open the airway of an unconscious victim?

B. If after opening the airway and delivering two breaths there is no air movement, what is the next appropriate step in rescue breathing?

C. What artery is palpated to determine if there is a pulse in an adult? In an infant?

   Adult —

   Infant —

D. At what point may cardiopulmonary resuscitation (CPR) be discontinued?

E. What is the compression-to-breath rate for one-rescuer CPR on an adult victim? Two-rescuer CPR?

   One rescuer — _____ compressions, _____ breaths

   Two-rescuer — _____ compressions, _____ breaths

II. ADULT, CHILD, AND INFANT CPR MODIFICATIONS

A. What is the compression-to-breath rate on the child and infant during one-rescuer CPR?

   Child — _____ compressions, _____ breaths

Infant —_____ compressions, _____ breaths

B. If the victim has a pulse but is not breathing, at what rate should you ventilate the following victims?

Adult —_____

Child —_____

Infant —_____

III. CPR — SPECIAL CONSIDERATIONS

A. Compressions achieve only _____% to _____% of normal blood flow.

B. What is the best indication of adequate cerebral blood flow during CPR?

C. A patient with suspected neck injury should have the airway opened by which method?

D. List three hazards of CPR.

1.

2.

3.

E. What may lead to a fat embolism following CPR?

IV. MANUAL RESUSCITATORS

A. List three uses of manual resuscitators.

1.

2.

3.

B. Why is it important to use a reservoir attachment on a manual resuscitator?

C. List four criteria that will aid in delivering the highest oxygen percentage to the patient while using a manual resuscitator.

1.

2.

3.

4.

D. List four hazards of manual resuscitators.

1.

2.

3.

4.

E. Describe the characteristics of a gas-powered resuscitator.

V. PHARMACOLOGIC INTERVENTION DURING CPR

A. List four routes of drug administration during CPR.

1.

2.

3.

4.

B. List three drugs that are commonly instilled directly down the endotracheal tube.

1.

2.

3.

C. What is the only drug that may be directly injected into the myocardium?

D. List the indications for the use of the following drugs during CPR.

Epinephrine —

Lidocaine —

Atropine —

Procainamide —

Bretylium —

Propranolol —

Dobutamine —

Isoproterenol —

Dopamine —

Sodium nitroprusside —

Calcium chloride —

E. Why is sodium bicarbonate no longer recommended for use during CPR?

VI. DEFIBRILLATION AND CARDIOVERSION

A. Describe proper paddle placement during defibrillation of a patient.

B. What is the initial current delivered during defibrillation of the adult?

C. Should this current be inadequate in restoring the heart to normal rhythm, what is the maximum current that may be used?

D. How does defibrillation reverse ventricular fibrillation?

E. What two drugs may be administered to improve the success of defibrillation?

1.

2.

F. What is the difference between defibrillation and cardioversion?

G. List five arrhythmias that cardioversion is used to terminate.

1.

2.

3.

4.

5.

H. How much electric current is normally delivered during cardioversion?

I. List the respiratory therapist's duties when assisting with cardioversion.

1.

2.

3.

4.

VII. TRANSPORTING THE CRITICALLY ILL PATIENT

A. What effect does increasing altitudes during air transport have on a patient's PO_2?

B. List respiratory therapy equipment necessary for transporting a patient.

CHAPTER **23**

Intermittent Positive Pressure Breathing Therapy

I. INTRODUCTION TO INTERMITTENT POSITIVE PRESSURE BREATHING (IPPB) THERAPY

A. Define IPPB.

B. List four factors that make IPPB effective.

1.

2.

3.

4.

II. PHYSIOLOGIC EFFECTS OF IPPB

A. List seven physiologic effects of IPPB.

1.

2.

3.

4.

5.

6.

7.

B. Explain how airway resistance and lung compliance affect the delivered tidal volume when using a pressure-limited ventilator for IPPB.

C. The respiratory care practitioner should set the ventilator to deliver _____ ml/kg of body weight for the delivered tidal volume during IPPB.

D. List four reasons why IPPB may increase the patient's work of breathing.

1.

2.

3.

4.

E. The patient should not be required to generate more than _____ cm of water to cycle the IPPB unit into inspiration.

III. INDICATIONS FOR IPPB

A. List seven indications for IPPB therapy.

   1.

   2.

   3.

   4.

   5.

   6.

   7.

B. List two conditions that result in increased airway resistance.

   1.

   2.

IV. HAZARDS OF IPPB THERAPY

A. List eight hazards of IPPB therapy.

   1.

2.

3.

4.

5.

6.

7.

8.

B. What is a common complaint from a patient who is being excessively ventilated during IPPB?

C. Give a set of arterial blood gas results that would indicate the patient's hypoxic drive was being knocked out during IPPB.

pH—

$PaCO_2$—

PaO_2—

D. Explain how IPPB may cause a decrease in cardiac output.

E. Explain how IPPB may cause an elevation in intracranial pressure (ICP).

F. What is the normal value for ICP?

G. How may the respiratory care practitioner decrease the potential of the ICP becoming elevated during IPPB therapy?

H. In what type of patient is it most common for a pneumothorax to be induced by IPPB?

V. CONTRAINDICATIONS FOR IPPB

A. List two **absolute** contraindications of IPPB.

   1.

   2.

B. List eight **relative** contraindications of IPPB.

   1.

   2.

   3.

   4.

   5.

   6.

7.

8.

VI. IPPB IN THE TREATMENT OF PULMONARY EDEMA

A. How does IPPB aid in the treatment of pulmonary edema?

VII. PROPER ADMINISTRATION OF IPPB

A. List the proper steps involved in the proper administration of IPPB.

B. If the patient's pulse increases more than _____ beats/min during IPPB therapy, the treatment should be stopped immediately and the physician notified.

C. Following IPPB therapy, what information should be recorded in the patient's chart?

VIII. CHARACTERISTICS OF SPECIFIC IPPB UNITS

A. Once gas enters the Bird Mark 7 unit, what is the first control to which it travels?

B. What determines the degree of sensitivity for the patient to cycle the unit into inspiration on the Bird Mark 7?

C. Describe the flow characteristics at end inspiration on the Bird Mark 7.

D. What liter flow is available on the Bird Mark 7 when air mix is used and when it is not used?

E. How does increasing the flowrate on the Bird Mark 7 affect the inspiratory time?

F. What kind of flow waveform occurs when the Bird Mark 7 is set on 100% and on air mix?

    1. 100% —

    2. Air mix —

G. What ends inspiration on the Bird Mark 7?

H. What ends inspiration on the Bennett PR-2?

I. What is the terminal flow control used for on the Bennett PR-2?

J. When the terminal flow control is used on the Bennett PR-2, what is the effect on the FIO_2?

IX. IMPORTANT FACTORS TO CONSIDER WHEN VENTILATING A PATIENT WITH A PRESSURE-LIMITED IPPB MACHINE

A. What effect do the following conditions have on the delivered tidal volume (increase or decrease)?

    Increased airway resistance —

    Decreased airway resistance —

    Increased lung compliance —

    Decreased lung compliance —

    Increased peak pressure —

Decreased peak pressure—

Increased flowrate—

Decreased flowrate—

B. What effect do the following conditions have on the inspiratory time (increase or decrease)?

Increased airway resistance—

Decreased airway resistance—

Increased lung compliance—

Decreased lung compliance—

Increased flowrate—

Decreased flowrate—

X. PROBLEMS ENCOUNTERED WHILE ADMINISTERING IPPB AND CORRECTIVE ACTIONS

A. List six corrective actions to take if the patient is having difficulty cycling the IPPB machine off.

1.

2.

3.

4.

5.

6.

B. If the patient complains of tingling in the fingers or dizziness during an IPPB treatment, what corrective action should be taken?

C. List five corrective actions to take if no nebulization of medications is occurring?

1.

2.

3.

4.

5.

D. You notice that during inspiration the manometer needle remains in the negative area for half of the inspiration before moving to the positive area for the last half of the inspiration. What machine adjustment would correct this?

E. While the patient is exhaling, the IPPB machine cycles into inspiration. How may this be corrected?

CHAPTER 24

Chest Physiotherapy/ Incentive Spirometry

I. CHEST PHYSIOTHERAPY

A. List four goals of chest physiotherapy.

1.

2.

3.

4.

B. List six indications for chest physiotherapy.

1.

2.

3.

4.

5.

6.

C. Describe how the patient should be positioned to drain the anterior basal segment of the right lower lobe.

D. Describe how the patient should be positioned to drain the anterior segment of the right upper lobe.

E. Describe how the patient should be positioned to drain the apical segment of the left upper lobe.

F. Describe how the patient should be positioned to drain the superior and inferior lingular segments of the left lung.

G. Percussion should be applied over a specified area for what length of time?

H. List six areas over which percussion should not be performed.

1.

2.

3.

4.

5.

6.

I. Describe how manual vibration should be performed on a patient.

J. List seven complications of chest physiotherapy.

    1.

    2.

    3.

    4.

    5.

    6.

    7.

K. How may hypoxemia be minimized during chest physiotherapy?

L. What modification in postural drainage position should be implemented on a patient with a closed head injury?

M. Describe the proper cough technique.

II. INCENTIVE SPIROMETRY (SUSTAINED MAXIMAL INSPIRATORY THERAPY)

A. List six goals of incentive spirometry.

    1.

2.

3.

4.

5.

6.

B. List four hazards of incentive spirometry.

1.

2.

3.

4.

C. List four guidelines for effective incentive spirometry.

1.

2.

3.

4.

D. Describe the proper positioning of the patient for the most effective incentive spirometry.

E. What is the proper inspiratory pattern the patient should perform in order to obtain effective incentive spirometry?

CHAPTER 25
Cardiac Monitoring

I. ELECTROCARDIOGRAPHY

A. Describe the role each of the following play in the conduction system of the heart.

1. Sinoatrial node —

2. Atrioventricular node —

3. Bundle of His —

4. Purkinje fibers —

B. Describe the lead placement positions for a 12-lead electrocardiogram (EKG).

C. Each small square on EKG graph paper represents ———— seconds.

D. Describe what each of the following EKG waves represents and its normal time interval.

1. P wave

2. Q wave

3. QRS complex

4. T wave

5. P-R interval

6. S-T segment

E. Describe three types of artifacts seen on EKG strips.

1.

2.

3.

F. Describe how to calculate a patient's heart rate on an EKG graph.

G. Describe how to determine if a patient's EKG reading is regular or irregular.

H. Describe the characteristics of the following cardiac arrhythmias.

1. Sinus bradycardia

a. Rate—

b. Rhythm—

c. Wave pattern abnormalities—

d. Causes—

    e. Treatment—

2. Sinus tachycardia

    a. Rate—

    b. Rhythm—

    c. Wave pattern abnormalities—

    d. Causes—

    e. Treatment—

3. Sinus arrhythmia

    a. Rate—

    b. Rhythm—

    c. Wave pattern abnormalities—

    d. Causes—

    e. Treatment—

4. Premature atrial contractions

    a. Rate—

b. Rhythm—

c. Wave pattern abnormalities—

d. Causes—

e. Treatment—

5. Premature ventricular contractions

a. Rate—

b. Rhythm—

c. Wave pattern abnormalities—

d. Causes—

e. Treatment—

6. Atrial fibrillation

a. Rate—

b. Rhythm—

c. Wave pattern abnormalities—

d. Causes—

    e. Treatment —

7. Atrial flutter

    a. Rate —

    b. Rhythm —

    c. Wave pattern abnormalities —

    d. Causes —

    e. Treatment —

8. Ventricular tachycardia

    a. Rate —

    b. Rhythm —

    c. Wave pattern abnormalities —

    d. Causes —

    e. Treatment —

9. Ventricular fibrillation

    a. Rate —

     b. Rhythm—

     c. Wave pattern abnormalities—

     d. Causes—

     e. Treatment—

10. First-degree heart block

     a. Rate—

     b. Rhythm—

     c. Wave pattern abnormalities—

     d. Causes—

     e. Treatment—

11. Second-degree heart block

     a. Rate—

     b. Rhythm—

     c. Wave pattern abnormalities—

     d. Causes—

e. Treatment—

12. Third-degree heart block

a. Rate—

b. Rhythm—

c. Wave pattern abnormalities—

d. Causes—

e. Treatment—

II. HEMODYNAMIC MONITORING

A. Where are the most common sites for the insertion of arterial line catheters?

1.

2.

3.

B. What type of transducer is most commonly connected to the arterial line system to display the pressure waveform?

C. What is pulse pressure?

D. List four complications of arterial catheters.

1.

2.

3.

4.

E. List the causes and ways to correct the following problems associated with arterial catheters.

1. "Damped" pressure tracing

a. Causes:

(1)

(2)

(3)

(4)

b. Corrected by:

(1)

(2)

(3)

(4)

2. Abnormally high or low pressure readings

    a. Causes:

        (1)

        (2)

    b. Corrected by:

        (1)

        (2)

3. No pressure reading

    a. Causes:

        (1)

        (2)

    b. Corrected by:

        (1)

        (2)

F. Describe the four-channel Swan-Ganz catheter and the pressures it is used to measure.

G. Describe the proper insertion technique of a Swan-Ganz catheter.

H. Central venous pressure (CVP) is a measurement of what portion of the heart?

I. Normal CVP is _____.

J. List 11 conditions that increase CVP.

1.

2.

3.

4.

5.

6.

7.

8.

9.

10.

11.

K. List four conditions that decrease CVP.

1.

2.

3.

4.

L. What is the normal value for pulmonary artery pressure (PAP)?

M. List three conditions that increase PAP.

1.

2.

3.

N. List two conditions that decrease PAP.

1.

2.

O. Pulmonary artery wedge pressure (PAWP) is a measurement of which area of the heart?

P. Describe how wedge pressure is obtained.

Q. Normal PAWP is _____ torr.

R. How do cardiogenic and noncardiogenic pulmonary edema affect PAWP?

S. List four conditions that increase PAWP.

    1.

    2.

    3.

    4.

T. List two conditions that decrease PAWP.

    1.

    2.

U. List seven complications of Swan-Ganz catheter insertion.

    1.

    2.

    3.

    4.

    5.

    6.

7.

    V. Write the equation for calculating cardiac output.

    W. Normal cardiac output is ——————— L/min.

    X. Calculate the cardiac output of a patient who has an oxygen consumption (Vo_2) of 240 ml/min and an arterial-venous oxygen content difference of 6 vol% (see answer at bottom of page).

    Y. Calculate the arterial-venous oxygen content difference given the following information:
PaO_2	82 torr
SaO_2	95%
PvO_2	37 torr
SvO_2	72%
Hb	14 vol% (g%)

    Z. In a normal, healthy person, the percentage of the cardiac output making up intrapulmonary shunting is ———————%.

  AA. List four conditions that increase physiologic shunting.

      1.

      2.

      3.

      4.

  BB. Write the equation for calculating clinical shunt.

Answer to Question X: 6 L/min

Answer to Question Y: 4.4 vol% (g%)

CC. Write the modified shunt equation.

DD. Given the following information, calculate the patient's percentage of shunt:

pH   7.39
$PaCO_2$ 40 torr
PaO_2 122 torr
FIO_2 0.50
P_B 747 torr

(See answer at bottom of page.)

EE. Explain the significance of the following shunt values.

<10% —

10% to 20% —

20% to 30% —

>30% —

FF. Write the equation for calculating cardiac index.

GG. The normal range for cardiac index is _____ $L/min/m^2$ to _____ $L/min/m^2$.

HH. What is meant by cardiac index?

II. List four factors that increase cardiac index.

1.

2.

Answer to Question DD: 11% shunt

3.

4.

JJ. List eight factors that decrease cardiac index.

1.

2.

3.

4.

5.

6.

7.

8.

KK. Define stroke volume and write the equation for calculating it.

LL. Normal stroke index is _____ to _____ ml/beat.

MM. Define systemic vascular resistance (SVR).

NN. Write the equation for calculating SVR.

OO. Write the normal values for SVR.

PP. List four factors that increase SVR.

    1.

    2.

    3.

    4.

QQ. List three factors that decrease SVR.

    1.

    2.

    3.

RR. Define pulmonary vascular resistance (PVR).

SS. Write the equation for calculating PVR.

TT. Write the normal values for PVR.

UU. List eight factors that increase PVR.

    1.

    2.

    3.

    4.

    5.

    6.

    7.

    8.

VV. List three factors that decrease PVR.

    1.

    2.

    3.

WW. Define oxygen consumption and give the normal value.

XX. Calculate the oxygen consumption given the following information:

Q_T 4.5 L/min

CaO_2 19 vol%

CvO_2 14 vol%

(See answer at bottom of page.)

YY. List four factors that increase oxygen consumption.

1.

2.

3.

4.

ZZ. List three factors that decrease oxygen consumption.

1.

2.

3.

CHAPTER 26

Arterial Blood Gas Interpretation

I. ARTERIAL BLOOD GAS ANALYSIS

A. What blood gas value is used to determine the following:

1. Alveolar ventilation —

2. Arterial oxygenation —

3. Oxygen delivery to the tissues —

4. Acid-base status of the blood —

B. Where is mixed venous blood obtained and by what method is it obtained?

C. Describe how to perform the modified Allen test. Why is it performed?

II. ARTERIAL OXYGENATION

A. What is the PaO_2 a measurement of?

B. For every 1 torr of PaO_2 there is _____ ml of oxygen dissolved in the plasma.

C. Write the equation used to calculate alveolar oxygen tension (PAO_2).

D. Given the following data calculate the patient's A-a gradient.

pH	7.35
FIO_2	1.0
$PaCO_2$	44 torr
HCO_3	26 mEq/L
PaO_2	135 torr
Barometric pressure	747 torr

(See answer at bottom of page.)

E. Define the term A-a gradient.

F. If the oxyhemoglobin dissociation curve is shifted to the right, what does this indicate?

G. What conditions will shift the curve to the right?

H. If the curve is shifted to the left, what does this indicate?

I. What conditions will shift the curve to the left?

J. Explain the Haldane effect.

K. Explain the Bohr effect.

L. List the normal PaO_2 levels according to age.

Age	*PaO_2 (torr)*
<60	
60	
65	
70	
75	
80	

Answer to Question D:

$$(700 \times 1) - (44 \times 1.25) =$$
$$700 \quad - \quad 55 \quad = 645 \text{ torr}$$

A-a gradient $= 645 - 135 = 510$ torr

O. Define the levels of hypoxemia.

60 to 79 torr ———————————

40 to 59 torr ———————————

<40 torr ———————————

N. What is the normal value for arterial oxygen saturation (SaO_2)?

III. CARBON DIOXIDE TRANSPORT AND ALVEOLAR VENTILATION

A. By what mechanism does carbon dioxide enter the blood?

B. What percentage of the atmosphere is composed of carbon dioxide?

C. List three ways that carbon dioxide is carried in the blood.

1.

2.

3.

D. What is the normal $PaCO_2$ level?

E. What effect does hyperventilation have on the $PaCO_2$?

F. What effect does hypoventilation have on the $PaCO_2$?

G. Define the terms:

1. Hypocapnia—

2. Hypercapnia—

H. What three mechanisms affect $PaCO_2$?

1.

2.

3.

IV. ACID-BASE BALANCE (pH)

A. Write the Henderson-Hasselbach equation.

B. From the Henderson-Hasselbach equation determine the following:

1. If base decreases and acid remains the same the pH will _____.

2. If base increases and acid remains the same the pH will _____.

3. If acid increases and base remains the same the pH will _____.

4. If acid decreases and base remains the same the pH will _____.

C. The ratio of bicarbonate to carbonic acid (H_2CO_3) is _____ when the pH is 7.4.

D. What is the normal value for arterial blood pH?

E. Define acidemia.

F. Define alkalemia.

G. Upon reviewing blood gas results acidemia is present. What two blood gas abnormalities would cause this pH change?

H. What is the normal value for blood bicarbonate?

I. What does the term compensation refer to in relation to arterial blood gas interpretation?

V. ARTERIAL BLOOD GAS INTERPRETATION

A. pH   7.21
   PaCO₂   66 torr
   HCO₃   24 mEq/L
   PaO₂   68 torr
   B.E.   0
   Acid-base status —

   Ventilatory status —

   Metabolic status —

   Oxygenation status —

   Interpretation —

   Corrective measures —

B. pH   7.55
   PaCO₂   24 torr
   HCO₃   23 mEq/L
   PaO₂   94 torr
   B.E.   −1
   Acid-base status —

   Ventilatory status —

Metabolic status—

Oxygenation status—

Interpretation—

Corrective measures—

C. pH   7.24
   PaCO₂   41 torr
   HCO₃   16 mEq/L
   PaO₂   86 torr
   B.E.   −8

Acid-base status—

Ventilatory status—

Metabolic status—

Oxygenation status—

Interpretation—

Corrective measures—

D. pH   7.42
   PaCO₂   43 torr
   HCO₃   25 mEq/L
   PaO₂   51 torr
   B.E.   +1

Acid-base status—

Ventilatory status—

Metabolic status—

Oxygenation status—

Interpretation—

Corrective measures—

E. pH   7.36
   PaCO₂   62 torr
   HCO₃   36 mEq/L
   PaO₂   58 torr
   B.E.   +12

Acid-base status—

Ventilatory status—

Metabolic status—

Oxygenation status—

Interpretation—

Corrective measures—

F. pH   7.19
    $PaCO_2$ 23 torr
    HCO_3 11 mEq/L
    PaO_2 88 torr
    B.E.   −13

Acid-base status—

Ventilatory status—

Metabolic status—

Oxygenation status—

Interpretation—

Corrective measures—

VI. BLOOD GAS ANALYZERS

A. Identify what each electrode measures:

    1. Sanz electrode—

    2. Severinghaus electrode—

    3. Clark electrode—

CHAPTER 27

Ventilator Management

I. NEGATIVE- VERSUS POSITIVE-PRESSURE VENTILATORS

A. List two types of negative-pressure ventilators and give the advantages and disadvantages of each.

1.
   Advantages:

   Disadvantages:

2.
   Advantages:

   Disadvantages:

B. List the two types of positive-pressure ventilators.

1.

2.

C. What type of ventilator is used on neonates and what effect do lung compliance and airway resistance have on delivered tidal volumes?

II. VENTILATOR CONTROLS

A. Describe the following modes of ventilation.

1. Control mode—

2. Assist mode—

3. Assist/control mode—

B. At what level should the sensitivity be set on the ventilator for the patient to cycle it into inspiration?

C. List the two types of intermittent mandatory ventilation (IMV) setups.

1.

2.

D. What should the sensitivity be set at on the ventilator (Bennett MA-1) during the IMV mode?

E. Describe how to determine if adequate IMV flows are being delivered on both kinds of IMV setups.

F. During a spontaneous breath on IMV, you notice the manometer needle is deflecting to -5 cm of water during inspiration. What action should be taken?

G. What does the term breath-stacking indicate?

H. Describe synchronized intermittent mandatory ventilation.

I. Describe pressure support ventilation.

J. Describe continuous positive airway pressure (CPAP).

K. As the oxygenation status of a patient worsens on an oxygen mask, at what point should CPAP be employed?

L. How do you determine what initial tidal volume setting should be used on a ventilated patient?

M. What is minute ventilation (volume) and how is it determined?

N. Calculate the ventilator tubing compliance when the volume is set at 300 ml (0.3 L) generating a pressure in the tubing of 60 cm of water (see answer at bottom of page).

O. Using the tubing compliance in Question N, calculate the corrected tidal volume when the patient is on 800 ml tidal volume and has a peak inspiratory pressure of 28 cm of water (see answer at bottom of page).

P. How is anatomic deadspace calculated?

Q. List the potential sources of leaks on the ventilator that will affect delivered tidal volume.

R. If the spirometer bellows on the Bennett MA-1 ventilator rises during inspiration, what is the most likely problem?

S. On initial ventilator setup, the respiratory rate should be set within what range?

Answer to Question N: 5 ml/cm of water

Answer to Question O: 660 ml

T. Explain the effect inspiratory flowrate has on the inspiratory time.

U. What is the normal inspiratory:expiratory (I:E) ratio for adults and infants? Write the equation for calculating I:E ratio.

Adults—

Infants—

I:E ratio—

V. List the three ventilator controls that alter the I:E ratio and what effect they have on the inspiratory and expiratory time when they are increased or decreased.

W. A patient has been set up with an inverse I:E ratio. How would you adjust the flowrate (increase or decrease) to place the patient on a 1:2 I:E ratio?

X. Describe the use of expiratory retard.

Y. What is the proper method for setting sigh volume?

Z. Describe positive end-expiratory pressure (PEEP).

AA. List six indications for PEEP.

1.

2.

3.

4.

5.

6.

BB. List four hazards of PEEP.

1.

2.

3.

4.

CC. What is optimal PEEP?

DD. If the mixed venous PO_2 drops to less than _____ torr after the initiation of PEEP, this would indicate a drop in cardiac output and reduced oxygen delivery to the tissues.

III. VENTILATOR ALARMS AND MONITORING

A. Describe the proper setting for the low-pressure alarm and ways it may be activated.

B. Describe the proper setting for the high-pressure alarm and ways it may be activated.

C. Describe the proper setting for the low PEEP/CPAP alarm and ways it may be activated.

D. Define mean airway pressure.

E. List eight factors that affect mean airway pressure.

    1.

    2.

    3.

    4.

    5.

    6.

    7.

    8.

F. Write the equation for calculating mean airway pressure.

G. What is meant by the term optimal mean airway pressure?

H. Normal end-tidal carbon dioxide is _____% to _____% or _____ torr to _____ torr.

I. List four conditions that result in a decreased end-tidal carbon dioxide reading.

    1.

    2.

3.

4.

J. List two conditions that result in an increased end-tidal carbon dioxide reading.

1.

2.

IV. INDICATIONS FOR MECHANICAL VENTILATION

A. List four indications for mechanical ventilation.

1.

2.

3.

4.

B. A $PaCO_2$ of greater than _____ torr indicates ventilatory failure and a need for mechanical ventilator assistance.

V. COMMON CRITERIA FOR INITIATION OF MECHANICAL VENTILATORY SUPPORT

A. List six criteria that would indicate mechanical ventilatory assistance is necessary.

1.

2.

3.

4.

5.

6.

B. What is a normal deadspace : tidal volume ratio?

C. What does an inadequate negative inspiratory force indicate physiologically?

VI. GOALS OF MECHANICAL VENTILATION

A. List five goals of mechanical ventilation.

1.

2.

3.

4.

5.

B. How does mechanical ventilation increase alveolar ventilation?

VII. COMPLICATIONS OF MECHANICAL VENTILATION

A. List eight complications of mechanical ventilation.

1.

2.

3.

4.

5.

6.

7.

8.

B. What causes patients on mechanical ventilators to be more prone to respiratory infections?

C. What are the two causes of decreased urinary output in patients on mechanical ventilators?

1.

2.

D. What effects can malnutrition have on ventilated patients?

VIII. DEADSPACE

A. Define the three types of deadspace.

1.

2.

3.

B. A tracheostomy reduces the amount of deadspace by _____%.

C. What is the purpose of adding mechanical deadspace to the ventilator circuit?

D. Mechanical deadspace should be added **only** in which ventilator modes?

IX. LUNG COMPLIANCE

A. Define compliance.

B. Define dynamic lung compliance and write the equation for calculating it.

C. Define static lung compliance and write the equation for calculating it.

D. Calculate the static lung compliance given the following data:

Tidal volume	750 ml
Flowrate	50 L/min
PEEP	8 cm of water
Peak inspiratory pressure	46 cm of water
Plateau pressure	28 cm of water

(See answer at bottom of page.)

E. What does a decreasing lung compliance indicate about the patient's pulmonary status?

F. List eight conditions that would lead to a decreased lung compliance.

1.

2.

3.

4.

5.

6.

7.

8.

G. What is a normal lung compliance in a ventilated patient?

Answer to Question D: $750/20 = 37.5$ ml/cm of water

X. VENTILATION OF THE HEAD TRAUMA PATIENT

A. How should the flowrate be altered in a head trauma patient and why?

B. What should the $Paco_2$ levels be maintained at on a head trauma patient and why?

XI. WEANING FROM THE MECHANICAL VENTILATOR

A. List nine criteria for weaning patients from mechanical ventilation.

1.

2.

3.

4.

5.

6.

7.

8.

9.

B. Before a patient is extubated, the FIO_2 should be _____ or less.

C. List two types of weaning techniques.

1.

2.

XII. HIGH-FREQUENCY VENTILATION

A. List the ventilator rates available and tidal volume setting (according to mean body weight) when ventilating with high-frequency positive pressure ventilation.

B. High-frequency jet ventilation uses respiratory rates of _____ to _____ cycles/min.

C. High-frequency oscillation delivers small tidal volumes at a rate of _____ to _____/min.

D. List four advantages of high-frequency ventilation over conventional ventilation.

1.

2.

3.

4.

XIII. ESTIMATING DESIRED VENTILATOR PARAMETER CHANGES

A. The following data are from a patient on a volume ventilator in the control mode:

pH	7.37
$PaCO_2$	37 torr
PaO_2	60 torr
Tidal volume	700 ml
Rate	12 breaths/min
FIO_2	0.3

In order to increase this patient's PaO_2 to 80 torr, what change to the FIO_2 must be made? (See answer at bottom of page.)

B. The following data were collected from a patient on a ventilator in the control mode.

pH	7.28
$PaCO_2$	55 torr
PaO_2	68 torr
Tidal volume	650 ml
Rate	8 breaths/min
FIO_2	0.4

In order to decrease this patient's $PaCO_2$ to 40 torr, what change must be made to the ventilator rate? (See answer at bottom of page.)

C. The following data were collected from a patient on a volume ventilator in the control mode.

pH	7.24
$PaCO_2$	60 torr
PaO_2	66 torr
Tidal volume	700 ml
Rate	10 breaths/min
FIO_2	0.4

In order to decrease this patient's $PaCO_2$ to 45 torr, what must the minute volume be changed to? (See answer at bottom of page.)

Answer to Question A: $\dfrac{80 \times 0.3}{60} = 0.4$

Answer to Question B: $\dfrac{8 \times 55}{40} = 11/min$

Answer to Question C: $\dfrac{7 \times 60}{45} = 9.3 \text{ L}$

D. The following data were collected from a patient on a ventilator in the control mode.

pH	7.5
$PaCO_2$	30 torr
Tidal volume	850 ml
Rate	10 breaths/min
PaO_2	92 torr
FIO_2	0.35
Anatomic VD	150 ml

In order to increase this patient's $PaCO_2$ to 40 torr, what change in alveolar ventilation must be made? (See answer at bottom of page.)

XIV. PRACTICE VENTILATOR PROBLEMS

A. A 65-kg (143-lb) patient is on an assist/control rate of 10 breaths/min, tidal volume of 1000 ml (1 L), and an FIO_2 of 0.5. ABG results are as follows:

pH	7.58
$PaCO_2$	25 torr
PaO_2	99 torr

What is the appropriate recommendation at this time?

A. Increase the respiratory rate

B. Decrease the tidal volume

C. Decrease the sensitivity

D. Increase the FIO_2

E. Increase the flowrate

(See answer at bottom of page.)

Answer to Question D: $\dfrac{7 \times 30}{40} = 5.25$ L

Answer to Question A: B

B. A spontaneously breathing 44-year-old patient is on a 60% oxygen mask with the following ABG results:

pH   7.46
PaCO$_2$ 34 torr
PaO$_2$ 56 torr

What is the appropriate measure to take?

A. Place on 90% nonrebreather

B. Place on assist/control ventilation

C. Place on control ventilation

D. Place on CPAP

E. No change is necessary at this time.
(See answer at bottom of page.)

C. A 36-year-old woman is on the following ventilator settings:

Assist/control rate   10 breaths/min
Tidal volume   650 ml (0.65 L)
FIO$_2$ 0.4

ABG results:

pH   7.22
PaCO$_2$ 61 torr
PaO$_2$ 75 torr
HCO$_3$ 26 mEq/L
B.E.   +1

What is the appropriate ventilator change at this time?

A. Decrease rate

B. Decrease tidal volume

C. Increase tidal volume

D. Increase FIO$_2$

E. Add PEEP
(See answer at bottom of page.)

Answer to Question B: D

Answer to Question C: C

D. A 65-kg (143-lb) patient is on a ventilator on the following settings:

Control mode
Rate   6 breaths/min
Tidal volume   800 ml
FIO_2 0.4

ABG results:

pH   7.26
$PaCO_2$ 59 torr
PaO_2 80 torr
HCO_3 23 mEq/L
B.E.   −1

What is the appropriate recommendation at this time?

A. Increase rate

B. Increase tidal volume

C. Decrease tidal volume

D. Increase FIO_2

E. Give sodium bicarbonate
   (See answer at bottom of page.)

E. A 45-year-old woman with adult respiratory distress syndrome is being ventilated on the following settings:

Assist/control mode
Rate   12 breaths/min
Tidal volume   700 ml
FIO_2 0.8
PEEP   10 cm of water

ABG results:

pH   7.41
$PaCO_2$ 37 torr
PaO_2 158 torr

What is the appropriate recommendation at this time?

A. Decrease FIO_2

B. Decrease PEEP

C. Decrease tidal volume

D. Decrease rate

E. Increase tidal volume
   (See answer at bottom of page.)

Answer to Question D: A

Answer to Question E: A

XV. VENTILATOR FLOW WAVE CAPABILITIES

A. List the four types of flow patterns and describe their characteristics.

1.

2.

3.

4.

B. Which type of flow pattern would benefit a patient with increased airway resistance?

XVI. CHARACTERISTICS OF SPECIFIC MECHANICAL VENTILATORS

A. The PEEP valve on the Bennett MA-1 is capable of producing a maximum of _____ cm of water of PEEP.

B. What type of flow wave pattern does the Bennett MA-1 produce?

C. What are some of the major differences between the Bennett MA-1 and the Bennett MA-2 ventilators?

D. What type of flow wave patterns may be accomplished with the Bennett 7200 ventilator?

E. Describe what occurs when the 100% oxygen suction button is depressed on the Bennett 7200.

F. What is meant by the Bennett 7200 being compliance-compensated?

G. Describe how the tidal volume is determined on the Siemens Servo 900 C ventilator.

H. Describe how the inspiratory flowrate is determined when using the Servo 900 C.

I. Which of the ventilators covered in this section operate on the principle of fluidics?

J. Write the equation for calculating the approximate tidal volume using the Sechrist IV-100B infant ventilator.

CHAPTER 28

Disorders of the
Respiratory System

I. CHRONIC OBSTRUCTIVE PULMONARY DISEASE (COPD)

A. What diseases are classified as COPD?

1.

2.

3.

4.

5.

B. Define emphysema.

C. Which type of emphysema is usually associated with alpha$_1$-antitrypsin deficiency?

D. What is a bleb?

E. What causes a COPD patient to have an increased functional residual capacity?

F. Is a COPD patient's lung compliance normal, increased, or decreased?

G. List nine signs and symptoms of emphysema.

1.

2.

3.

4.

5.

6.

7.

8.

9.

H. What is characteristic about the chest x-ray film of an emphysema patient?

I. Which pulmonary function values would be **decreased** in a COPD patient?

J. Which oxygen delivery device is most acceptable for use in a patient with emphysema who is chronically hypoxemic?

K. What should the PaO₂ be maintained at in a patient with COPD who is chronically hypoxemic?

L. Define chronic bronchitis.

M. In which type of COPD is there an increase in the size of mucous glands and an increase in the number of goblet cells?

N. Describe cor pulmonale and what causes it.

O. List clinical signs and symptoms of cor pulmonale.

P. How does oxygen therapy help prevent or treat cor pulmonale?

Q. Define asthma.

R. Describe the difference between extrinsic and intrinsic asthma.

S. When mast cells in the airway are stimulated, what five substances are released?

1.

2.

3.

4.

5.

T. The release of the substances in Question S results in:

1.

2.

3.

4.

5.

U. What does the term paradoxical pulse indicate?

V. Write a set of arterial blood gas values that would be normal for a chronic emphysema patient and one for an asthmatic patient in mild to moderate acute distress.

Emphysema	*Asthma*
pH	pH
$PaCO_2$	$PaCO_2$
PaO_2	PaO_2
Bicarbonate	Bicarbonate
B.E.	B.E.

W. What type of white blood cell is characteristically elevated in the sputum of an asthmatic patient?

X. What does cromolyn sodium do and when is it to be administered?

Y. What bronchodilator is commonly administered intravenously for the treatment of status asthmaticus?

Z. What does the term status asthmaticus refer to?

AA. List the proper treatment modalities for emphysema.

BB. List the proper treatment modalities for asthma.

CC. Define bronchiectasis.

DD. List four causes of bronchiectasis.

    1.

    2.

    3.

    4.

EE. List nine clinical signs and symptoms of bronchiectasis.

    1.

    2.

    3.

    4.

    5.

    6.

7.

8.

9.

FF. What is characteristic about the sputum produced by patients with bronchiectasis?

GG. List treatment modalities for bronchiectasis.

II. LOWER RESPIRATORY TRACT INFECTIONS

A. Define pneumonia.

B. What decreased airway defense mechanisms may lead to the invasion of pathogenic organisms?

C. What causes the consolidation of specific lung areas with pneumonia?

D. List seven signs and symptoms of pneumonia.

1.

2.

3.

4.

5.

6.

7.

E. List five types of bacterial pneumonia. Which type is the most common?

1.

2.

3.

4.

5.

F. What condition is *Pneumocystis carinii* pneumonia most commonly associated with?

G. What medication is *P. carinii* pneumonia treated with?

H. List the proper treatment modalities for pneumonia.

I. Define lung abscess.

J. What is the most common microorganism responsible for lung abscesses?

K. List the signs and symptoms of lung abscess.

L. List the treatment modalities for lung abscess.

M. Define tuberculosis.

N. How is tuberculosis spread?

O. How is tuberculosis diagnosed?

P. List clinical signs and symptoms of tuberculosis.

Q. List treatment modalities for tuberculosis.

III. OTHER LUNG DISORDERS

A. Define cardiogenic pulmonary edema.

B. List four causes of cardiogenic pulmonary edema.

1.

2.

3.

4.

C. What are two forces that maintain fluid in the capillaries?

    1.

    2.

D. Which one of these forces, when increased, causes pulmonary edema?

E. Define orthopnea.

F. Define paroxysmal nocturnal dyspnea.

G. List the signs and symptoms of pulmonary edema.

H. What chest x-ray findings are characteristic for a patient with pulmonary edema?

I. List the treatment modalities for pulmonary edema.

J. Define pulmonary embolism.

K. List three causes for pulmonary embolism.

    1.

    2.

    3.

L. List the signs and symptoms of pulmonary embolism.

M. List the treatment modalities for pulmonary embolism.

N. Define adult respiratory distress syndrome (ARDS).

O. List the various causes of ARDS.

P. What effect does decreased surfactant production have on the lung compliance of a patient with ARDS?

Q. List the signs and symptoms of ARDS.

R. List the treatment modalities for ARDS.

S. What effect does the lung compliance of a patient with ARDS have on ventilator peak inspiratory pressure?

T. Define pneumothorax.

U. Define tension pneumothorax and appropriate action to take should it occur.

V. List the signs and symptoms of a pneumothorax.

W. What are characteristic features of a pneumothorax on chest x-ray film?

X. List the treatment modalities for a pneumothorax.

Y. Define pleural effusion.

z. List the signs and symptoms of a pleural effusion.

AA. What are characteristic features of a pleural effusion on chest x-ray film?

BB. List the treatment modalities for pleural effusion.

CC. Describe obstructive sleep apnea.

DD. What is the most effective method for treating obstructive sleep apnea?

EE. What is the difference between respiratory effort observed in a patient with obstructive sleep apnea and one with central sleep apnea?

FF. List five symptoms of obstructive sleep apnea.

   1.

   2.

   3.

   4.

   5.

GG. Describe central sleep apnea.

HH. With what disorders are obstructive sleep apnea and central sleep apnea associated?

Obstructive   **Central**

II. List four symptoms of central sleep apnea.

1.

2.

3.

4.

JJ. What is the purpose of performing sleep studies?

KK. What is a polysomnograph?

LL. List six things that are recorded continuously on a polysomnogram.

1.

2.

3.

4.

5.

6.

CHAPTER 29

Neonatal/Pediatric Respiratory Care

I. NEONATAL RESPIRATORY CARE

A. Describe what the term high-risk infant means.

B. List eight **maternal** factors involved with high-risk infants.

1.

2.

3.

4.

5.

6.

7.

8.

C. List seven other factors, related to the delivery, that are associated with high-risk infants.

1.

2.

3.

4.

5.

6.

7.

D. Describe the Dubowitz scoring system and its purpose.

E. Normal gestational age is _____ to _____ weeks.

F. What do the following abbreviations represent?

1. AGA—

2. SGA—

3. LGA—

G. What five conditions are assessed in the APGAR score?

   1.

   2.

   3.

   4.

   5.

H. When is an APGAR test performed?

I. Given the following APGAR scores, describe appropriate intervention.

   0 to 3—

   4 to 6—

   7 to 10—

J. What does the term acrocyanosis refer to?

K. What does the Silverman test determine?

L. List five areas that are assessed in the Silverman test.

   1.

2.

3.

4.

5.

M. What is often the first sign of respiratory distress in the infant?

N. What is the normal respiratory rate and blood pressure for the infant?

Respiratory rate —

Blood pressure —

O. What are normal arterial blood gas values for an infant?

pH —

$PaCO_2$ —

PaO_2 —

Bicarbonate —

B.E. —

P. Describe oxygen delivery with the use of an incubator (Isolette).

Q. What is the recommended method of delivering oxygen to an infant?

R. Describe oxygen delivery using a hood.

S. List six indications for nasal continuous positive airway pressure (CPAP).

1.

2.

3.

4.

5.

6.

T. List five complications of nasal CPAP.

1.

2.

3.

4.

5.

U. List two hazards of oxygen therapy in the neonate.

1.

2.

V. In order to decrease the potential of retrolental fibroplasia, the infant's PaO_2 should be maintained at no higher than _____ torr.

W. If the infant has a ductal shunt, where should arterial blood gases be drawn if there is concern for elevated PaO_2 to the retinal arteries?

X. Describe where the tip of the umbilical artery catheter should rest when properly positioned.

Y. List four advantages of an umbilical artery catheter.

1.

2.

3.

4.

Z. List four complications of umbilical artery catheters.

1.

2.

3.

4.

AA. Umbilical artery catheters should be left in no longer than _____ to _____ days.

BB. List four sites at which peripheral artery puncture may be performed in the neonate.

1.

2.

3.

4.

CC. Describe the use of the transilluminator in relation to peripheral artery puncture.

DD. Describe the proper procedure for peripheral artery puncture in the neonate.

EE. Describe the procedure for obtaining capillary blood from the neonate.

FF. How reliable are capillary blood gas values in relation to arterial blood gas values?

GG. Describe the use of transcutaneous monitoring of a neonate's PaO_2 and $PaCO_2$.

HH. List three disadvantages of transcutaneous monitoring.

1.

2.

3.

II. What is a thermal neutral environment?

JJ. Describe the process of nonshivering thermogenesis in the neonate.

KK. Describe the use of a radiant warmer.

II. NEONATAL CARDIOPULMONARY DISORDERS

A. Define respiratory distress syndrome (RDS).

B. A lecithin : sphingomyelin ratio of less than _____ indicates immature lung surfactant.

C. List six clinical manifestations associated with respiratory distress syndrome.

1.

2.

3.

4.

5.

6.

D. Describe the chest x-ray findings in an infant with RDS.

E. List the treatment modalities for RDS.

F. Define bronchopulmonary dysplasia (BPD).

G. What causes BPD?

H. List nine clinical manifestations of BPD.

1.

2.

3.

4.

5.

6.

7.

8.

9.

I. Describe chest x-ray findings in infants with BPD.

J. List the treatment modalities for BPD.

K. Define meconium aspiration.

L. Describe the causes of meconium aspiration.

M. List eight clinical manifestations of meconium aspiration.

1.

2.

3.

4.

5.

6.

7.

8.

N. Describe chest x-ray findings in infants with meconium aspiration.

O. List the treatment modalities for meconium aspiration.

P. Define persistent fetal circulation (PFC).

Q. Describe normal fetal circulation.

R. List eight conditions associated with PFC.

1.

2.

3.

4.

5.

6.

7.

8.

S. List five clinical manifestations of PFC.

1.

2.

3.

4.

5.

T. Describe chest x-ray findings in infants with PFC.

U. List the treatment modalities for PFC.

III. AIRWAY DISORDERS OF THE PEDIATRIC PATIENT

A. Define epiglottitis.

B. List the causes of epiglottitis.

C. List 12 clinical manifestations of epiglottitis.

1.

2.

3.

4.

5.

6.

7.

8.

9.

10.

11.

12.

D. Describe the characteristic x-ray finding for diagnosing epiglottitis.

E. List the treatment modalities for epiglottitis.

F. Define laryngotracheobronchitis (croup).

G. List the causes for croup.

H. List 10 clinical manifestations of croup.

1.

2.

3.

4.

5.

6.

7.

8.

9.

10.

I. Describe the characteristic x-ray finding of croup.

J. List the treatment modalities for croup.

K. Define foreign body aspiration.

L. What are the most common objects children aspirate?

M. Once the object is aspirated, what pathologic effects occur?

N. List five clinical manifestations of foreign body aspiration.

1.

2.

3.

4.

5.

O. Describe the x-ray findings of foreign body aspiration.

P. List the treatment modalities for foreign body aspiration.

Q. Define bronchiolitis.

R. What is the most common cause of bronchiolitis?

S. List nine clinical manifestations of bronchiolitis.

1.

2.

3.

4.

5.

     6.

     7.

     8.

     9.

T. Describe chest x-ray findings associated with bronchiolitis.

U. List the treatment modalities for bronchiolitis.

V. Define cystic fibrosis.

W. Describe the cause of cystic fibrosis.

X. Describe the pathology of the mucus production in cystic fibrosis.

Y. List 12 clinical manifestations of cystic fibrosis.

     1.

     2.

     3.

     4.

5.

6.

7.

8.

9.

10.

11.

12.

Z. Describe chest x-ray findings for cystic fibrosis.

AA. List the treatment modalities for cystic fibrosis.

CHAPTER **30**

Respiratory
Medications

I. CLASSIFICATIONS OF RESPIRATORY MEDICATIONS

A. List four types of diluents and what each is used for.

  1.

  2.

  3.

  4.

B. What type of medication is acetylcysteine (Mucomyst) and what is its primary use?

C. List the side effects of acetylcysteine.

D. Identify three receptors that are stimulated by sympathomimetic drugs and give their locations and responses to stimulation.

  1.

  2.

  3.

E. When is racemic epinephrine most commonly used?

F. Which of the following medications are considered sympathomimetic bronchodilators?

	YES	NO
Acetylcysteine	_____	_____
Isoetharine	_____	_____
Atropine	_____	_____
Isoproterenol	_____	_____
Albuterol	_____	_____
Theophylline	_____	_____
Terbutaline	_____	_____

G. Which sympathomimetic bronchodilator is the strongest beta$_2$ receptor stimulator?

H. What is the most common side effect of isoproterenol?

I. To what classification of bronchodilator does atropine belong?

J. What other conditions is atropine used for?

K. Give an example of a phosphodiesterase inhibitor.

L. What type of patient is most commonly administered theophylline?

M. What is the purpose of administering ethanol to a patient with pulmonary edema?

N. Describe the use of cromolyn sodium for asthma.

O. List three neuromuscular blocking agents and what purposes they are used for in respiratory care.

    1.

2.

3.

P. Which of the three neuromuscular blockers release histamine?

Q. The paralyzing effects of nondepolarizing agents may be reversed with the administration of what two drugs?

1.

2.

R. List five antibiotics that are aerosolized and the conditions that they are indicated for.

1.

2.

3.

4.

5.

S. List three corticosteroids that are aerosolized and the conditions that they are indicated for.

1.

2.

3.

T. List the side effects of steroid therapy.

II. DRUG CALCULATIONS

A. Calculate the percentage strength of a 1:1000 solution (see answer at bottom of page).

B. What is the ratio strength of a 20% solution? (See answer at bottom of page.)

C. How many milligrams of a 1:100 preparation of isoproterenol are in 0.25 ml of the drug? (See answer at bottom of page.)

D. How many milligrams is 0.3 ml of a 5% solution of metaproterenol? (See answer at bottom of page.)

E. Write the two equations used to calculate children's doses of medications and identify both by name.

Answer to Question A: $1/1000 = 0.001 \times 100 = 0.1\%$

Answer to Question B: $20/100 = 1:5$ ratio

Answer to Question C: 2.5 mg

Answer to Question D: 15 mg

CHAPTER 31

Respiratory Home Care

I. HOME REHABILITATION

A. List the four goals of rehabilitation.

1.

2.

3.

4.

B. List the various conditions requiring pulmonary rehabilitation.

II. CARE OF THE REHABILITATION PATIENT

A. List 10 treatment modalities that are part of the patient home care plan.

1.

2.

3.

4.

5.

6.

7.

8.

9.

10.

B. List five periodic evaluations that should be performed on the home care patient.

1.

2.

3.

4.

5.

C. Describe pursed-lip breathing and what the advantages are of this breathing exercise.

D. Describe how to instruct a patient in diaphragmatic breathing exercises and the advantages that will be gained from performing it.

E. A vital capacity of less than _____ ml/kg of ideal body weight indicates an inadequate volume to achieve an effective cough.

F. Describe the steps in performing an effective cough maneuver.

G. List the four disadvantages of using oxygen cylinders in home oxygen administration.

  1.

  2.

  3.

  4.

H. Explain why liquid oxygen is more advantageous for home oxygen administration.

I. What is an oxygen concentrator and how does it work?

J. List the two types of oxygen concentrators and the oxygen percentage available on both.

  1.

  2.

K. What types of evaluations should be made on the oxygen concentrator by the respiratory care practitioner on routine visitations?

L. Describe how nondisposable humidifiers and nebulizers should be cleaned in the home setting.

M. List the seven responsibilities of the respiratory care practitioner in caring for the pulmonary patient in the home.

1.

2.

3.

4.

5.

6.

7.

CHAPTER 32

Pulmonary Function Testing

I. LUNG VOLUMES AND CAPACITIES

A. Define the following volumes and give their normal values:

    1. Tidal volume (V_T)—

    2. Residual volume (RV)—

    3. Inspiratory reserve volume (IRV)—

    4. Expiratory reserve volume (ERV)—

B. Describe how the following volumes are measured and give examples of diseases or conditions that may lead to a decrease or increase in the volume.

    1. V_T—

    2. RV—

    3. IRV—

    4. ERV—

C. Define the following capacities and give their normal values:

1. Functional residual capacity (FRC) —

2. Inspiratory capacity (IC) —

3. Vital capacity (VC) —

4. Forced vital capacity (FVC) —

5. Total lung capacity (TLC) —

D. Describe how each of the capacities is measured and give examples of diseases or conditions that may lead to a decrease or increase in the capacity.

1. FRC —

2. IC —

3. VC —

4. FVC —

5. TLC —

E. Which capacity is used to measure flow studies such as forced expiratory volume $(FEV)_{0.5}$, forced expiratory flow $(FEF)_{25-75}$, and $FEF_{200-1200}$?

F. Describe three ways to measure FRC.

1.

2.

3.

F. What is the normal RV:TLC ratio; give an example of a condition in which it is increased.

G. List four conditions in which minute volume would be increased.

   1.

   2.

   3.

   4.

H. What is the normal range for minute volume?

I. What ratio is the best indicator for differentiating an obstructive disorder from a restrictive one?

J. List the normal values for the FEV:FVC ratio percentage.
   _____% of the FVC is exhaled in 0.5 seconds.
   _____% of the FVC is exhaled in 1 second.
   _____% of the FVC is exhaled in 2 seconds.
   _____% of the FVC is exhaled in 3 seconds.

K. Define FEV.

L. Define $FEF_{200-1200}$ and give the normal value.

M. An FEV_1:FVC ratio of < _____ % indicates an obstructive disease.

N. Define FEF$_{25\%-75\%}$.

O. Define peak flow and give the normal value.

P. Define maximum voluntary ventilation (MVV) and explain its significance.

Q. What five values may be measured on a flow volume loop?

1.

2.

3.

4.

5.

R. Write the equation to calculate diffusion capacity.

S. What is the normal value for diffusion capacity?

T. List five conditions in which diffusion capacity is decreased.

1.

2.

3.

4.

5.

U. What type of study is done to determine the distribution of gas and pulmonary perfusion in the lung?

II. OBSTRUCTIVE VERSUS RESTRICTIVE DISEASES

A. List five obstructive diseases.

1.

2.

3.

4.

5.

B. What is the characteristic pulmonary function finding in determining an obstructive process?

C. List six restrictive diseases or disorders.

1.

2.

3.

4.

5.

6.

D. What is the characteristic pulmonary function finding in determining a restrictive process?

E. Pulmonary function predicted values are determined by what five factors?

1.

2.

3.

4.

5.

III. MISCELLANEOUS PULMONARY FUNCTION STUDIES

A. What does a before-and-after bronchodilator study determine?

B. After a bronchodilator is administered, the flow studies must show an increase of at least _____% to prove significant reversibility of airway obstruction.

C. What does the negative inspiratory force (NIF) represent?

D. Describe the proper procedure for obtaining an NIF on a patient.

E. What is the normal value for NIF?

F. An NIF of less than −_____ indicates inadequate respiratory muscle strength to cough and maintain a patent airway.

G. Describe the procedure for obtaining a maximal expiratory pressure (MEP) measurement on a patient.

H. What is the normal value for MEP?

I. List six parameters that should be obtained from a patient prior to exercise stress testing.

1.

2.

3.

4.

5.

6.

J. List eight contraindications to stress testing.

1.

2.

3.

4.

5.

6.

7.

8.

K. List the emergency equipment that should be present during a stress test.

1.

2.

3.

4.

5.

6.

7.

L. List 12 values that are measured during a cardiopulmonary stress test.

   1.

   2.

   3.

   4.

   5.

   6.

   7.

   8.

   9.

  10.

  11.

  12.

M. List nine signs and symptoms a patient may exhibit that would indicate the stress test should be discontinued.

1.

2.

3.

4.

5.

6.

7.

8.

9.

IV. INTERPRETATION CHART SUMMARY

A. Determine if the following pulmonary function tests would be normal, increased, or decreased in an **obstructive disorder**:

1. FVC	Normal _____	Increased _____	Decreased _____
2. V_T	Normal _____	Increased _____	Decreased _____
3. FRC	Normal _____	Increased _____	Decreased _____
4. RV	Normal _____	Increased _____	Decreased _____
5. RV:TLC	Normal _____	Increased _____	Decreased _____
6. FEV_1	Normal _____	Increased _____	Decreased _____
7. FEV:FVC	Normal _____	Increased _____	Decreased _____
8. FEF_{25-75}	Normal _____	Increased _____	Decreased _____
9. MVV	Normal _____	Increased _____	Decreased _____

B. Determine if the following pulmonary function tests would be normal, increased, or decreased in a **restrictive disorder**:

1. FVC   Normal _____   Increased _____   Decreased _____
2. VT   Normal _____   Increased _____   Decreased _____
3. FRC   Normal _____   Increased _____   Decreased _____
4. RV   Normal _____   Increased _____   Decreased _____
5. RV : TLC   Normal _____   Increased _____   Decreased _____
6. FEV_1 Normal _____   Increased _____   Decreased _____
7. FEV : FVC   Normal _____   Increased _____   Decreased _____
8. FEF_{25-75} Normal _____   Increased _____   Decreased _____
9. MVV   Normal _____   Increased _____   Decreased _____

VI. FLOW-SENSING DEVICES

A. Describe the operation of a Wright's respirometer.

B. What parameters may be measured using the Wright's respirometer?

C. List three types of pneumotachometers.

1.

2.

3.

CHAPTER 33

Clinical Simulation Practice Problems

This chapter is intended to prepare the individual for successful completion of the National Board for Respiratory Care (NBRC) Clinical Simulation Examination. Three practice simulations, which are similar to those found on the NBRC examination, are presented in this chapter. Although the NBRC examination requires the use of a latent image marker to reveal information, I have modified the material in this chapter so that the information chosen by the user is revealed on the next page.

Let us now discuss the two content areas in the simulations and how they are to be worked in my modified format. Each simulation has an information-gathering section and a decision-making section. These sections are preceded by a case scenario about the particular patient that we are about to assess and recommend treatment modalities for. Once you have read the scenario about the patient you will go to Section A (Selections), which is an information-gathering section. This section will have a list of options to choose from in order to assess the patient's condition. Go through the list and **place check marks beside each choice you feel is important** to evaluate this patient's condition. (On the NBRC examination you will use a latent image marker to reveal the information from the options you have chosen.) Be sure and choose only those options you feel are necessary to evaluate the patient. Each option has been assessed a specific point value ranging from −3 to +3. Options of **greatest importance** for the patient's evaluation at that time are worth **3 points**, with **2 points** and **1 point given for options that are less important but still important to assess**. Those options that are **detrimental** at the time of assessment are worth **−3 points for most detrimental** and −2 or −1 point for less serious detrimental choices. In other words, points will be deducted from your score if these options are chosen. Options given 0 points are those that do not necessarily help in assessing the patient but at the same time are not harmful.

Once you have placed check marks next to the options you feel are important to evaluate, locate Section A (Responses) to reveal the information from the options you have chosen. Circle the ones you selected from the previous page so that they will stand out from those you did not select. After doing that, find the directive that tells you which section to go to next. Each information-gathering section will work in this manner.

During the simulation you will be directed to decision-making sections in which you will be asked to make certain decisions in therapy based on the information you have gathered. The decision options are also given points ranging from −3 to +3. Again, the most appropriate decisions will add points to your total score, whereas detrimental decisions will deduct points from your total score. The better the choice, the more points added; the more detrimental, the more points deducted. **In the decision-making sections, only one choice is made unless you are directed to make another selection.** Place a check mark next to the choice you feel is most appropriate. Locate the responses section of that section to reveal the information given from the decision option you selected. **Look only at the choice you selected.** Follow the instructions that apply to that decision. You will be told either that the physician agrees and to proceed to another section or that the physician disagrees and to make another selection. There may be more than one appropriate selection just as there are different treatment modalities that benefit the patient. In this case, you may choose an appropriate option only to see that the physician disagrees and that you are directed to make another selection. You will not be penalized for this selection but you then need to choose another option that is appropriate. If an incorrect choice of therapy is chosen that may not be beneficial and only mildly harmful, you will be sent to a section that deals with the resulting complications. At that point, you can rectify your mistake and get back on track in the problem. If you do not make appropriate selections to correct the complications, you may be further directed to another section in which the patient is in more trouble. Choices that are seriously harmful to the patient may also be included, but if they are chosen, you will be instructed to make another selection and will not be allowed to pursue this detrimental decision.

Follow the directives throughout the simulation until the statement "End of problem" is revealed. This signifies that the simulation has been completed.

At the end of the simulation you will find a score sheet to tabulate the selections you have made throughout the simulation, along with the maximum possible score and the minimum passing score. Go back through the problem and check the options you chose with the points each selection is worth based on the point scale at the end of each simulation. This will determine your score on each clinical simulation. **Subtract all negative responses from all positive responses in each section to obtain your "Total Section Score," then compare this to the maximum points available and the minimum passing score.**

While doing these three clinical simulations, please do not look ahead in the problem or look at information you did not select. It is obvious that with this format, with all the information available, whether you selected it or not, right in front of you, the temptation to look at that information is great. Resist this temptation. Remember, you want to discover the areas in which you need more work and in the areas in which you excel. The best way to determine this is to work the problem just as if it were the actual NBRC examination (minus latent image marker).

Also included at the end of the simulation is the optimal pathway through the sections that should have been followed, and if they were not, how it was possible to reenter that pathway. By taking the optimal pathway, less points would have been deducted for making inappropriate decision-making selections. By making inappropriate decision-making choices, and being sent to alternate sections, more points will be deducted. Check the pathway you followed and compare it with the optimal pathway to see what mistakes you made.

Clinical simulation examinations are fun, although I am sure you will want to experience this fun with the NBRC only once. While grading these simulations, pay very close attention to what information was considered important, unimportant, harmful, or detrimental by noting the points given to each individual choice. After grading the simulation, note the points given to the choices you did not select. This will give you an overall picture of the patient's assessment, evaluation, and treatment and the appropriateness of each selection.

NOTE: The system I have used to grade the simulations in this text may be somewhat different than the one used by the NBRC. However, I feel strongly that if you score high on these simulations you should perform well on the actual examination. A minimal passing score or lower may indicate a need for more practice with clinical simulations.

For more practice with clinical simulations, the NBRC offers packets of simulations that closely resemble those given on the actual examination. The best way to feel comfortable with this unique test is to practice several simulations prior to the examination, and it is my sincere hope that what I have covered in this text will increase your confidence level on both the Written Registry and the Clinical Simulation Examination.

CLINICAL SIMULATION NO. 1

Patient: Sally Cook—Age 44 Years

You are the evening shift supervisor at your hospital and have just been paged to the emergency room. Sally Cook, a 44-year-old woman, has just arrived in the emergency room following a motor vehicle accident. The emergency room physician wants your assistance in assessing and managing Ms. Cook. **GO TO SECTION A (SELECTIONS).**

Section A (Selections)

Which of the following would you assess in order to best evaluate Ms. Cook's cardiopulmonary status? Place a check mark next to as many as you feel are indicated in this section.

———— A-1. Color

———— A-2. Pupillary reaction

———— A-3. Respiratory rate and pattern

———— A-4. Deep pain response

———— A-5. Sputum culture

———— A-6. Spinal tap

———— A-7. Level of consciousness

———— A-8. Pulse and blood pressure

———— A-9. General appearance

———— A-10. Urine culture

———— A-11. Chest auscultation

———— A-12. Bowel sounds

———— A-13. Electrocardiogram (EKG)

———— A-14. Arterial blood gases (ABGs)

———— A-15. Spontaneous tidal volume

After completing your selections, go to Section A (Responses) to obtain responses from the selections you have made. **LOOK ONLY AT THE SELECTIONS YOU CHOSE.**

Section A (Responses)

Place a check mark next to the responses that correspond to the selections you made.

_____ A-1. Dusky

_____ A-2. Sluggish response to light

_____ A-3. 28 breaths/min and labored

_____ A-4. Normal

_____ A-5. Not evaluated

_____ A-6. Not evaluated

_____ A-7. Semiconscious and combative

_____ A-8. 130 beats/min and 110/65

_____ A-9. Anxious with bleeding from head laceration

_____ A-10. Not evaluated

_____ A-11. Bilateral breath sounds diminished in the bases

_____ A-12. Normal

_____ A-13. Sinus tachycardia, rate of 130 breaths /min

_____ A-14. pH—7.3, PCO_2—50 torr, PO_2—69 torr, HCO_3—25 mEq/L

_____ A-15. 250 ml

After placing a check mark next to your selections, **GO TO SECTION E (SELECTIONS).**

Section B (Selections)

Which of the following would you recommend at this time? (Select only one unless directed to "Make another selection in this section.")

Place a check mark next to the selection you feel is most appropriate, then go to Section B (Responses) to obtain the response from the selections you made.

_____ B-1. Increase rate to 12 breaths/min.

_____ B-2. Increase FIO_2 to 0.7.

_____ B-3. Decrease tidal volume to 400 ml.

_____ B-4. Increase tidal volume to 550 ml.

_____ B-5. Decrease FIO_2 to 0.4.

Section B (Responses)

B-1. Physician disagrees. Make another selection in this section.

B-2. Physician disagrees. Make another selection in this section.

B-3. Physician disagrees. Make another selection in this section.

B-4. Physician agrees. **GO TO SECTION J (SELECTIONS).**

B-5. Physician disagrees. Make another selection in this section.

Section C (Selections)

Ms. Cook remains combative and disoriented. To facilitate intubation, which of the following would you recommend at this time? (Select only one unless directed to "Make another selection in this section.")

Place a check mark next to the selection you feel is most appropriate, then go to Section C (Responses) to obtain the response from the selection you made.

_____ C-1. Use restraints to immobilize the patient.

_____ C-2. Insert an oropharyngeal airway.

_____ C-3. Sedate patient and administer 2 mg of succinylcholine.

_____ C-4. Administer a bolus of lidocaine.

_____ C-5. Perform blind nasal intubation.

Section C (Responses)

C-1. Physician disagrees. Make another selection in this section.

C-2. Physician disagrees. Make another selection in this section.

C-3. Physician agrees. **GO TO SECTION I (SELECTIONS).**

C-4. Physician disagrees. Make another selection in this section.

C-5. Physician disagrees. Make another selection in this section.

Section D (Selections)

Twenty-four hours later, you are performing ventilator checks on Ms. Cook's ventilator when the high-pressure alarm begins to sound with each breath. Ms. Cook is in respiratory distress with a respiratory rate of 32 breaths/min. Which of the following would you assess to evaluate this problem?

Place a check mark next to as many as you feel are indicated in this section.

_____ D-1. Vital capacity

_____ D-2. Ventilator function

———— D-3. Ability to pass suction catheter

———— D-4. Breath sounds

———— D-5. Pupillary reaction

———— D-6. Negative inspiratory force (NIF)

———— D-7. Chest percussion

———— D-8. Ability to manually ventilate

———— D-9. Maximal expiratory pressure

———— D-10. Chest excursion

———— D-11. Body temperature

———— D-12. Gag reflex

———— D-13. Heart rate

After completing your selections, go to Section D (Responses) to obtain responses from the selections you have made. **LOOK ONLY AT THE SELECTIONS YOU CHOSE.**

Section D (Responses)

Place a check mark next to the responses that correspond to the selections you made.

———— D-1. 200 ml

———— D-2. Ventilator is functioning normally with appropriately set parameters

———— D-3. No obstruction as suction catheter is inserted into endotracheal tube

———— D-4. None on right side

———— D-5. Normal

———— D-6. Not evaluated

———— D-7. Hyperresonant sound over right lung field

———— D-8. Increased resistance with difficulty ventilating

———— D-9. Not evaluated

———— D-10. Asymmetric chest movement with left lung expanding more than right lung

———— D-11. 37°C

———— D-12. Intact

———— D-13. 130 beats/min

After placing a check mark next to your selections, **GO TO SECTION H (SELECTIONS)**

Section E (Selections)

The physician wants your recommendation concerning Ms. Cook's care. Which of the following would you recommend at this time? (Select only one unless directed to "Make another selection in this section.")

Place a check mark next to the selection you feel is most appropriate, then go to Section E (Responses) to obtain the response from the selection you made.

———— E-1. Place patient on a continuous positive airway pressure (CPAP) mask of 5 cm of water and 50% oxygen.

———— E-2. Intubate patient and institute mechanical ventilation.

———— E-3. Administer oxygen via a nonrebreathing mask.

———— E-4. Administer a bronchodilator via a hand-held nebulizer followed by postural drainage and percussion.

———— E-5. Administer oxygen via a 30% Venturi mask.

Section E (Responses)

E-1. Physician disagrees. Make another selection in this section.

E-2. Physician agrees. **GO TO SECTION C (SELECTIONS).**

E-3. Done. **GO TO SECTION G (SELECTIONS).**

E-4. Physician disagrees. Make another selection in this section.

E-5. Physician disagrees. Make another selection in this section.

Section F (Selections)

Which of the following would you recommend at this time? (Select only one unless directed to "Make another selection in this section.")

Place a check mark next to the selection you feel is most appropriate, then go to Section F (Responses) to obtain the response from the selection you made.

———— F-1. Increase the ventilator rate.

———— F-2. Decrease the FIO_2.

———— F-3. Decrease the ventilator rate.

———— F-4. Maintain present settings.

———— F-5. Decrease the tidal volume.

Section F (Responses)

F-1. Physician agrees. **GO TO SECTION D (SELECTIONS).**

F-2. Physician disagrees. Make another selection in this section.

F-3. Physician disagrees. Make another selection in this section.

F-4. Done. **GO TO SECTION N (SELECTIONS).**

F-5. Physician disagrees. Make another selection in this section.

Section G (Selections)

After being placed on a 100% nonrebreathing mask, Ms. Cook's ABG values are pH — 7.23, PCO_2 — 59 torr, PO_2 — 68 torr, bicarbonate — 26 mEq/L. Based on this information, which of the following would you now recommend? (Select only one unless directed to "Make another selection in this section.")

Place a check mark next to the selection you feel is most appropriate, then go to Section G (Responses) to obtain the response from the selection you made.

_____ G-1. Place patient on CPAP mask of 5 cm of water and 100% oxygen.

_____ G-2. Maintain present therapy.

_____ G-3. Administer intermittent positive pressure breathing (IPPB) with 0.3 ml of metaproterenol in 2 ml of normal saline.

_____ G-4. Intubate patient and institute mechanical ventilation.

_____ G-5. Intubate and place patient on CPAP of 10 cm of water.

Section G (Responses)

G-1. Physician disagrees. Make another selection in this section.

G-2. Physician disagrees. Make another selection in this section.

G-3. Physician disagrees. Make another selection in this section.

G-4. Physician agrees. **GO TO SECTION C (SELECTIONS).**

G-5. Physician disagrees. Make another selection in this section.

Section H (Selections)

Which of the following would you recommend at this time? (Select only one unless directed to "Make another selection in this section.")

Place a check mark next to the selection you feel is most appropriate, then go to Section H (Responses) to obtain the response from the selection you made.

_____ H-1. Increase the high-pressure limit.

_____ H-2. Increase the FIO_2.

_____ H-3. Decrease the ventilator rate.

_____ H-4. Place a chest tube in the second intercostal space.

_____ H-5. Place a chest tube in the sixth intercostal space.

Section H (Responses)

H-1. Physician disagrees. Make another selection in this section.

H-2. Done. **GO TO SECTION K (SELECTIONS).**

H-3. Physician disagrees. Make another selection in this section.

H-4. Done. **GO TO SECTION L (SELECTIONS).**

H-5. Physician disagrees. Make another selection in this section.

Section I (Selections)

Ms. Cook has been successfully intubated and the physician wants your recommendation for ventilator settings. Ms. Cook weighs 50 kg (110 lb). (Select only one unless directed to "Make another selection in this section.")

Place a check mark next to the selection you feel is most appropriate, then go to Section I (Responses) to obtain the response from the selection you made.

I-1. Control mode, rate — 10 breaths/min, tidal volume — 450 ml, FIO_2 — 0.5

I-2. Assist/control mode, rate — 10 breaths/min, tidal volume — 550 ml, FIO_2 — 0.5

I-3. Intermittent mandatory ventilation (IMV) mode, rate — 6 breaths/min, tidal volume — 700 ml, FIO_2 — 0.6

I-4. Control mode, rate — 10 breaths/min, tidal volume — 550 ml, FIO_2 — 0.5

I-5. Assist/control mode, rate — 4 breaths/min, tidal volume — 750 ml, FIO_2 — 0.5

I-6. IMV mode, rate — 10 breaths/min, tidal volume — 550 ml, FIO_2 — 0.5

I-7. IMV mode, rate — 10 breaths/min, tidal volume — 450 ml, FIO_2 — 0.5

Section I (Responses)

I-1. Thirty minutes later ABG results are pH — 7.28, PCO_2 — 56 torr, PO_2 — 70 torr, HCO_3 — 26 mEq/L. **GO TO SECTION B (SELECTIONS).**

I-2. Thirty minutes later ABG results are pH—7.39, PCO$_2$—40 torr, PO$_2$—86 torr, HCO$_3$—25 mEq/L. **GO TO SECTION J (SELECTIONS).**

I-3. Physician disagrees. Make another selection in this section.

I-4. Thirty minutes later ABG results are pH—7.39, PCO$_2$—40 torr, PO$_2$—86 torr, HCO$_3$—25 mEq/L. **GO TO SECTION J (SELECTIONS).**

I-5. Physician disagrees. Make another selection in this section.

I-6. Thirty minutes later ABG results are pH—7.39, PCO$_2$—40 torr, PO$_2$—86 torr, HCO$_3$—25 mEq/L. **GO TO SECTION J (SELECTIONS).**

I-7. Thirty minutes later ABG results are pH—7.28, PCO$_2$—56 torr, PO$_2$—70 torr, HCO$_3$—26 mEq/L. **GO TO SECTION B (SELECTIONS).**

Section J (Selections)

Two hours later Ms. Cook has stabilized. Which of the following would you assess to monitor the effects of the ventilator on Ms. Cook?

Place a check mark next to as many as you feel are indicated in this section.

_____ J-1. Pulse and blood pressure

_____ J-2. Intracranial pressure

_____ J-3. Serum electrolytes

_____ J-4. Peak expiratory pressure

_____ J-5. Static lung compliance

_____ J-6. ABGs

_____ J-7. Gag reflex

_____ J-8. Chest x-ray

_____ J-9. Functional residual capacity

_____ J-10. Vital capacity

After completing your selections, go to Section J (Responses) to obtain responses from the selections you have made. **LOOK ONLY AT THE SELECTIONS YOU CHOSE.**

Section J (Responses)

Place a check mark next to the responses that correspond to the selections you made.

_____ J-1. 88 beats/min and 122/80

_____ J-2. 20 torr

_____ J-3. Noted

_____ J-4. Noted

_____ J-5. 40 ml/cm of water

_____ J-6. pH—7.39, PCO$_2$—38 torr, PO$_2$—89 torr, HCO$_3$—24 mEq/L

_____ J-7. Noted

_____ J-8. Lungs clear bilaterally, endotracheal tube 3 cm above carina

_____ J-9. Not determined

_____ J-10. 200 ml

After placing a check mark next to your selections, **GO TO SECTION F (SELECTIONS).**

Section K (Selections)

Ms. Cook becomes anxious and complains of shortness of breath. Her oxygen saturation, according to the continuous pulse oximeter, has dropped from 98% before the episode to 81%. At this time which of the following would you recommend? (Select only one unless directed to "Make another selection in this section.")

Place a check mark next to the selection you feel is most appropriate, then go to Section K (Responses) to obtain the response from the selection you made.

_____ K-1. Increase the FIO$_2$.

_____ K-2. Place a chest tube in the second intercostal space of the right lung.

_____ K-3. Increase the tidal volume.

_____ K-4. Increase the flowrate.

_____ K-5. Place a chest tube in the sixth intercostal space of the right lung.

Section K (Responses)

K-1. Physician disagrees. Make another selection in this section.

K-2. Done. **GO TO SECTION L (SELECTIONS).**

K-3. Physician disagrees. Make another selection in this section.

K-4. Physician disagrees. Make another selection in this section.

K-5. Physician disagrees. Make another selection in this section.

Section L (Selections)

One week later, Ms. Cook remains on the ventilator in the assist/control mode with a tidal volume of 750 ml and an FIO$_2$ of 0.35. On these settings her ABG results are pH—7.42, PCO$_2$—41 torr, PO$_2$—90 torr, HCO$_3$—24 mEq/L. Her chest x-ray study is normal and her intracranial pressure is 5 torr. The physician would like to begin weaning Ms. Cook from the ventilator and wants your recommendations for assessing her ability to be weaned at this time. Which of the following would best evaluate this?

Place a check mark next to as many as you feel are indicated in this section.

_____ L-1. Vital capacity
_____ L-2. Temperature
_____ L-3. Functional residual capacity
_____ L-4. NIF
_____ L-5. Spontaneous tidal volume and rate
_____ L-6. $V_D:V_T$ ratio
_____ L-7. A-a gradient on 100% oxygen
_____ L-8. Maximal voluntary ventilation (MVV)
_____ L-9. Diffusion capacity
_____ L-10. Bowel sounds

After completing your selections, go to Section L (Responses) to obtain the responses from the selections you have made. **LOOK ONLY AT THE SELECTIONS YOU CHOSE.**

Section L (Responses)

Place a check mark next to the responses that correspond to the selections you made.

_____ L-1. 1100 ml
_____ L-2. 37°C
_____ L-3. Not evaluated
_____ L-4. −31 cm of water
_____ L-5. 350 ml and 14 breaths/min
_____ L-6. 38%
_____ L-7. 80 torr
_____ L-8. Not evaluated
_____ L-9. Not evaluated
_____ L-10. Normal

After placing a check mark next to your selections, **GO TO SECTION M (SELECTIONS).**

Section M (Selections)

At this time you would recommend which of the following? (Select only one unless directed to "Make another selection in this section.")

Place a check mark next to the selection you feel is most appropriate, then go to Section M (Responses) to obtain the response from your selection.

_____ M-1. Maintain present settings.
_____ M-2. Place patient on flow-by and 50% oxygen.
_____ M-3. Place patient on synchronized intermittent mandatory ventilation (SIMV), rate—10 breaths/min, tidal volume—750 ml, FIO_2—0.4.
_____ M-4. Extubate and place patient on 40% aerosol mask.
_____ M-5. Place patient on SIMV, rate—4 breaths/min, tidal volume—700 ml, FIO_2—0.3.

Section M (Responses)

M-1. Physician disagrees. Make another selection in this section.

M-2. Physician disagrees. Make another selection in this section.

M-3. Done. End of problem.

M-4. Physician disagrees. Make another selection in this section.

M-5. Physician disagrees. Make another selection in this section.

Section N (Selections)

Ms. Cook's intracranial pressure has increased to 24 torr. At this time which of the following would you recommend? (Select only one unless directed to "Make another selection in this section.")

Place a check mark next to the selection you feel is most appropriate, then go to Section N (Responses) to obtain the response from the selection you made.

_____ N-1. Increase the FIO_2.
_____ N-2. Increase the ventilator rate.
_____ N-3. Decrease the tidal volume.
_____ N-4. Add 5 cm of water of PEEP.
_____ N-5. Decrease the flowrate.

Section N (Responses)

N-1. Physician disagrees. Make another selection in this section.

N-2. Physician agrees. **GO TO SECTION D (SELECTIONS).**

N-3. Physician disagrees. Make another selection in this section.

N-4. Physician disagrees. Make another selection in this section.

N-5. Physician disagrees. Make another selection in this section.

Clinical Simulation No. 1

Score Evaluation

Section A — Information Gathering

A-1. +1	A-9. +1
A-2. 0	A-10. −1
A-3. +2	A-11. +2
A-4. −1	A-12. −1
A-5. −1	A-13. +1
A-6. −2	A-14. +2
A-7. +1	A-15. +1
A-8. +2	

Total (+) responses = _____
Total (−) responses = − _____
Total Section Score = _____
Maximum points available: 13
Minimum passing score: 8

Section B — Decision-making

B-1. −1
B-2. −1
B-3. −2
B-4. +2
B-5. −2
Total (+) responses = _____
Total (−) responses = − _____
Total Section Score = _____
Maximum points available: 2
Minimum passing score: 1

Section C — Decision-making

C-1. −1
C-2. −3
C-3. +2
C-4. −2
C-5. −1
Total (+) responses = _____
Total (−) responses = − _____
Total Section Score = _____
Maximum points available: 2
Minimum passing score: 2

Section D — Information Gathering

D-1. −2	D-8. +2
D-2. +2	D-9. −1
D-3. +2	D-10. +2
D-4. +2	D-11. −1
D-5. −1	D-12. −2
D-6. −2	D-13. +1
D-7. +1	

Total (+) responses = _____
Total (−) responses = − _____
Total Section Score = _____
Maximum points available: 12
Minimum passing score: 9

Section E — Decision-making

E-1. −1
E-2. +2
E-3. 0
E-4. −1
E-5. −1
Total (+) responses = _____
Total (−) responses = − _____
Total Section Score = _____
Maximum points available: 2
Minimum passing score: 0

Section F — Decision-making

F-1. +2
F-2. −1
F-3. −2
F-4. 0
F-5. −2
Total (+) responses = _____
Total (−) responses = − _____
Total Section Score = _____
Maximum points available: 2
Minimum passing score: 0

Section G — Decision-making

G-1. −1
G-2. −2
G-3. −1
G-4. +1
G-5. −1
Total (+) responses = _____
Total (−) responses = − _____
Total Section Score = _____
Maximum points available: 1
Minimum passing score: 1

Section H — Decision-making

H-1. −1
H-2. −1
H-3. −1
H-4. +2
H-5. −2
Total (+) responses = _____
Total (−) responses = − _____
Total Section Score = _____
Maximum points available: 2
Minimum passing score: 1

Section I — Decision-making

I-1. −1
I-2. +2
I-3. −2
I-4. +2
I-5. −2
I-6. +2
I-7. −1
Total (+) responses = _____
Total (−) responses = − _____
Total Section Score = _____
Maximum points available: 2
Minimum passing score: 2

Section J — Information Gathering

J-1. +1   J-6. +2
J-2. +2   J-7. −1
J-3. 0   J-8. +2
J-4. −1   J-9. −2
J-5. +2   J-10. −1
Total (+) responses = _____
Total (−) responses = − _____
Total Section Score = _____
Maximum points available: 9
Minimum passing score: 7

Section K — Decision-making

K-1. −1
K-2. +1
K-3. −2
K-4. −1
K-5. −2
Total (+) responses = _____
Total (−) responses = − _____
Total Section Score = _____
Maximum points available: 1
Minimum passing score: 0

Section L — Information Gathering

L-1. +2   L-6. +1
L-2. 0   L-7. +2
L-3. −2   L-8. −1
L-4. +2   L-9. −1
L-5. +2   L-10. −1
Total (+) responses = _____
Total (−) responses = − _____
Total Section Score = _____
Maximum points available: 9
Minimum passing score: 7

Section M — Decision-making

M-1. −1
M-2. −2
M-3. +2
M-4. −3
M-5. −2
Total (+) responses = _____
Total (−) responses = − _____
Total Section Score = _____
Maximum points available: 2
Minimum passing score: 1

Section N — Decision-making

N-1. −1
N-2. +1
N-3. −2
N-4. −2
N-5. −2
Total (+) responses = _____
Total (−) responses = − _____
Total Section Score = _____
Maximum points available: 1
Minimum passing score: 1

Maximum points available in Information Gathering sections: 43
Minimum passing score in Information Gathering sections: 31 (72%)
Your total Information Gathering points:
_____

Maximum points available in Decision-making sections: 12
Minimum passing score in Decision-making sections: 9 (75%)
Your total Decision-making points: _____

OPTIMAL SECTION ROUTE THROUGH THE SIMULATION: A,E,C,I,J,F,D,H,L,M

CLINICAL SIMULATION NO. 2

Patient: Phil Brown — Age 57 Years

You are the evening shift supervisor and have been called to go check on a patient, Phil Brown, a 57-year-old man who was admitted to your hospital earlier in the day complaining of mild respiratory distress. He is currently on a 2-L/min nasal cannula and is still in mild to moderate respiratory distress. The physician would like your help in evaluating Mr. Brown's condition and helping with his treatment regimen. **GO TO SECTION A (SELECTIONS).**

Section A (Selections)

Which of the following would you assess in order to best evaluate Mr. Brown's cardiopulmonary status?

Place a check mark next to as many as you feel are indicated in this section.

_____ A-1. Breath sounds

_____ A-2. Bowel sounds

_____ A-3. Respiratory rate

_____ A-4. Heart rate

_____ A-5. Complete blood count

_____ A-6. Chest x-ray study

_____ A-7. Gag reflex

_____ A-8. Babinski's reflex

_____ A-9. Color of lips and nailbeds

_____ A-10. Chest configuration

_____ A-11. Temperature

_____ A-12. Urine culture

_____ A-13. ABG values

_____ A-14. Smoking history

_____ A-15. Peak expiratory flow

_____ A-16. Lactic acid level

After completing your selections, go to Section A (Responses) to obtain responses from the selections you have made. **LOOK ONLY AT THE SELECTIONS YOU CHOSE.**

Section A (Responses)

Place a check mark next to the responses on this page that correspond to the selections you made on the previous page.

_____ A-1. Diminished in the bases with right upper lobe rales

_____ A-2. Normal

_____ A-3. 22 breaths/min

_____ A-4. 110 beats/min

_____ A-5. Hb—18 vol%, red blood cells—6.8/mm³, white blood cells—16,000/mm³, hematocrit—52%

_____ A-6. Hyperinflation with bullous disease and consolidation in right upper lobe

_____ A-7. Normal

_____ A-8. None

_____ A-9. Cyanotic

_____ A-10. Barrel chest

_____ A-11. 38.5°C

_____ A-12. Not evaluated

_____ A-13. pH—7.32, PCO_2—58 torr, PO_2—40 torr, HCO_3—34 mEq/L

_____ A-14. 40 pack years

_____ A-15. Not evaluated

_____ A-16. Not evaluated

After placing a check mark next to your selections, **GO TO SECTION D (SELECTIONS).**

Section B (Selections)

One hour later the patient is in more respiratory distress, with the following ABG results: pH—7.23, PCO_2—69 torr, PO_2—49 torr, HCO_3—35 mEq/L. Which of the following changes would you make at this time? (Select only one unless directed to "Make another selection in this section.")

Place a check mark next to the selection you feel is most appropriate, then go to Section B (Responses) to obtain the response from the selection you made.

_____ B-1. Change to a 100% nonrebreathing mask.

_____ B-2. Place patient on a CPAP mask at 5 cm of water.

_____ B-3. Intubate and place patient on a mechanical ventilator.

_____ B-4. Place patient on a 50% aerosol mask.

_____ B-5. Make no changes now, but obtain ABG values in 1 hour.

Section B (Responses)

B-1. Done. **GO TO SECTION C (SELECTIONS).**

B-2. Physician disagrees. Make another selection in this section.

B-3. Physician agrees. **GO TO SECTION L (SELECTIONS).**

B-4. Physician disagrees. Make another selection in this section.

B-5. Physician disagrees. Make another selection in this section.

Section C (Selections)

One hour later the patient is in severe respiratory distress with the following ABG results: pH—7.2, PCO_2—73 torr, PO_2—42 torr, HCO_3—35 mEq/L. Which of the following would you recommend at this time? (Select only one unless directed to "Make another selection in this section.")

Place a check mark next to the selection you feel is most appropriate, then go to Section C (Responses) to obtain the response from the selection you made.

_____ C-1. Intubate and place patient on mechanical ventilation.

_____ C-2. Place patient on a CPAP mask of 5 cm of water.

_____ C-3. Begin IPPB every 2 hours with normal saline and albuterol (Ventolin).

_____ C-4. Intubate and place patient on CPAP of 5 cm of water.

_____ C-5. Start chest physiotherapy TID.

Section C (Responses)

C-1. Physician agrees. **GO TO SECTION L (SELECTIONS).**

C-2. Physician disagrees. Make another selection in this section.

C-3. Physician disagrees. Make another selection in this section.

C-4. Physician disagrees. Make another selection in this section.

C-5. Physician disagrees. Make another selection in this section.

Section D (Selections)

The physician wants your recommendation on Mr. Brown's treatment plan. Which of the following is most appropriate at this time? (Select only one unless directed to "Make another selection in this section.")

Place a check mark next to the selection you feel is most appropriate, then go to Section D (Responses) to obtain the response from the selection you made.

_____ D-1. Change to a 35% Venturi mask.

_____ D-2. Decrease cannula flow to 1 L/min.

_____ D-3. Increase cannula flow to 4 L/min.

_____ D-4. Begin incentive spirometry every hour.

_____ D-5. Make no change at this time, but monitor closely.

Section D (Responses)

D-1. Done. **GO TO SECTION G (SELECTIONS).**

D-2. Physician disagrees. Make another selection in this section.

D-3. Done. **GO TO SECTION G (SELECTIONS).**

D-4. Physician disagrees. Make another selection in this section.

D-5. Physician disagrees. Make another selection in this section.

Section E (Selections)

You are called to Mr. Brown's room where the inspiratory:expiratory (I:E) ratio alarm is sounding on his volume ventilator. Which of the following would you check to determine what is causing this problem?

Place a check mark next to as many as you feel are indicated in this section.

_____ E-1. Positive end-expiratory pressure (PEEP) level setting

_____ E-2. Sensitivity control setting

_____ E-3. Inflation hold setting

_____ E-4. Tidal volume setting

_____ E-5. Sigh volume setting

_____ E-6. Rate setting

_____ E-7. Humidifier water level

_____ E-8. Flowrate setting

_____ E-9. Expiratory resistance setting

_____ E-10. High-pressure alarm setting

After completing your selections, go to Section E (Responses) to obtain responses from the selections you have made. **LOOK ONLY AT THE SELECTIONS YOU CHOSE.**

Section E (Responses)

Place a check mark next to the responses that correspond to the selections you made.

_____ E-1. Zero PEEP

_____ E-2. −2 cm of water

_____ E-3. Off

_____ E-4. 800 ml

_____ E-5. 1200 ml

_____ E-6. 12 breaths/min

_____ E-7. At maximum fill level

_____ E-8. 20 L/min

_____ E-9. Off

_____ E-10. 10 cm of water above peak inspiratory pressure

After placing a check mark next to your selections, **GO TO SECTION I (SELECTIONS).**

Section F (Selections)

After 5 days on the ventilator, Mr. Brown has been successfully weaned and extubated. For the next 4 days Mr. Brown's PaO_2 on room air was in the mid-40s, so a 2 L/min nasal cannula was started that maintained his PaO_2 at greater than 50 torr. His chest x-ray study reveals scattered infiltrates, hyperinflated lung fields, and a flattened diaphragm. He is to be discharged in 2 days, and the physician wants your recommendations for Mr. Brown's respiratory care after he returns home. Which of the following would you recommend?

Place a check mark next to as many as you feel are indicated in this section.

_____ F-1. Antibiotics daily

_____ F-2. Diaphragmatic breathing exercises

_____ F-3. Aerosolized bronchodilator daily

_____ F-4. Reduce or quit smoking

_____ F-5. Oxygen via concentrator at 2 L/min

_____ F-6. Drink plenty of fluids daily

_____ F-7. Pursed-lip breathing exercises

_____ F-8. IPPB daily

_____ F-9. Chest percussion and postural drainage daily

_____ F-10. Bed rest

_____ F-11. Cromolyn sodium daily

After completing your selections, go to Section F (Responses) to obtain responses from the selections you have made. **LOOK ONLY AT THE SELECTIONS YOU CHOSE.**

Section F (Responses)

_____ F-1. Noted

_____ F-2. Noted

_____ F-3. Noted

_____ F-4. Noted

_____ F-5. Noted

_____ F-6. Noted

_____ F-7. Noted

_____ F-8. Noted

_____ F-9. Noted

_____ F-10. Noted

After placing a check mark next to your selections, **GO TO SECTION N (SELECTIONS).**

Section G (Selections)

Thirty minutes later, Mr. Brown's ABG results are pH—7.3, PCO_2—60 torr, PO_2—47 torr, HCO_3—35 mEq/L. His respiratory rate is 24 breaths/min. Which of the following recommendations is appropriate at this time? (Select only one unless directed to "Make another selection in this section.")

Place a check mark next to the selection you feel is most appropriate, then go to Section G (Responses) to obtain the response from the selection you made.

_____ G-1. Change to a 5-L/min nasal cannula.

_____ G-2. Begin Q1 chest physiotherapy.

_____ G-3. Make no changes at this time. Continue to monitor.

_____ G-4. Change to a 40% Venturi mask.

_____ G-5. Intubate patient and place on mechanical ventilation.

Section G (Responses)

G-1. Done. **GO TO SECTION B (SELECTIONS).**

G-2. Physician disagrees. Make another selection in this section.

G-3. Physician disagrees. Make another selection in this section.

G-4. Done. **GO TO SECTION B (SELECTIONS).**

G-5. Physician agrees. **GO TO SECTION L (SELECTIONS).**

Section H (Selections)

Mr. Brown has been on the ventilator for 24 hours. At this time what recommendations would you make to assess Mr. Brown's cardiopulmonary status?

Place a check mark next to as many as you feel are indicated in this section.

_____ H-1. Static lung compliance

_____ H-2. Forced expiratory volume in 1 second (FEV_1)

_____ H-3. Deep tendon reflexes

_____ H-4. ABG values

_____ H-5. Chest x-ray study

_____ H-6. Sputum production

_____ H-7. Electroencephalogram

_____ H-8. Spinal tap

_____ H-9. Closing volume

_____ H-10. Heart rate and blood pressure

_____ H-11. Fiberoptic bronchoscopy

After completing your selections, go to Section H (Responses) to obtain responses from the selections you have made. **LOOK ONLY AT THE SELECTIONS YOU CHOSE.**

Section H (Responses)

Place a check mark next to the responses on this page that correspond to the selections you made on the previous page.

_____ H-1. 41 ml/cm of water

_____ H-2. Not evaluated

_____ H-3. Not evaluated

_____ H-4. pH—7.36, PCO_2—52 torr, PO_2—54 torr, HCO_3—34 mEq/L

_____ H-5. Consolidation in right lower lobe, endotracheal tube 3 cm of water above the carina

_____ H-6. Moderate amount of thick and purulent sputum

_____ H-7. Not evaluated

_____ H-8. Not evaluated

_____ H-9. Not evaluated

_____ H-10. 94 beats/min and 122/78

_____ H-11. Not evaluated

After placing a check mark next to your selections, **GO TO SECTION J (SELECTIONS).**

Section I (Selections)

Which of the following would you recommend at this time? (Select only one unless directed to "Make another selection in this section.")

Place a check mark next to the selection you feel is most appropriate, then go to Section I (Responses) to obtain the response from the selection you made.

_____ I-1. Increase the tidal volume to 900 ml.

_____ I-2. Decrease the flowrate to 10 L/min.

_____ I-3. Increase the respiratory rate to 16/min.

_____ I-4. Increase the sensitivity level.

_____ I-5. Increase the flowrate to 50 L/min.

Section I (Responses)

I-1. Physician disagrees. Make another selection in this section.

I-2. Physician disagrees. Make another selection in this section.

I-3. Physician disagrees. Make another selection in this section.

I-4. Physician disagrees. Make another selection in this section.

I-5. Physician agrees. **GO TO SECTION M (SELECTIONS).**

Section J (Selections)

The physician has ordered antibiotic therapy and wants your recommendation for other therapy at this time. Which of the following would you recommend for Mr. Brown's continuing care? (Select only one unless directed to "Make another selection in this section.")

Place a check mark next to the selection you feel is most appropriate, then go to Section J (Responses) to obtain the response from the selection you made.

_____ J-1. Normal saline in-line via nebulizer every 4 hours

_____ J-2. Cromolyn sodium in-line via nebulizer every 6 hours

_____ J-3. In-line bronchodilator via nebulizer followed by postural drainage and percussion every 4 hours.

_____ J-4. Suction airway every hour.

_____ J-5. No therapy indicated at this time.

Section J (Responses)

J-1. Physician disagrees. Make another selection in this section.

J-2. Physician disagrees. Make another selection in this section.

J-3. Ordered. **GO TO SECTION E (SELECTIONS).**

J-4. Physician disagrees. Make another selection in this section.

J-5. Physician disagrees. Make another selection in this section.

Section K (Selections)

One hour later ABG results are pH—7.56, PCO_2—32 torr, PO_2—59 torr, HCO_3—34 mEq/L. Which of the following would you recommend at this time? (Select only one unless directed to "Make another selection in this section.")

Place a check mark next to the selection you feel is most appropriate, then go to Section K (Responses) to obtain the response from the selection you made.

_____ K-1. Place on CPAP of 10 cm of water.

_____ K-2. Decrease rate to 12 breaths/min and tidal volume to 800 ml.

_____ K-3. Increase rate to 20 breaths/min.

_____ K-4. Place patient on 50% flow-by.

_____ K-5. Maintain present settings.

Section K (Responses)

K-1. Physician disagrees. Make another selection in this section.

K-2. Physician agrees. **GO TO SECTION H (SELECTIONS).**

K-3. Physician disagrees. Make another selection in this section.

K-4. Physician disagrees. Make another selection in this section.

K-5. Physician disagrees. Make another selection in this section.

Section L (Selections)

The physician wants your recommendation for ventilator settings. Mr. Brown weighs 80 kg. You would recommend which of the following at this time? (Select only one unless directed to "Make another selection in this section.")

Place a check mark next to the selection you feel is most appropriate, then go to Section L (Responses) to obtain the response from the selection you made.

_____ L-1. Assist/control mode, rate—12 breaths/min, tidal volume—800 ml, FIO_2—0.4

_____ L-2. IMV mode, rate—6 breaths/min, tidal volume—700 ml, FIO_2—0.6

_____ L-3. SIMV mode, rate—12 breaths/min, tidal volume—800 ml, FIO_2—0.4

_____ L-4. Control mode, rate—18 breaths/min, tidal volume—850 ml, FIO_2—0.3

_____ L-5. Assist/control mode, rate—18 breaths/min, tidal volume—850 ml, FIO_2—0.3

Section L (Responses)

L-1. Physician agrees. **GO TO SECTION H (SELECTIONS).**

L-2. Physician disagrees. Make another selection in this section.

L-3. Physician agrees. **GO TO SECTION H (SELECTIONS).**

L-4. Done. **GO TO SECTION K (SELECTIONS).**

L-5. Done. **GO TO SECTION K (SELECTIONS).**

Section M (Selections)

While performing chest percussion and vibration on Mr. Brown in the Trendelenburg position, he becomes dusky and his respiratory rate increases with a drop in his blood pressure to 100/64. Which of the following would you recommend at this time? (Select only one unless directed to "Make another selection in this section.")

Place a check mark next to the selection you feel is most appropriate, then go to Section M (Responses) to obtain the response from the selection you made.

_____ M-1. Leave patient in Trendelenburg position and perform endotracheal suctioning.

_____ M-2. Leave patient in Trendelenburg position and place him on his right side.

_____ M-3. Place Mr. Brown in semi-Fowler's position and when he is stable, continue therapy in this position.

_____ M-4. Increase the FIO_2 by 5%.

_____ M-5. Decrease the ventilator tidal volume.

Section M (Responses)

M-1. No change in patient's status. Make another selection in this section.

M-2. No change in patient's status. Make another selection in this section.

M-3. Done. **GO TO SECTION F (SELECTIONS).**

M-4. No change in patient's status. Make another selection in this section.

M-5. No change in patient's status. Make another selection in this section.

Section N (Selections)

Prior to discharge, you discuss with Mr. Brown the proper equipment cleaning techniques he should use in his home. Which of the following should you recommend to him to ensure his equipment is cleaned adequately? (Select only one unless directed to "Make another selection in this section.")

Place a check mark next to the selection you feel is most appropriate, then go to Section N (Responses) to obtain the response from the selection you made.

_____ N-1. Wash in soap and water every 3 days.

_____ N-2. Soak in disinfectant solution for 5 minutes after each use.

_____ N-3. Wash in soap and water after each use and soak in vinegar for 4 hours each night.

_____ N-4. Soak in vinegar each week for 15 minutes.

_____ N-5. Hold over boiling water for 10 minutes after each use.

Section N (Responses)

N-1. Done. End of problem.

N-2. Done. End of problem.

N-3. Done. End of problem.

N-4. Done. End of problem.

N-5. Done. End of problem.

Clinical Simulation No. 2

Score Evaluation

Section A — Information Gathering

A-1. +2	A-9. +2
A-2. −1	A-10. +1
A-3. +2	A-11. 0
A-4. +2	A-12. −1
A-5. +1	A-13. +2
A-6. +2	A-14. +1
A-7. −2	A-15. −1
A-8. −1	A-16. −1

Total (+) responses = _____

Total (−) responses = − _____

Total Section Score = _____

Maximum points available: 15

Minimum passing score: 13

Section B — Decision-making

B-1. −2

B-2. −2

B-3. +1

B-4. −2

B-5. −3

Total (+) responses = _____

Total (−) responses = − _____

Total Section Score = _____

Maximum points available: 1

Minimum passing score: 1

Section C — Decision-making

C-1. +2

C-2. −2

C-3. −2

C-4. −2

C-5. −2

Total (+) responses = _____

Total (−) responses = − _____

Total Section Score = _____

Maximum points available: 2

Minimum passing score: 2

Section D — Decision-making

D-1. +2

D-2. −2

D-3. +2

D-4. −1

D-5. −2

Total (+) responses = _____

Total (−) responses = − _____

Total Section Score = _____

Maximum points available: 2

Minimum passing score: 1

Section E — Information Gathering

E-1. −1

E-2. −1

E-3. +2

E-4. +2

E-5. −1

E-6. +2

E-7. −1

E-8. +2

E-9. −1

E-10. −1

Total (+) responses = _____

Total (−) responses = − _____

Total Section Score = _____

Maximum points available: 8

Minimum passing score: 6

Section F — Information Gathering

F-1. −1	F-7. +1
F-2. +1	F-8. −1
F-3. +1	F-9. +1
F-4. +1	F-10. −2
F-5. +2	F-11. −1
F-6. +1	

Total (+) responses = _____

Total (−) responses = − _____

Total Section Score = _____

Maximum points available: 8

Minimum passing score: 5

Section G — Decision-making

G-1. 0

G-2. −2

G-3. −2

G-4. 0

G-5. +2

Total (+) responses = _____

Total (−) responses = − _____

Total Section Score = _____

Maximum points available: 2

Minimum passing score: 0

Section H—Information Gathering

H-1. +2	H-7. −1
H-2. −1	H-8. −3
H-3. −1	H-9. −1
H-4. +2	H-10. +2
H-5. +1	H-11. −2
H-6. +1	

Total (+) responses = _____
Total (−) responses = − _____
Total Section Score = _____
Maximum points available: 8
Minimum passing score: 5

Section I—Decision-making

I-1. −1
I-2. −1
I-3. −1
I-4. −1
I-5. +1
Total (+) responses = _____
Total (−) responses = − _____
Total Section Score = _____
Maximum points available: 1
Minimum passing score: 1

Section J—Decision-making

J-1. 0
J-2. −1
J-3. +2
J-4. −2
J-5. 0
Total (+) responses = _____
Total (−) responses = − _____
Total Section Score = _____
Maximum points available: 2
Minimum passing score: 2

Section K—Decision-making

K-1. −2
K-2. +1
K-3. −2
K-4. −2
K-5. −1
Total (+) responses = _____
Total (−) responses = − _____
Total Section Score = _____
Maximum points available: 1
Minimum passing score: 0

Section L—Decision-making

L-1. +2
L-2. −2
L-3. +2
L-4. −1
L-5. −1

Total (+) responses = _____
Total (−) responses = − _____
Total Section Score = _____
Maximum points available: 2
Minimum passing score: 2

Section M—Decision-making

M-1. −2
M-2. −1
M-3. +1
M-4. −2
M-5. −1
Total (+) responses = _____
Total (−) responses = − _____
Total Section Score = _____
Maximum points available: 2
Minimum passing score: 1

Section N—Decision-making

N-1. −2
N-2. −1
N-3. +1
N-4. −2
N-5. −1
Total (+) responses = _____
Total (−) responses = − _____
Total Section Score = _____
Maximum points available: 1
Minimum passing score: 1

Maximum points available in Information Gathering Sections: 39
Minimum passing score in Information Gathering Sections: 29 (74%)
Your total Information Gathering points: _____

Maximum points available in Decision-making Sections: 12
Minimum passing score in Decision-making Sections: 9 (75%)
Your total Decision-making points: _____

OPTIMAL SECTION ROUTE THROUGH THE SIMULATION: A,D,G,L,H,J,E,I,M,F,N

CLINICAL SIMULATION NO. 3

Patient: Craig Johnson—Age 56 Years

You are a staff therapist in the intensive care unit of your hospital. You have been assigned to care for Craig Johnson, a 56-year-old, 75-kg man who was admitted 2 days ago with congestive heart failure and pulmonary edema. **GO TO SECTION A (SELECTIONS).**

Clinical Simulation Practice Problems ↓ **391**

Section A (Selections)

Mr. Johnson is on a volume ventilator with the following settings: assist/control mode, rate—12 breaths/min, tidal volume—800 ml, FIO_2—0.6. A Swan-Ganz catheter is in place and reveals the following cardiac pressures: pulmonary artery wedge pressure—16 torr, pulmonary artery pressure—26 torr, and central venous pressure—11 cm of water. To further assess Mr. Johnson's cardiopulmonary status, which of the following would you evaluate at this time?

Place a check mark next to as many as you feel are indicated in this section.

_____ A-1. Heart rate and blood pressure
_____ A-2. Deep tendon reflex
_____ A-3. Temperature
_____ A-4. ABG values
_____ A-5. Urinalysis
_____ A-6. Spontaneous tidal volume and rate
_____ A-7. Static lung compliance
_____ A-8. Gag reflex
_____ A-9. Sputum production
_____ A-10. Functional residual capacity
_____ A-11. Pupillary reaction

After completing your selections, go to Section A (Responses) to obtain responses from the selections you

have made. **LOOK ONLY AT THE SELECTIONS YOU CHOSE.**

Section A (Responses)

Place a check mark next to the responses that correspond to the selections you made.

_____ A-1. 108 beats/min, 148/98
_____ A-2. Not evaluated
_____ A-3. 37.5°C
_____ A-4. pH—7.41, PCO_2—42 torr, PO_2—57 torr, bicarbonate—22 mEq/L
_____ A-5. Normal
_____ A-6. 150 ml, 24 breaths/min
_____ A-7. 26 ml/cm of water
_____ A-8. Not evaluated
_____ A-9. Small amount of pink, frothy secretions
_____ A-10. Not evaluated
_____ A-11. Normal

After placing a check mark next to your selections, **GO TO SECTION D (SELECTIONS).**

Section B (Selections)

Mr. Johnson's EKG strip shows the following:

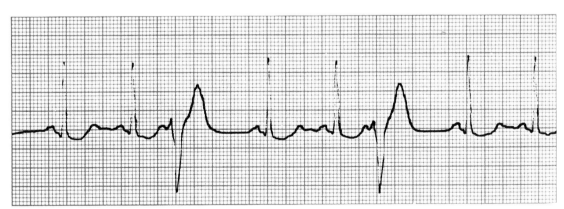

From Davis D. *Differential Diagnosis of Arrhythmias.* Philadelphia: WB Saunders; 1992.

You notice that Mr. Johnson's intravenous solution has infiltrated. What would you recommend at this time? (Select only one unless directed to "Make another selection in this section.")

Place a check mark next to the selection you feel is most appropriate, then go to Section B (Responses) to obtain the response from the selection you made.

———— B-1. Inject epinephrine into the myocardium.

———— B-2. Instill lidocaine directly down the endotracheal tube.

———— B-3. Begin cardiac compressions.

———— B-4. Increase PEEP to 10 cm of water.

———— B-5. Instill atropine directly down the endotracheal tube.

Section B (Responses)

B-1. Physician disagrees. Make another selection in this section.

B-2. Done. **GO TO SECTION E (SELECTIONS).**

B-3. Physician disagrees. Make another selection in this section.

B-4. Physician disagrees. Make another selection in this section.

B-5. Physician disagrees. Make another selection in this section.

Section C (Selections)

Which of the following would you recommend at this time? (Select only one unless directed to "Make another selection in this section.")

Place a check mark next to the selection you feel is most appropriate, then go to Section C (Responses) to obtain the response from the selection you made.

———— C-1. Place patient on 40% flow-by.

———— C-2. Place patient on IMV, rate—10 breaths/min, tidal volume—800 ml, FIO_2—0.5.

———— C-3. Place patient on IMV, rate—4 breaths/min, tidal volume—700 ml, FIO_2—0.4.

———— C-4. Extubate patient and place on 40% aerosol mask.

———— C-5. Maintain present ventilator settings.

Section C (Responses)

C-1. Physician disagrees. Make another selection in this section.

C-2. Done. **GO TO SECTION J (SELECTIONS).**

C-3. Physician disagrees. Make another selection in this section.

C-4. Physician disagrees. Make another selection in this section.

C-5. Physician agrees. **GO TO SECTION G (SELECTIONS).**

Section D (Selections)

Which of the following ventilator changes would you recommend at this time? (Select only one unless directed to "Make another selection in this section.")

Place a check mark next to the selection you feel is most appropriate, then go to Section D (Responses) to obtain the response from the selection you made.

———— D-1. Decrease the tidal volume to 700 ml.

———— D-2. Increase the FIO_2 to 0.7.

———— D-3. Add 5 cm of water of PEEP.

———— D-4. Add 100 cc of mechanical deadspace.

———— D-5. Increase rate to 15 breaths/min.

Section D (Responses)

D-1. Physician disagrees. Make another selection in this section.

D-2. Done. **GO TO SECTION F (SELECTIONS).**

D-3. Physician agrees. **GO TO SECTION H (SELECTIONS).**

D-4. Physician disagrees. Make another selection in this section.

D-5. Physician disagrees. Make another selection in this section.

Section E (Selections)

The following day, the physician wants Mr. Johnson's PEEP level increased from 5 cm of water to 8 cm of water. After making the change, mixed venous blood gases are drawn, indicating a drop in the $P\bar{v}O_2$ from 39 to 33 torr. Which of the following would you recommend at this time? (Select only one unless directed to "Make another selection in this section.")

Place a check mark next to the selection you feel is most appropriate, then go to Section E (Responses) to obtain the response from the selection you made.

———— E-1. Increase the oxygen 10%.

———— E-2. Make no change at this time.

_____ E-3. Decrease the PEEP back to 5 cm of water.

_____ E-4. Discontinue PEEP.

_____ E-5. Decrease the oxygen 10%.

Section E (Responses)

E-1. Physician disagrees. Make another selection in this section.

E-2. Physician disagrees. Make another selection in this section.

E-3. Done. **GO TO SECTION I (SELECTIONS).**

E-4. Physician disagrees. Make another selection in this section.

E-5. Physician disagrees. Make another selection in this section.

Section F (Selections)

Mr. Johnson's ABG results are now pH—7.4, PCO_2—39 torr, PO_2—59 torr, HCO_3—23 mEq/L. Which of the following ventilator changes would you recommend at this time? (Select only one unless directed to "Make another selection in this section.")

Place a check mark next to the selection you feel is most appropriate, then go to Section F (Responses) to obtain the response from the selection you made.

_____ F-1. Increase the FIO_2 to 0.9.

_____ F-2. Increase the tidal volume to 900 ml.

_____ F-3. Decrease the flowrate.

_____ F-4. Maintain the present ventilator settings.

_____ F-5. Add 5 cm of water of PEEP.

Section F (Responses)

F-1. Physician disagrees. Make another selection in this section.

F-2. Physician disagrees. Make another selection in this section.

F-3. Physician disagrees. Make another selection in this section.

F-4. Physician disagrees. Make another selection in this section.

F-5. Done. **GO TO SECTION H (SELECTIONS).**

Section G (Selections)

Over the next 6 days, Mr. Johnson is weaned to flow-by of 30% through the ventilator. His spontaneous tidal volume is 400 ml, vital capacity is 1500 ml, and respiratory rate is 14 breaths/min. ABG values are pH —7.38, PCO_2—41 torr, PO_2—86 torr, HCO_3—25 mEq/L. Which of the following would you recommend at this time? (Select only one unless directed to "Make another selection in this section.")

Place a check mark next to the selection you feel is most appropriate, then go to Section G (Responses) to obtain the response from the selection you made.

_____ G-1. Add 4 cm of water of CPAP.

_____ G-2. Extubate patient and place on nonrebreathing mask.

_____ G-3. Extubate patient and place on 30% aerosol mask.

_____ G-4. Place patient on IMV rate of 4 breaths/min.

_____ G-5. Increase FIO_2 to 0.4.

Section G (Responses)

G-1. Physician disagrees. Make another selection in this section.

G-2. Physician disagrees. Make another selection in this section.

G-3. Done. **GO TO SECTION K (SELECTIONS).**

G-4. Physician disagrees. Make another selection in this section.

G-5. Physician disagrees. Make another selection in this section.

Section H (Selections)

Mr. Johnson's ABG results are pH—7.39, PCO_2—41 torr, PO_2—87 torr, HCO_3—23 mEq/L. Two hours later, following endotracheal suctioning, you observe the following on Mr. Johnson's EKG monitor:

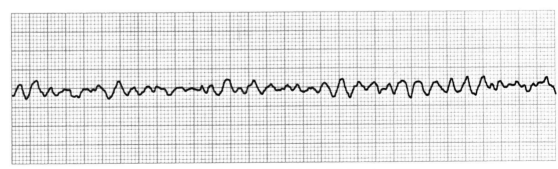

From Davis D. *Differential Diagnosis of Arrhythmias.* Philadelphia: WB Saunders; 1992.

Which of the following would you recommend at this time? (Select only one unless directed to "Make another selection in this section.")

Place a check mark next to the selection you feel is most appropriate, then go to Section H (Responses) to obtain the response from the selection you made.

———— H-1. Begin cardiac compression.
———— H-2. Defibrillate.
———— H-3. Administer atropine.
———— H-4. Administer sodium bicarbonate.
———— H-5. Administer intracardiac epinephrine.

Section H (Responses)

H-1. Physician disagrees. Make another selection in this section.

H-2. Done. **GO TO SECTION B (SELECTIONS).**

H-3. Physician disagrees. Make another selection in this section.

H-4. Physician disagrees. Make another selection in this section.

H-5. Physician disagrees. Make another selection in this section.

Section I (Selections)

Two days later, the physician wants to try weaning Mr. Johnson from the ventilator. Which of the following should be assessed to evaluate whether or not the weaning process should be attempted on Mr. Johnson?

Place a check mark next to as many as you feel are indicated in this section.

———— I-1. Current ventilator settings
———— I-2. Blood pressure
———— I-3. Temperature
———— I-4. Closing volume
———— I-5. Spontaneous rate and tidal volume
———— I-6. Chest x-ray film
———— I-7. ABG values
———— I-8. Gag reflex
———— I-9. Heart rate
———— I-10. Deep pain response
———— I-11. Vital capacity
———— I-12. MVV
———— I-13. Urine culture
———— I-14. NIF

After completing your selections, go to Section I (Responses) to obtain responses from the selections you have made. **LOOK ONLY AT THE SELECTIONS YOU CHOSE.**

Section I (Responses)

Place a check mark next to the responses that correspond to the selections you made.

———— I-1. Assist/control mode, rate—12 breaths /min, tidal volume—800 ml, FIO_2—0.4
———— I-2. 128/90
———— I-3. 36.8°C
———— I-4. Not evaluated
———— I-5. 22 breaths/min, 200 ml
———— I-6. Scattered infiltrates in right middle lobe
———— I-7. pH—7.37, PCO_2—43 torr, PO_2—81 torr, HCO_3—24 mEq/L
———— I-8. Intact
———— I-9. 84 beats/min
———— I-10. Not evaluated
———— I-11. 400 ml
———— I-12. Not evaluated
———— I-13. Not evaluated
———— I-14. —16 cm of water

After placing a check mark next to your selections, **GO TO SECTION C (SELECTIONS).**

Section J (Selections)

Two hours later, Mr. Johnson's respiratory rate is 32 breaths/min and he complains of shortness of breath. Arterial blood gases are drawn and reveal the following: pH—7.29, PCO_2—51 torr, PO_2—72 torr, HCO_3—26 mEq/L. Which of the following would you recommend at this time? (Select only one unless directed to "Make another selection in this section.")

Place a check mark next to the selection you feel is most appropriate, then go to Section J (Responses) to obtain the response from the selection you made.

———— J-1. Place patient back on assist/control mode and previous settings.
———— J-2. Increase the FIO_2 to 0.6.
———— J-3. Decrease the IMV rate to 8 breaths/min.

_____ J-4. Place patient on 5 cm of water of PEEP.

_____ J-5. Maintain present ventilator settings.

Section J (Responses)

J-1. Physician agrees. **GO TO SECTION G (SELECTIONS).**

J-2. Physician disagrees. Make another selection in this section.

J-3. Physician disagrees. Make another selection in this section.

J-4. Physician disagrees. Make another selection in this section.

J-5. Physician disagrees. Make another selection in this section.

Section K (Selections)

Immediately following extubation Mr. Johnson experiences increased work of breathing with inspiratory stridor. What would you recommend at this time? (Select only one unless directed to "Make another selection in this section.")

Place a check mark next to the selection you feel is most appropriate, then go to Section K (Responses) to obtain the response from the selection you made.

_____ K-1. Reintubate immediately.

_____ K-2. Perform emergency tracheotomy.

_____ K-3. Place on 40% aerosol mask and monitor closely.

_____ K-4. Deliver hypotonic saline with a handheld nebulizer.

_____ K-5. Deliver racemic epinephrine and saline with a hand-held nebulizer.

Section K (Responses)

K-1. Physician disagrees. Make another selection in this section.

K-2. Physician disagrees. Make another selection in this section.

K-3. Physician disagrees. Make another selection in this section.

K-4. Physician disagrees. Make another selection in this section.

K-5. Done. End of problem.

Clinical Simulation No. 3

Score Evaluation

Section A — Information Gathering

A-1. +2
A-2. −1
A-3. 0
A-4. +2
A-5. −1
A-6. +1
A-7. +2
A-8. −1
A-9. +1
A-10. −2
A-11. −1
Total (+) responses = _____
Total (−) responses = − _____
Total Section Score = _____
Maximum points available: 8
Minimum passing score: 6

Section B — Decision-making

B-1. −2
B-2. +2
B-3. −2
B-4. −2
B-5. −2
Total (+) responses = _____
Total (−) responses = − _____
Total Section Score = _____
Maximum points available: 2
Minimum passing score: 2

Section C — Decision-making

C-1. −2
C-2. 0
C-3. −2
C-4. −2
C-5. +2
Total (+) responses = _____
Total (−) responses = − _____
Total Section Score = _____
Maximum points available: 2
Minimum passing score: 0

Section D — Decision-making

D-1. −2
D-2. 0
D-3. +2
D-4. −3
D-5. −1
Total (+) responses = _____
Total (−) responses = − _____
Total Section Score = _____

Maximum points available: 2
Minimum passing score: 0

Section E—Decision-making

E-1. −1
E-2. −1
E-3. +2
E-4. −2
E-5. −2
Total (+) responses = _____
Total (−) responses = − _____
Total Section Score = _____
Maximum points available: 2
Minimum passing score: 2

Section F—Decision-making

F-1. −1
F-2. −1
F-3. −2
F-4. −2
F-5. +2
Total (+) responses = _____
Total (−) responses = − _____
Total Section Score = _____
Maximum points available: 2
Minimum passing score: 2

Section G—Decision-making

G-1. −1
G-2. −1
G-3. +2
G-4. −1
G-5. −1
Total (+) responses = _____
Total (−) responses = − _____
Total Section Score = _____
Maximum points available: 2
Minimum passing score: 2

Section H—Decision-making

H-1. −1
H-2. +2
H-3. −2
H-4. −2
H-5. −2
Total (+) responses = _____
Total (−) responses = − _____
Total Section Score = _____
Maximum points available: 2
Minimum passing score: 2

Section I—Information Gathering

I-1. +1
I-2. +1
I-3. 0
I-4. −2
I-5. +2
I-6. +1
I-7. +2
I-8. −2
I-9. +1
I-10. −1
I-11. +2
I-12. −1
I-13. −1
I-14. +2
Total (+) responses = _____
Total (−) responses = − _____
Total Section Score = _____
Maximum points available: 12
Minimum passing score: 8

Section J—Decision-making

J-1. +1
J-2. −1
J-3. −2
J-4. −2
J-5. −2
Total (+) responses = _____
Total (−) responses = − _____
Total Section Score = _____
Maximum points available: 1
Minimum passing score: 1

Section K—Decision-making

K-1. −1
K-2. −2
K-3. −1
K-4. −2
K-5. +2
Total (+) responses = _____
Total (−) responses = − _____
Total Section Score = _____
Maximum points available: 2
Minimum passing score: 2

Maximum points available in Information Gathering sections: 20
Minimum passing score in Information Gathering sections: 14 (70%)
Your total Information Gathering points: _____

Maximum points available in Decision-making sections: 14
Minimum passing score in Decision-making sections: 10 (71%)
Your total Decision-making points: _____

OPTIMAL SECTION ROUTE THROUGH THE SIMULATION: A,D,H,B,E,I,L,G,K

Equations You Need to Know

1. Calculating the minutes remaining in an oxygen cylinder

$$\frac{\text{cylinder pressure} \times \text{cylinder factor}}{\text{flowrate}}$$

Cylinder factors:

E cylinder — 0.28 L/psig
H cylinder — 3.14 L/psig

2. Air : oxygen entrainment ratios:
   24% — 25 : 1
   28% — 10 : 1
   30% — 8 : 1
   35% — 5 : 1
   40% — 3 : 1
   50% — 1.7 : 1
   60% — 1 : 1

3. Calculating air : oxygen entrainment ratios

$$\frac{100 - x}{x - 20^*} = \frac{\text{parts air entrained}}{\text{1 part oxygen}}$$

*Note: use 21 when calculating percentages less than 40%.

4. Calculating total flow

   Add the total ratio parts (of air : oxygen ratio) and multiply by the flowrate on the flowmeter.

5. Calculating FIO_2

$$FIO_2 = \frac{O_2 \text{ flow} + (\text{air flow} \times 0.2)}{\text{total flow}}$$

6. Calculating relative humidity

$$\text{R.H.} = \frac{\text{absolute humidity}}{\text{capacity}} \times 100$$

7. Calculating body humidity

$$\text{B.H.} = \frac{\textbf{absolute humidity}}{\textbf{44 mg/L}} \times \textbf{100}$$

8. Calculating humidity deficit

44 mg/L − absolute humidity

9. Calculating static lung compliance

$$\frac{\textbf{volume}}{\textbf{static pressure − PEEP}}$$

10. Calculating minute ventilation (minute volume)

Respiratory rate × tidal volume

11. Calculating alveolar PO_2 and A-a gradient

Alveolar air equation:

$$\textbf{PAO}_2 = [(\textbf{Pb − 47 torr})(\textbf{FIO}_2)] − \textbf{PaCO}_2 \times \textbf{1.25}$$

$$\textbf{A-a gradient} = \textbf{PAO}_2 − \textbf{PaO}_2$$

12. Calculating I:E ratio

$$\frac{\text{inspiratory flowrate}}{\text{minute ventilation}} − 1 \text{ (for inspiration)}$$

After subtracting 1 from the answer, the remainder is expiration.

13. Calculating mean airway pressure (MAP)

0.5 [PIP − PEEP × (inspiratory time/total respiratory cycle)]

PIP = peak inspiratory pressure

PEEP = positive end-expiratory pressure

14. $VD:VT$ ratio $= \dfrac{PaCO_2 − PECO_2}{PaCO_2}$

15. Estimation of FIO_2 changes

$$\text{Desired } FIO_2 = \frac{PaO_2 \text{ (desired)} \times FIO_2 \text{ (current)}}{PaO_2 \text{ (current)}}$$

16. Estimation of ventilator rate changes

$$\text{Desired rate} = \frac{\text{rate (current)} \times \text{PaCO}_2 \text{ (current)}}{\text{PaCO}_2 \text{ (desired)}}$$

17. Estimation of minute volume changes

$$\text{Desired } \dot{V}_E = \frac{\dot{V}_E \text{ (current)} \times \text{PaCO}_2 \text{ (current)}}{\text{PaCO}_2 \text{ (desired)}}$$

18. Calculating cardiac output

$$\dot{Q}_T = \frac{\dot{V}_{O_2}}{[\text{CaO}_2 - \text{C}\overline{\text{v}}\text{O}_2] \times 10}$$

$\dot{Q}_T$ = cardiac output (L/min)

$\dot{V}_{O_2}$ = oxygen consumption (ml/min)

19. Calculating total oxygen content

   arterial oxygen content:

$1.34 \times \text{SaO}_2 \times \text{Hb} = \text{O}_2$ bound to hemoglobin
$0.003 \times \text{PaO}_2 = \text{O}_2$ dissolved in the plasma

   These two added together equal arterial oxygen content (CaO_2)

   venous oxygen content:

$1.34 \times \text{S}\overline{\text{v}}\text{O}_2 \times \text{Hb}$
$0.003 \times \text{P}\overline{\text{v}}\text{O}_2$

   These two added together equal venous oxygen content ($\text{C}\overline{\text{v}}\text{O}_2$)

$\text{CaO}_2 - \text{C}\overline{\text{v}}\text{O}_2$ = arterial to venous content difference

20. Calculating intrapulmonary shunting

$$\frac{\dot{Q}_S}{\dot{Q}_T} = \frac{\text{PAO}_2 - \text{PaO}_2 \, (0.003)}{\text{CaO}_2 - \text{C}\overline{\text{v}}\text{O}_2 + (\text{PAO}_2 - \text{PaO}_2) \, (0.003)}$$

$\dot{Q}_S$ = shunted blood
$\dot{Q}_T$ = total blood flow (cardiac output)

21. Modified shunt equation

$$\frac{\dot{Q}_S}{\dot{Q}_T} = \frac{(\text{PAO}_2 - \text{PaO}_2) \, (0.003)}{(4.5 \text{ vol \%}) + (\text{PAO}_2 - \text{PaO}_2) \, (0.003)}$$

22. Calculating cardiac index(CI)

$$CI = \frac{\text{cardiac output (L/min)}}{\text{body surface area (m}_2)}$$

23. Calculating stroke volume (SV)

$$SV = \frac{\text{cardiac output (ml/min)}}{\text{heart rate (beats/min)}}$$

24. Calculating systemic vascular resistance (SVR)

$$SVR = \frac{\text{MSAP} - \text{CVP (torr)}}{\text{QT (L/min)}}$$

MSAP = mean systemic arterial pressure
CVP = central venous pressure
QT = cardiac output

25. Calculating pulmonary vascular resistance (PVR)

$$PVR = \frac{\text{MPAP} - \text{PAWP (torr)}}{\text{QT (L/min)}}$$

MPAP = mean pulmonary artery pressure
PAWP = pulmonary artery wedge pressure

26. Calculating oxygen consumption

$$Vo_2 = Q_T [C(a - v)o_2] \times 10$$

$C(a - v)o_2$ = arterial − venous oxygen content

Written Registry Review Posttest

Directions: Each of the questions or incomplete statements below are followed by five suggested answers or completions. Choose the best answer and circle it on the test.

1. Which protective airway reflex is responsible for eliciting a gag response?

   A. Pharyngeal reflex
   B. Laryngeal reflex
   C. Tracheal reflex
   D. Vagal reflex
   E. Carinal reflex

2. The first heart sound (S_1) represents which of the following?

   A. Opening of the aortic valve
   B. Closing of the aortic valve
   C. Opening of the semilunar valves
   D. Closing of the atrioventricular valves
   E. Closing of the semilunar valves

3. Normal gestational age is:

   A. 30 to 32 weeks
   B. 32 to 34 weeks
   C. 34 to 38 weeks
   D. 38 to 42 weeks
   E. 40 to 44 weeks

4. A patient presenting with a productive cough consisting of purulent, foul-smelling sputum that settles into several layers most likely has which of the following lung disorders?

   A. Asthma
   B. Bronchiectasis
   C. Emphysema
   D. Pulmonary edema
   E. Pleural effusion

5. Which of the following are indications for bronchoscopy?

   I. Treatment of pulmonary hemorrhage
   II. Removal of foreign objects
   III. Removal of mucous plugs
   IV. Difficult tracheal intubation

   A. I and II only
   B. II and III only
   C. I, II, and IV only
   D. II, III, and IV only
   E. I, II, III, and IV

6. During a routine ventilator check, the high-pressure alarm begins to sound. The respiratory care practitioner should do which of the following to determine why the alarm is sounding?

   A. Check to see if the patient has become disconnected from the ventilator.
   B. Make sure the expiratory drive line is properly connected.
   C. Listen to the patient's breath sounds to determine if the patient needs to be suctioned.
   D. Increase the high-pressure limit.
   E. Increase the patient's tidal volume.

7. The most common cause of epiglottitis is:

   A. *Pseudomonas aeruginosa*
   B. *Streptococcus*
   C. *Haemophilus influenzae*
   D. *Pneumococcus*
   E. *Escherichia coli*

8. While assisting with a thoracentesis it is noted that purulent fluid is drained from the pleural space. The respiratory care practitioner should suspect which of the following?

   A. Chylothorax
   B. Empyema
   C. Hydrothorax
   D. Pneumothorax
   E. Pleural effusion

9. While assessing a patient you notice he exhibits pedal edema. You would suspect which of the following?

   A. Pleural effusion
   B. Pneumonia
   C. Asthma
   D. Cor pulmonale
   E. Bronchiectasis

10. A patient on the Servo 900 C ventilator has a blood pressure of 175/100. The respiratory care practitioner should recommend which of the following?

    A. Administration of sodium nitroprusside (nitropride)
    B. Decreasing the tidal volume
    C. Administration of lidocaine
    D. Defibrillation
    E. Adding positive end-expiratory pressure (PEEP)

11. While performing cardiopulmonary resusitation (CPR) on a patient, the electrocardiogram strip indicates the patient is in ventricular fibrillation. Defibrillation with 250 joules is administered with no change in the electrocardiogram reading. The respiratory care practitioner should recommend which of the following?

    A. Repeat defibrillation with 500 joules.
    B. Inject epinephrine into the pericardial sac.
    C. Administer sodium nitroprusside via intravenous (IV) line.
    D. Suction the patient's airway.
    E. Repeat defibrillation with 350 joules.

12. The following is a list of data obtained from a patient on the Bennett 7200A ventilator in the control mode.

Ventilator Settings		Arterial Blood Gas (ABG) Results	
FIO_2	0.7	pH	7.42
Tidal volume (VT)	800 ml	$PaCO_2$	43 torr
Rate	12/min	HCO_3	23 mEq/L
PEEP	8 cm H_2O	PaO_2	172 torr

    Based on this information, the respiratory care practitioner should recommend which of the following?

    A. Decrease FIO_2 to 0.6
    B. Increase tidal volume to 900 ml
    C. Decrease rate to 8 breaths/min
    D. Decrease PEEP to 4 cm of water
    E. Increase FIO_2 to 0.9

13. The type of breathing pattern associated with a diabetic patient in ketoacidosis is which of the following?

    A. Bradypnea
    B. Kussmaul's respiration
    C. Biot's respiration
    D. Cheyne-Stokes respiration
    E. Hypopnea

14. Upon entering a patient's room to administer chest physiotherapy you notice the patient is cyanotic and not breathing. After calling for help, your next action should be which of the following?

    A. Deliver four back blows.
    B. Administer an intermittent positive pressure breathing (IPPB) treatment immediately.
    C. Deliver two breaths and check for a pulse.
    D. Open the patient's airway.
    E. Begin chest compressions.

15. In order to maintain a patent upper airway in an unconscious drug-overdose patient, the respiratory care practitioner should recommend the use of which one of the following devices?

    A. Continuous positive airway pressure (CPAP) mask
    B. Nasopharyngeal airway
    C. Oropharyngeal airway
    D. Esophageal obturator airway
    E. Tracheostomy tube

16. A chest x-ray film from a spontaneously breathing neonate in a 60% oxygen hood reveals right upper and middle lobe atelectasis. ABG results follow:

pH	7.36
$PaCO_2$	39 torr
HCO_3	22 mEq/L
PaO_2	38 torr

    In order to increase this infant's PaO_2, the respiratory therapist should recommend a change to which of the following devices?

    A. Oxygen tent
    B. Incubator with oxygen
    C. Nasal CPAP
    D. Nasal catheter
    E. Mechanical ventilator

17. While performing your routine ventilator check you hear an audible leak around the patient's endotracheal (E-T) tube. After instilling air, you determine it takes 40 torr to seal the leak. Which of the following actions should the respiratory therapist recommend?

    A. Deflate the cuff to less than 20 torr regardless of the leak.

B. Deflate the cuff to less than 20 torr and compensate with the ventilator.
C. Maintain the cuff pressure at 40 torr.
D. Replace the E-T tube with a larger one.
E. Replace E-T tube with a talking tracheostomy tube.

18. The physician would like for a tracheostomy patient to be able to talk yet still maintain the airway for suctioning. He wants your recommendation for the airway that would cause the least amount of airway resistance. The best choice would be which of the following?

A. Tracheostomy button
B. Uncuffed tracheostomy tube
C. Fenestrated tracheostomy tube
D. Talking tracheostomy
E. Cuffed tracheostomy tube

19. The inspiratory:expiratory ratio alarm is sounding on the Bear 2 ventilator on a patient in the intensive care unit. Which of the following ventilator changes would correct this problem?

A. Increase the flowrate.
B. Decrease the flowrate.
C. Add PEEP.
D. Increase the tidal volume.
E. Increase the respiratory rate.

20. Digital clubbing is the result of which of the following?

A. Acute hypoxemia
B. Acute hypercapnia
C. Chronic hypoxemia
D. Chronic hypercapnia
E. Acute respiratory acidosis

21. The following data have been collected from a patient on the Bennett 7200 ventilator.

VT	0.8 L
Peak inspiratory pressure	42 cm H_2O
PEEP	5 cm H_2O
Plateau pressure	23 cm H_2O

Based on these data, the patient's static lung compliance is which of the following?

A. 19 ml/cm H_2O
B. 22 ml/cm H_2O
C. 35 ml/cm H_2O
D. 44 ml/cm H_2O
E. 52 ml/cm H_2O

22. On chest x-ray film you notice the patient's E-T tube is resting at the level of the fifth rib. The tube most likely has entered the

A. Left mainstem bronchus
B. Right mainstem bronchus
C. Esophagus
D. Right upper lobe bronchiole
E. Left upper lobe bronchiole

23. The following data were collected from a patient on a volume ventilator in the control mode.

Ventilator Settings		*ABG Results*	
VT	800 ml (0.8 L)	pH	7.29
Rate	10 breaths/min	$PaCO_2$	50 torr
FIO_2	0.4	HCO_3	27 mEq/L
		PaO_2	77 torr

Which of the following ventilator settings would decrease the patient's $PaCO_2$ to 40 torr?

A. Tidal volume—850 ml, rate—10 breaths/min
B. Tidal volume—900 ml, rate—15 breaths/min
C. Tidal volume—800 ml, rate—8 breaths/min
D. Tidal volume—1000 ml, rate—10 breaths/min
E. Tidal volume—800 ml, rate—12 breaths/min

24. While monitoring a patient's chest tube you notice it is obstructed with a blood clot. The first action that should be taken is to

A. "Milk" the tubing from the chest tube.
B. Clamp off the drainage tube.
C. Remove the chest tube.
D. Increase the suction pressure.
E. Decrease the level of water in the water seal bottle.

25. A patient breathing 30 times/min with a tidal volume that fluctuates between 300 and 600 ml is ordered placed on 30% oxygen. The respiratory therapist should recommend which oxygen delivery device?

A. Nasal catheter at 2 L/min
B. Nasal cannula at 3 L/min
C. Venturi mask
D. Simple mask at 6 L/min
E. Nasal cannula at 4 L/min

26. Which of the following are **absolute** contraindications for IPPB?

    I. Pulmonary hemorrhage
    II. Untreated pneumothorax
    III. Closed head injury
    IV. Bullous disease

    A. I and II only
    B. II and III only
    C. II, III, and IV only
    D. I, II, and III only
    E. I, II, III, and IV

27. A patient is set up on a 35% Venturi mask and you discover the patient's inspiratory flow exceeds the flow output of the mask. The respiratory therapist should do which of the following?

    A. Change to a nasal cannula at 5 L/min.
    B. Decrease the size of the entrainment port.
    C. Increase the flow to the mask.
    D. Change to a nonrebreathing mask.
    E. Decrease the flow to the mask.

28. A "damped" pressure tracing on an arterial line may be caused by which of the following?

    I. Catheter tip resting against the wall of the vessel
    II. A clot occluding the catheter
    III. A clot in the transducer
    IV. Air bubbles in the line

    A. I and II only
    B. II and III only
    C. I, II, and IV only
    D. II, III, and IV only
    E. I, II, III, and IV

29. Central venous pressure is a measurement of which of the following?

    A. Left atrial pressure
    B. Left ventricular preload
    C. Pulmonary capillary pressure
    D. Pulmonary artery pressure
    E. Right atrial pressure

30. Which of the following are considered immediate complications of a tracheostomy?

    I. Pneumothorax
    II. Air embolism
    III. Tracheoesophageal fistula

    A. I only
    B. II only
    C. I and II only
    D. II and III only
    E. I, II, and III

31. The following data pertain to a patient on the Bear 2 ventilator in the control mode.

Ventilator Settings		*ABG Results*	
VT	800 ml	pH	7.41
Rate	10 breaths/min	$PaCO_2$	37 torr
FIO_2	0.6	HCO_3	25 mEq/L
Flow	50 L/min	PaO_2	53 torr

Based on this information, the respiratory therapist should recommend which of the following ventilator changes?

    A. Increase tidal volume to 900 ml.
    B. Increase rate to 12 breaths/min.
    C. Increase flow to 60 L/min.
    D. Add 5 cm of water PEEP.
    E. Increase FIO_2 to 0.75.

32. A 5-year-old boy presents to the emergency room with shortness of breath, fever of 38.8°C, sore throat, and drooling. The most likely diagnosis would be which of the following?

    A. Epiglottitis
    B. Croup
    C. Asthma
    D. Cystic fibrosis
    E. Bronchiolitis

33. While performing chest wall percussion on a ventilated patient, you notice an area of hyperresonance. This is diagnostic for which of the following conditions?

    A. Pulmonary edema
    B. Pneumothorax
    C. Pleural effusion
    D. Consolidation
    E. Massive atelectasis

34. While ventilating a patient with a manual resuscitator at 12 breaths/min and 10 L/min of oxygen flow to the bag, arterial blood gas results reveal a PaO_2 of 52 torr. Which of the following will increase the FIO_2 being delivered by the bag?

    I. Increase the flow to 15 L/min.
    II. Increase the ventilation rate to 20/min.
    III. Add an oxygen reservoir to the bag.

A. I only
B. I and II only
C. I and III only
D. II and III only
E. I, II, and III

35. While performing CPR on a patient, the physician has difficulty inserting an IV line to administer lidocaine. What is the **first** action the respiratory therapist should recommend at this time?

    A. Administer the drug by intracardiac injection.
    B. Instill the drug down the E-T tube.
    C. Attempt to place an IV line in the subclavian vein.
    D. Administer the drug with a hand-held nebulizer.
    E. Administer the drug by intramuscular injection.

36. While you are administering IPPB, the patient suddenly complains of chest pain and shortness of breath and you notice that the left lung is not expanding as well as the right lung. The respiratory therapist should do which of the following?

    A. Continue the treatment as ordered.
    B. Continue the treatment but decrease the peak pressure.
    C. Stop the treatment for a brief rest period.
    D. Stop the treatment and use a hand-held nebulizer to continue the medication delivery.
    E. Stop the treatment and recommend a chest x-ray study immediately.

37. An increased pulmonary artery wedge pressure may be the result of which of the following conditions?

    I. Pulmonary hypertension
    II. Cor pulmonale
    III. Left ventricular failure
    IV. Mitral valve stenosis

    A. I and II only
    B. II and III only
    C. III and IV only
    D. I, II, and III only
    E. II, III, and IV only

38. An active 3-year-old child with croup has been ordered placed on 40% oxygen. Which oxygen delivery device would be most appropriate in this situation?

    A. Oxygen tent

B. Oxygen hood
C. Aerosol mask
D. Venturi mask
E. Nasal catheter

39. An elevated blood urea nitrogen level is indicative of which of the following?

    A. Respiratory failure
    B. Renal failure
    C. Pulmonary edema
    D. Pleural effusion
    E. Increased intracranial pressure

40. In the normal individual, what percentage of the cardiac output makes up intrapulmonary (anatomic) shunting?

    A. 0% to 2%
    B. 2% to 5%
    C. 5% to 10%
    D. 8% to 12%
    E. 10% to 15%

41. Which of the following values would indicate that a patient is ready to begin weaning from the ventilator?

    I. $V_D : V_T$ ratio of 0.7
    II. Negative inspiratory force of -30 cm H_2O
    III. A-a gradient of 100 torr on 100% oxygen

    A. I only
    B. II only
    C. III only
    D. I and II only
    E. II and III only

42. Cardiogenic pulmonary edema may be distinguished from the noncardiogenic type by determining which value?

    A. Central venous pressure
    B. Pulmonary artery wedge pressure
    C. Pulmonary artery pressure
    D. Right atrial pressure
    E. Right ventricular pressure

43. While administering IPPB, the patient has difficulty cycling the machine off. Which of the following could be the cause of the problem?

    I. Sensitivity set too low
    II. Leak in the circuit
    III. Malfunctioning exhalation valve

A. I only
B. II only
C. I and III only
D. II and III only
E. I, II, and III

44. Which of the following values represents the normal value for central venous pressure?

    A. 0 to 2 torr
    B. 4 to 10 torr
    C. 15 to 20 torr
    D. 20 to 25 torr
    E. 30 to 40 torr

45. Immediately following E-T extubation, the patient experiences inspiratory stridor. This is most likely the result of which of the following?

    A. Tracheomalacia
    B. Glottic edema
    C. Laryngeal web
    D. Tracheal stenosis
    E. Vocal cord ulceration

46. Which of the following are true in regard to mechanical ventilation of a head trauma patient?

    A. Tidal volumes of 20 ml/kg of body weight should be used.
    B. The inspiratory flow should be set at 10 to 20 L/min.
    C. $PaCO_2$ levels should be maintained at 15 to 20 torr.
    D. PaO_2 levels should be maintained at 50 to 60 torr.
    E. $PaCO_2$ levels should be maintained at 25 to 30 torr.

47. While analyzing the oxygen concentration on a 40% aerosol mask you notice the polarographic analyzer is reading 65%. What is the appropriate action to take at this time?

    A. Increase the nebulizer flow.
    B. Decrease the nebulizer flow.
    C. Drain the water from the aerosol tubing.
    D. Add a heater to the nebulizer.
    E. Shorten the aerosol tubing.

48. Carbon monoxide poisoning is an example of which type of hypoxia?

    A. Circulatory hypoxia
    B. Hypoxemic hypoxia
    C. Anemic hypoxia
    D. Stagnant hypoxia
    E. Histotoxic hypoxia

49. A disoriented, combative ventilated patient is on 80% oxygen and a PEEP of 15 cm of water in order to maintain acceptable PaO_2 levels. The patient has disconnected himself from the ventilator on numerous occasions even with restraints in use, which leads to cardiac arrhythmias. The respiratory therapist should recommend which of the following to improve this situation?

    A. Extubate and place patient on a nonrebreathing mask.
    B. Increase the PEEP level to 25 cm of water.
    C. Decrease the inspiratory flowrate.
    D. Sedate the patient and paralyze him with a neuromuscular blocking agent.
    E. Place the patient on flow-by and 100% oxygen to attempt weaning.

50. The following data pertain to a patient on the Bennett 7200 ventilator in the control mode.

Ventilator Settings		ABG Results	
VT	750 ml	pH	7.52
Rate	12 breaths/min	$PaCO_2$	27 torr
Flow	50 L/min	HCO_3	26 mEq/L
FIO_2	0.5	PaO_2	98 torr

Based on this information, which of the following changes could be made to correct this alkalemia?

    I. Decrease the tidal volume.
    II. Increase the flowrate.
    III. Add mechanical deadspace.
    IV. Increase the FIO_2.

    A. I and II only
    B. I and III only
    C. III and IV only
    D. I, III, and IV
    E. II, III, and IV

51. In order to prevent pulmonary infarction from occurring during the measurement of pulmonary artery wedge pressure, the cuff on the tip of the Swan-Ganz catheter should remain inflated for no longer than

    A. 5 seconds
    B. 10 to 15 seconds
    C. 15 to 20 seconds
    D. 20 to 30 seconds
    E. 45 to 60 seconds

52. The following is a set of ABG values obtained from a patient in the intensive care unit who is on a 2-L nasal cannula.

pH	7.22
$PaCO_2$	27 torr
HCO_3	12 mEq/L
PaO_2	78 torr

The correct interpretation of these ABG results is which of the following?

A. Partially compensated metabolic acidosis
B. Uncompensated metabolic acidosis
C. Fully compensated respiratory acidosis
D. Uncompensated respiratory alkalosis
E. Partially compensated respiratory alkalosis

53. The heater on a patient's 40% aerosol mask malfunctions, delivering 26 mg of water/L of air. The patient's humidity deficit is which of the following?

A. 18 mg/L
B. 24 mg/L
C. 37 mg/L
D. 44 mg/L
E. 47 mg/L

54. Which of the following are considered hazards to sustained maximal inspiratory therapy?

I. Hyperventilation
II. Pneumothorax
III. Bradycardia

A. I only
B. II only
C. I and III only
D. II and III only
E. I, II, and III

55. A patient with orthopnea resulting from pulmonary edema may best be treated by placing him/her in which of the following positions?

A. Supine
B. Trendelenburg
C. Supine on the left side
D. Fowler's
E. Prone

56. Which one of the following is **not** a goal of pulmonary rehabilitation?

A. To help the patient become independent

B. To help the patient set realistic goals for life and help him/her attain them
C. To help reverse the patient's disease process
D. To help the patient gain an understanding of the disease and the limitations that result from the disease
E. To help decrease the frequency of hospitalizations

57. Which of the following methods may be used to measure functional residual capacity?

I. Helium dilution test
II. Nitrogen washout test
III. Body plethsmography

A. I only
B. II only
C. I and II only
D. II and III only
E. I, II, and III

58. The proper suctioning level for adults is which of the following?

A. −40 to −60 torr
B. −60 to −80 torr
C. −80 to −120 torr
D. −100 to −140 torr
E. −120 to −160 torr

59. Which of the following devices, when calibrated to room air, should read zero?

A. Capnograph
B. Oxygen analyzer
C. Nitrogen analyzer
D. Transcutaneous oxygen monitor
E. Barometer

60. Which of the following aerosolized medications is indicated for the treatment of *Pneumocystis carinii* pneumonia?

A. Ribavirin
B. Amoxicillin
C. Gentamicin
D. Pentamidine
E. Cromolyn sodium

61. After two unsuccessful attempts to intubate a combative patient in respiratory failure, which of the following medications will aid in the facilitation of intubation?

A. Dopamine

B. Cromolyn sodium
C. Lidocaine
D. Succinylcholine
E. Atropine

62. The following data were collected from a patient on a volume ventilator in the control mode.

TIME	PEEP (cm of water)	PaO_2	PvO_2
2:00 PM	4	62	36
4:00 PM	6	68	39
6:00 PM	8	74	43
8:00 PM	10	78	41
9:00 PM	12	83	38

Based on this information, which of the PEEP levels would be best for this patient?

A. 4 cm of water
B. 6 cm of water
C. 8 cm of water
D. 10 cm of water
E. 12 cm of water

63. While preparing to analyze a patient's aerosol mask, you notice water bubbling in the tubing. What effect would this have on the operation of this device?

A. Increase the FIO_2
B. Increase air entrainment into the nebulizer
C. Increase gas flow to the patient
D. Decrease the FIO_2
E. Has no effect

64. A patient with severe chronic obstructive pulmonary disease is admitted with fever, cough, and mild confusion. Oxygen is administered via a nasal cannula at 3 L/min. One-half hour later, the patient is less alert. ABG results follow:

	Room Air on Admission		Nasal Cannula (4 L/min)
pH	7.32	pH	7.21
$PaCO_2$	63 torr	$PaCO_2$	74 torr
HCO_3	33 mEq/L	HCO_3	34 mEq/L
PaO_2	39 torr	PaO_2	88 torr

Based on these data, the most appropriate change in this patient's treatment would be which of the following?

A. Switch to a nonrebreathing mask.
B. Institute mechanical ventilation.
C. Change to a Venturi mask at 40%.
D. Decrease the flow to 2 L/min on the nasal cannula.

E. Continue with present therapy and obtain blood gas values in 2 hours.

65. The ability of the patient to follow instructions would be indicated by which of the following?

A. Orientation to place
B. Performance of tasks when asked
C. Orientation to person
D. Ability to feed himself/herself
E. Awareness of time

66. To reduce the possibility of aspiration following the removal of an esophageal obturator airway (EOA), which of the following should be performed?

A. The patient should be intubated with an E-T tube immediately following removal of the EOA.
B. The patient should be intubated with an E-T tube prior to removal of the EOA.
C. The EOA should be removed as rapidly as possible.
D. The patient should be suctioned prior to removal of the EOA.
E. The patient should be suctioned immediately following the removal of the EOA.

67. A patient is breathing 18 breaths/min with a tidal volume of 500 ml. What is this patient's minute volume?

A. 5.5 L/min
B. 7 L/min
C. 9 L/min
D. 10.5 L/min
E. 12 L/min

68. The most reliable method of determining if a ventilated patient's lungs are getting stiffer and harder to ventilate is by measuring the

A. Dynamic lung compliance
B. PaO_2
C. $PaCO_2$
D. Spontaneous tidal volume
E. Static lung compliance

69. A patient's $PaCO_2$ decreases from 42 to 31 torr. All of the following could have increased *except*

A. Physiologic deadspace
B. Tidal volume
C. Minute ventilation
D. Respiratory rate

E. Alveolar ventilation

70. Chest physiotherapy is indicated in all of the following *except*:

A. Bronchiectasis
B. Cystic fibrosis
C. Pulmonary edema
D. Pneumonia
E. Chronic bronchitis

71. A patient is on intermittent mandatory ventilation on the Bennett MA-1 ventilator and you observe the reservoir bag collapsing during inspiration. To correct this, the respiratory therapist should do which of the following?

A. Increase the tidal volume.
B. Increase flow to the reservoir.
C. Decrease flow to the reservoir.
D. Place the ventilator on the assist/control mode.
E. Increase the sensitivity.

72. Prior to obtaining arterial blood gas values, the respiratory therapist performs an Allen's test on the patient's right wrist and determines that inadequate collateral circulation is present. What should the therapist do at this time?

A. Perform an Allen's test on the left wrist.
B. Obtain blood from the right brachial artery.
C. Obtain blood from the right femoral artery.
D. Obtain blood from the right radial artery.
E. Wait for the physician to evaluate collateral circulation.

73. In which of the following lung conditions would you find acid-fast bacilli in the sputum?

A. Chronic bronchitis
B. Tuberculosis
C. Cystic fibrosis
D. Bronchiectasis
E. Asthma

74. What is the minimum flowrate necessary on a simple oxygen mask to prevent the buildup of exhaled carbon dioxide?

A. 3 L/min
B. 6 L/min
C. 8 L/min
D. 10 L/min
E. 12 L/min

75. A diffusion capacity (D_L) is typically decreased in all of the following lung conditions **except**:

A. Emphysema
B. Oxygen toxicity
C. Sarcoidosis
D. Asbestosis
E. Asthma

76. The normal respiratory rate for a neonate is which of the following?

A. 10 to 20/min
B. 20 to 30/min
C. 40 to 60/min
D. 60 to 80/min
E. 80 to 100/min

77. Which of the following statements concerning an EOA are true?

I. The EOA should be used in unconscious or semiconscious patients only.
II. The airway should not be left in any longer than 2 hours.
III. Once inserted into the esophagus, the cuff of the EOA must be passed below the level of the carina.

A. I only
B. I and II only
C. I and III only
D. II and III only
E. I, II, and III

78. Sputum obtained from a patient with a *Pseudomonas* infection would typically consist of which of the following characteristics?

A. Thick and brown
B. Bright red
C. Pink and frothy
D. Green and foul smelling
E. White and stringy

79. After attaching a regulator to an E cylinder and turning it on, a whistling noise is heard coming from the cylinder. What may be the cause of this?

A. The plastic washer is missing.
B. The humidifier jar attached to the regulator is loose.
C. The plastic cover on the cylinder gauge is missing.
D. The regulator is uncompensated for pressure.
E. The cylinder is almost empty.

80. The following data were collected on a ventilated patient with the ventilator in the control mode.

    Oxygen consumption (V_{O_2}) = 200 ml/min
    $C_{aO_2} - C_{\bar{v}O_2}$ = 5 vol %
    Hb   14 vol %
    pH   7.43
    Pa_{CO_2} 37 torr
    Pa_{O_2} 85 torr
    V_T 850 ml
    Rate   10 breaths/min
    F_{IO_2} 0.45
    PEEP   6 cm of water

    This patient's cardiac output is which of the following?

    A. 2 L/min
    B. 3 L/min
    C. 4 L/min
    D. 5.5 L/min
    E. 6 L/min

81. A patient on mechanical ventilation complains of sudden chest pain and becomes tachycardic, and the high-pressure alarm begins to sound with each ventilator breath. Breath sounds are decreased on the right side, and on palpation the trachea is deviated to the left. The immediate action is which of the following?

    A. Recommend a chest x-ray study.
    B. Insert a needle in the third intercostal space.
    C. Institute PEEP.
    D. Decrease the machine sensitivity.
    E. Decrease the F_{IO_2}.

82. A small-particle aerosol generator (SPAG) is used to deliver which of the following medications?

    A. Acetylcysteine (Mucomyst)
    B. Ribavirin
    C. Cromolyn sodium
    D. Racemic epinephrine
    E. Atropine

·83. Immediately following extubation, the patient complains of difficulty in breathing, and stridor is heard during inspiration. The respiratory therapist should recommend which of the following?

    A. Chest x-ray study
    B. Hand-held nebulizer with racemic epinephrine

C. IPPB with acetylcysteine
D. Intubate and place patient on mechanical ventilation
E. Place patient on nasal CPAP

84. The data below were obtained from a patient on a 40% aerosol mask.

    ABG Results
    pH   7.37
    Pa_{CO_2} 42 torr
    Pa_{O_2} 83 torr
    Sa_{O_2} 96%

    Hb   14 vol %
    $P\bar{v}_{O_2}$ 39 torr
    $S\bar{v}_{O_2}$ 75%

    Based on this information, which of the following represents this patient's arterial-venous (A-V) content difference?

    A. 2.4 vol %
    B. 3.2 vol %
    C. 4.1 vol %
    D. 5.7 vol %
    E. 6.6 vol %

85. Which of the following are complications of a thoracentesis?

    I. Subcutaneous emphysema
    II. Bacterial infection
    III. Pneumothorax

    A. I only
    B. II only
    C. I and III only
    D. II and III only
    E. I, II, and III only

86. According to the American Heart Association, the compression to breath rate for two-rescuer CPR on an adult is which of the following?

    A. 15:2
    B. 5:2
    C. 15:1
    D. 5:1
    E. 4:2

87. The following data were collected from a 70-kg (154-lb) male patient on a volume ventilator in the control mode.

Ventilator Settings

VT	650 ml
Rate	12 breaths/min
FIO₂	0.45
Flow	45 L/min

ABG Results

pH	7.28
PaCO₂	58 torr
HCO₃	27 mEq/L
PaO₂	72 torr

Based on this information, the respiratory therapist should recommend which of the following?

A. Increase FIO₂ to 0.6.
B. Add 100 ml of deadspace.
C. Increase flow to 60 L/min.
D. Add 5 cm of water of PEEP.
E. Increase tidal volume to 750 ml.

88. A patient on a PEEP of 6 cm of water has a PvO₂ of 43 torr. The respiratory therapist receives an order to increase the PEEP level to 9 cm of water and after doing so, the PvO₂ drops to 34 torr. The respiratory therapist should recommend which of the following at this time?

A. Increase the PEEP to 12 cm of water and measure blood gases in 1 hour.
B. Increase the FIO₂.
C. Decrease the PEEP to 6 cm of water.
D. Discontinue PEEP.
E. Maintain PEEP at 9 cm of water and check blood gas values in 12 hours.

89. The physician writes an order for a patient to receive 15 L/min of a helium/oxygen mixture of 80%:20% from a premixed helium/oxygen (Heliox) cylinder using a nonrebreathing mask. In order for the patient to receive this flowrate through an oxygen flowmeter, the flow must be set at approximately

A. 8 L/min
B. 9 L/min
C. 12 L/min
D. 14 L/min
E. 15 L/min

90. Which of the following may result in a heart murmur?

I. Aortic stenosis
II. Tachycardia
III. Tricuspid valve insufficiency

A. I only
B. II only
C. I and III only
D. II and III only
E. I, II, and III

91. Cyanosis will be detected when

A. A patient's PaO₂ drops to 75 torr
B. There is more than 5 g of unsaturated hemoglobin/dl in the blood
C. The patient's heart rate increases 20 beats/min
D. The patient's hemoglobin level drops from 16 vol % to 14 vol %
E. The patient's SaO₂ drops to 95%

92. While administering IPPB with a Bird Mark 7, you notice the air mix control is inadvertently pushed in, delivering 100% oxygen. Which of the following would be affected by this?

A. Peak inspiratory pressure
B. Sensitivity
C. Nebulization
D. Inspiratory flow
E. Inlet pressure

93. Which of the following statements concerning a metered dose inhaler (MDI) is **false**?

A. The patient should hold the lips tightly around the delivery port.
B. The patient should hold the breath at peak inspiration for 5 to 10 seconds.
C. The MDI should be activated just after the patient has begun inhaling.
D. The patient should be instructed to inhale slowly and as deeply as possible.
E. The MDI should be activated during a sigh breath for patients on ventilators.

94. Amphotericin B is used for the treatment of which of the following?

A. *Candida albicans*
B. *Pseudomonas*
C. *Pneumocystis carinii*
D. Tuberculosis
E. Bronchiolitis

95. A lecithin:sphingomyelin ratio of which of the following indicates immature surfactant?

A. 3.5:1
B. 3:1
C. 2.5:1
D. 2:1
E. 1:1

96. The most effective therapy in the treatment of obstructive sleep apnea is which of the following?

A. Tracheostomy
B. Sleeping on right side
C. CPAP
D. Sleeping in Trendelenberg position
E. Sleeping in supine position

97. The percentage of the forced vital capacity exhaled in 1 second in a normal individual is which of the following?

    A. 30% to 50%
    B. 50% to 60%
    C. 75% to 85%
    D. 90% to 95%
    E. 95% to 97%

98. After turning an oxygen flowmeter completely off, you notice the water in the humidifier is still bubbling slightly. What is the most likely reason for this?

    A. The flowmeter is uncompensated.
    B. There is a crack in the humidifier jar.
    C. There is a faulty valve seat in the humidifier.
    D. The wall outlet is loose.
    E. The pop-off valve on the humidifier is malfunctioning.

99. A patient brought to the emergency room has just been rescued from a house fire. The respiratory therapist should recommend which oxygen delivery device to provide supplemental oxygen?

    A. Nasal cannula
    B. Simple oxygen mask
    C. Nasal catheter
    D. Nonrebreathing mask
    E. Partial rebreathing mask

100. A patient with severe chronic obstructive pulmonary disease presents to the emergency room complaining of shortness of breath. Arterial blood gas results on room air follow:

    pH   7.34
    $PaCO_2$ 58 torr
    PaO_2 46 torr

    The most appropriate recommendation for oxygen therapy is which of the following?

    A. Simple oxygen mask at 10 L/min
    B. Venturi mask at 28%
    C. Nasal cannula at 5 L/min
    D. Nonrebreathing mask at 15 L/min
    E. Simple oxygen mask at 4 L/min

WRITTEN REGISTRY REVIEW
POSTTEST ANSWER SHEET

Following each answer is the study guide chapter and section in which information relating to this answer may be found.

1. A	Ch. 4,	II	D 1b		
2. D	Ch. 3,	III	H		
3. D	Ch. 13,	I	B 1		
4. B	Ch. 3,	II	B		
5. E	Ch. 5,	I	C		
6. C	Ch. 11,	III	B		
7. C	Ch. 13,	III	A 2		
8. B	Ch. 5,	IV	B		
9. D	Ch. 3,	III	J 6		
10. A	Ch. 6,	V	B 10		
11. E	Ch. 6,	VI	A 3		
12. A	Ch. 11,	II	K 2		
13. B	Ch. 3,	III	A 7		
14 D	Ch. 6,	I	C		
15. C	Ch. 4,	II	A		
16. C	Ch. 13,	I	C 4		
17. D	Ch. 4,	III	A		
18. A	Ch. 4,	II	E 9		
19. A	Ch. 11,	II	E 6		
20. C	Ch. 3,	II	C 1		
21. D	Ch. 11,	IX	B 2		
22. B	Ch. 3,	III	I 2d		
23. D	Ch. 11,	XIII	C		
24. A	Ch. 5,	IV	E 3		
25. C	Ch. 1,	II	F 1g		
26. A	Ch. 7,	V			
27. C	Ch. 1,	II	G 5		
28. E	Ch. 9,	II	A 9		
29. E	Ch. 9,	II	C 1		
30. C	Ch. 4,	II	E 7		
31. D	Ch. 11,	II	K 2		
32. A	Ch. 13,	III	A 4		
33. B	Ch. 3,	III	F 2a		
34. C	Ch. 6,	IV	B 6		
35. B	Ch. 6,	V	A 3		
36. E	Ch. 7,	IV	E		
37. C	Ch. 9,	II	C 3e		
38. A	Ch. 1,	II	F 2f		
39. B	Ch. 3,	IV	B 4		
40. B	Ch. 9,	II	G 2		
41. E	Ch. 11,	XI	A		
42. B	Ch. 9,	II	C 3		
43. D	Ch. 7,	X	D		
44. B	Ch. 9,	II	C 1		
45. B	Ch. 4,	V	B 1		
46. E	Ch. 11,	X			
47. C	Ch. 1,	V	C 2		
48. C	Ch. 1,	II	E 2		
49. D	Ch. 14,	I	G 2 and 3		
50. B	Ch. 11,	II	B 4		
51. C	Ch. 9,	II	B 8e		
52. A	Ch. 10,	IV	E		
53. A	Ch. 2,	I	F		
54. E	Ch. 8,	II	B		
55. D	Ch. 12,	III	A 4a		
56. C	Ch. 15,	I	A		
57. E	Ch. 16,	I	B 1		
58. C	Ch. 4,	III	B 2		
59. A	Ch. 11,	III	F 7		
60. D	Ch. 14,	I	H 4		
61. D	Ch. 14,	I	G 1		
62. C	Ch. 11,	II	K 7d		
63. A	Ch. 2,	II	G 4		
64. D	Ch. 12,	I	A 7h		
65. B	Ch. 3,	III	M 3		
66. B	Ch. 4,	II	C 6		
67. C	Ch. 16,	II	A 3a		
68. E	Ch. 11,	IX	B 2		
69. A	Ch. 10,	III	E		
70. C	Ch. 8,	I	C		
71. B	Ch. 11,	II	A 4f		
72. A	Ch. 10,	I	E 1c		
73. B	Ch. 12,	II	C 4b		
74. B	Ch. 1,	II	F 1d		
75. E	Ch. 16,	II	B 8i		
76. C	Ch. 13,	I	B 4a		
77. D	Ch. 4,	II	C		
78. D	Ch. 3,	II	A 1b		
79. A	Ch. 1,	I	B 6e		
80. C	Ch. 9,	II	E 2		
81. B	Ch. 12,	III	D 3		
82. B	Ch. 2,	II	E 5a		
83. B	Ch. 4,	V	B 3		
84. C	Ch. 9,	II	F		
85. E	Ch. 5,	II	E		
86. D	Ch. 6,	I	D 2		
87. E	Ch. 11,	XIV	A		
88. C	Ch. 11,	II	K 7b to d		
89. A	Ch. 1,	III	A 4		
90. C	Ch. 3,	III	H 2c		
91. B	Ch. 3,	III	C 3		
92. D	Ch. 7,	VIII	A 3b		
93. A	Ch. 2,	II	E 4		
94. A	Ch. 14,	I	H 3		
95. E	Ch. 13,	II	A 2b		
96. C	Ch. 12,	III	C 1c		
97. C	Ch. 16,	II	B 2b		
98. C	Ch. 1,	I	B 8b(5)		
99. D	Ch. 1,	II	E 2a(2)		
100. B	Ch. 12,	I	A 7h		

INDEX

Note: Page numbers in *italics* refer to illustrations.